Springer Series on PSYCHIATRY
Carl Eisdorfer, PhD, MD, Series Editor

1982 **Stress and Human Health:** Analysis and Implications of Research
Glen R. Elliot, PhD, MD, and **Carl Eisdorfer, PhD, MD,** *Editors*
(out of print)

1982 **Treatment of Psychopathology in the Aging**
Carl Eisdorfer, PhD, MD, and **William E. Fann, MD,** *Editors*
(out of print)

1983 **Geropsychiatric Diagnostics and Treatment:** Multidimensional Approaches
Manfred Bergener, MD, *Editor* (out of print)

1991 **The Psychobiology of Obsessive-Compulsive Disorder**
Joseph Zohar, MD, Thomas Insel, MD, and **Steven Rasmussen, MD,** *Editors*

1994 **Stress in Psychiatric Disorders**
Robert Paul Liberman, MD, and **Joel Yager, MD,** *Editors*

1996 **The Schizophrenias:** A Biological Approach to the Schizophrenia Spectrum Disorders
Mary Coleman, MD, and **Christopher Gillberg, MD**

1998 **Advances in the Diagnosis and Treatment of Alzheimer's Disease**
Vinod Kumar, MD, and **Carl Eisdorfer, PhD, MD,** *Editors*

Vinod Kumar, M.D., M.R.C. Psych., D.P.M., is a Professor of Psychiatry and Neurology, Chief, Division of Geriatric Psychiatry and Co-Director of Alzheimer's Disease Program of the University of Illinois at Chicago, and Chief of Geriatric Psychiatry at the West Side Veteran's Administrative Medical Center in Chicago. He was trained in Psychiatry and Geriatric Psychiatry at the University of Leicester, England, West Midland Regional Health Authority, Birmingham University England and at the Neuropsychiatric Institute of University of California at Los Angeles. He has authored and co-authored several papers on Alzheimer's Disease and Pharmacology. He has been the Principal Investigator for several studies including Tacrine (Cognex), E2020 (Aricept), and Vitamin E and Depression studies. He is founding Editor in Chief of International Journal of Geriatric Psychopharmacology, and Associated Editor of Alzheimer's Disease and Associated Disorders an International Journal. He is also on the Editorial Board of International Journal of Geriatric Psychiatry and American Journal of Geriatric Psychiatry.

Recently he has been appointed to the International Advisory Committee of W.H.O. on the Early Diagnosis, Prevention and Treatment of Alzheimer's Disease. Dr. Kumar has equally devoted his time in Clinical Practice, Teaching and Research.

Dr. Eisdorfer holds his B.A., M.A. and Ph.D. from New York University and his medical degree from Duke University. He has served as Professor of Psychiatry and Head of Medical Psychology at Duke, where he also directed the Center on Aging and Human Development. He was Professor and Chair of the Department of Psychiatry and Behavioral Sciences at the University of Washington in Seattle, where he also founded its Institute on Aging. He later became CEO of Montifiore Medical Center and Professor at the Albert Einstein Medical School in New York.

He has authored over 280 books and articles including a major work on health care policy for the aged, published by John Hopkins Press for whom he is now writing another volume on the future of health care in the U.S. He has served as President of three national organizations—the Gerontological Society, the American Society on Aging, and the American Federation of Aging Research. Dr. Eisdorfer served on the Federal Council on Aging, the National Advisory Committee of the National Institute on Aging, and the Commission on the Future Veterans Health Care of the Office the Secretary.

Advances in the Diagnosis and Treatment of Alzheimer's Disease

VINOD KUMAR, MD, MRC, PSYCH
CARL EISDORFER, MD, PHD
EDITORS

Springer Publishing Company

Copyright © 1998 by Springer Publishing Company, Inc.

All rights reserved

No part of this publication may be reproduced, stored in a retrieval system, or transmitted in any form or by any means, electronic, mechanical, photocopying, recording, or otherwise, without the prior permission of Springer Publishing Company, Inc.

Springer Publishing Company, Inc.
536 Broadway
New York, NY 10012-3955

Cover design by: Margaret Dunin
Acquisitions Editor: Bill Tucker
Production Editor: Kathleen Kelly

98 99 00 01 02 / 5 4 3 2 1

Library of Congress Cataloging-in-Publication Data

Advances in the diagnosis and treatment of Alzheimer's / Vinod Kumar, Carl Eisdorfer, editors.
    p.   cm. — (Springer series on psychiatry)
  Includes bibliographical references and index.
  ISBN 0-8261-1167-X
  1. Alzheimer's disease. I. Kumar, Vinod. II. Eisdorfer, Carl. III. Series: Springer series on psychiatry (unnumbered).
  [DNLM: 1. Alzheimer's Disease—diagnosis. 2. Alzheimer's Disease—therapy.   WT 155 A244 1998]
RC523.A33   1998
616.8'31—dc21
DNLM/DLC
for Library of Congress   97-41352
                                                                            CIP

Printed in the United States of America

Contents

Editors and Contributors	ix
Preface	xiii
Vinod Kumar	
Carl Eisdorfer	

Part One: General Issues

1. Epidemiology of Alzheimer's Disease Jasenka Demirovic	3

2. Etiology and Neuropathogenesis
  of Alzheimer's Disease
  H. M. Wiesniewski
  T. Pirttilä
  J. Wegiel
	31

3. Neurobiological Systems Disrupted by Alzheimer's
  Disease and Molecular Biological Theories
  of Vulnerability
  J. Wesson Ashford
  Mark Mattson
  Vinod Kumar
	53

4. Genetics of Alzheimer's Disease Steven S. Matsuyama	90

Part Two: Diagnosis Updates

5. Diagnosis of Alzheimer's Disease
  J. Wesson Ashford
  Frederick Schmitt
  Vinod Kumar
	111

6. Neuropsychological Assessment of Alzheimer's Disease: An Examination of Important Issues Underlying Current Practice ... 152
   David A. Loewenstein
   Michele Quiroga

7. Uses of Neuroimaging Methods in the Diagnosis of Alzheimer's Disease Patients ... 170
   Ranjan Duara

8. Biological Test to Confirm the Diagnosis of Alzheimer's Disease in Cognitively Impaired Patients. A Fact or Fiction? ... 214
   P. D. Mehta
   T. Pirttilä
   H. M. Wiesniewski

Part Three: Treatment Updates

9. Diagnosis and Treatment of Alzheimer's Disease and Combined Depression ... 233
   Barnett S. Meyers
   Fughik Tirumalasetti

10. Diagnosis and Management of Paranoia, Delusion, Agitation, and Other Behavioral Problems in Alzheimer's Disease Patients ... 247
    J. Thad Lake
    George T. Grossberg

11. Noncholinergic Drugs in the Treatment of Memory Problems in Alzheimer's Disease Patients ... 264
    Maurice W. Dysken
    Kathleen M. Hoover

12. Cholinergic System Therapy for Alzheimer's Disease ... 298
    John S. Kennedy
    Joseph A. Kwentus
    Vinod Kumar
    Dennis Schmidt

13.	**Management of Families Caring for Relatives With Dementia: Issues and Interventions** *Donna Cohen* *Blake Andersen* *Richard Cairl*	351
14.	**Community Care of Alzheimer's Disease** *Kathleen Peterson* *Vinod Kumar*	376
15.	**Ethical and Medicolegal Issues in Alzheimer's Disease Treatment** *Panagiota V. Caralis* *Edwin J. Olsen*	391
16.	**Future Directions for the Research in Alzheimer's Disease** *Vinod Kumar* *Carl Eisdorfer*	409

Index   *417*

Editors and Contributors

Editors

Vinod Kumar, MD, MRC, Psych., DPM
Professor, Department of Psychiatry
Chief, Geriatric Psychiatry
Co-Director, Alzheimer's Disease Program
University of Illinois at Chicago
Chicago, IL

Carl Eisdorfer, MD, PhD
Chairman
Department of Psychiatry (D28)
University of Miami
School of Medicine
Miami, FL

Contributors

Blake Andersen, PhD
Assistant Professor
Department of Aging and Mental Health
Florida Mental Health Institute
University of South Florida
Tampa, FL

J. Wesson Ashford, MD, PhD
Associate Professor of Psychiatry and Neurology (and the Sanders-Brown Center on Aging and the Alzheimer's Disease Research Center)
University of Kentucky Medical Center
College of Medicine
Lexington, KY, and
Staff Psychiatrist
VA Medical Center
Lexington, KY

Richard Cairl, PhD
Associate Professor
Department of Aging and Mental Health
Florida Mental Health Institute
University of South Florida
Tampa, FL

Pangiota V. Caralis, MD, JD
Chief, General Medicine Section
Miami VA Medical Center, and
Professor of Medicine
Division of General Medicine
University of Miami School of Medicine
Miami, FL

Donna Cohen, PhD
Professor and Chairman
Department of Aging and Mental
 Health
Florida Mental Health Institute
University of South Florida
Tampa, FL

Jasenka Demirovic, MD, PhD
Associate Professor
Department of Epidemiology and
 Public Health and the
 Department of Medicine
School of Medicine
University of Miami
Miami, FL

Ranjan Duara, MD
Departments of Medicine,
 Neurology, and Psychiatry
University of Miami School
 of Medicine
Miami, FL and
Medical Director
Wien Center for Alzheimer's
 Disease and Memory
 Disorders
Miami Beach, FL

Maurice W. Dysken, MD
Director, GRECC
Program (11G)
Minneapolis VA Medical Center
One Veterans Drive
Minneapolis, MN, and
Professor of Psychiatry
University of Minnesota

George T. Grossberg, MD
Department of Psychiatry and
 Human Behavior
Division of Geriatric Psychiatry
Saint Louis University School
 of Medicine
St. Louis, MO

Kathleen M. Hoover, BA
Clinical Research Coordinator
Department of Psychiatry
St. Paul Ramsey Medical Center
St. Paul, MN

John S. Kennedy, MD, FRCP[c]
Assistant Professor of Psychiatry
Vanderbilt University School
 of Medicine
Nashville, TN

J. Thad Lake, MD
Department of Psychiatry and
 Human Behavior
Division of Geriatric Psychiatry
Saint Louis University School
 of Medicine
St. Louis, MO

David A. Loewenstein, PhD
Department of Psychiatry and
 Behavioral Sciences
University of Miami School
 of Medicine
Miami, FL

Steven S. Matsuyama, PhD
Associate Director
UCLA Alzheimer Disease Center
 and Chief, Psychogeriatric
 Laboratory
West Los Angeles VA Medical
 Center
Los Angeles, CA

Mark P. Mattson, PhD
Associate Professor of Anatomy
 and Neurobiology and the
 Sanders-Brown Center on
 Aging and the Alzheimer's
 Disease Research Center
University of Kentucky
Lexington, KY

P. D. Mehta, PhD
Institute for Basic Research in
 Developmental Disabilities
Staten Island, NY

Barnett S. Meyers, MD
Associate Professor of Clinical
 Psychiatry
Cornell University Medical
 College
The New York Hospital—
 Cornell Medical Center
Westchester Division
White Plains, NY

Edwin J. Olsen, MD, MBA
Professor of Clinical Psychiatry
University of Miami School of
 Medicine and Associate
 Director for Education
Miami Veterans Affairs Medical
 Center
GRECC
Miami, FL

Kathleen Peterson, MA, LCPC
Assistant Professor, Department
 of Psychiatry
Director, Community Support
 Network
Southern Illinois University
 School of Medicine
Springfield, IL

T. Pirttilä, MD, PhD
Institute for Basic Research in
 Developmental Disabilities
Staten Island, NY and
 Department of Neurology
 Medical School
University of Tampere
Tampere, Finland

Michele Quiroga, PhD
Department of Psychiatry and
 Behavioral Sciences
University of Miami School
 of Medicine
Miami, FL

Dennis Schmidt, PhD
Associate Research Professor
 of Psychiatry
Vanderbilt University School
 of Medicine
Nashville, TN

Frederick Schmitt, PhD
Associate Professor of Neurology
  and the Sanders-Brown Center
  on Aging
University of Kentucky Medical
  Center
College of Medicine
Lexington, KY

Fughik Tirumalasetti, MD
The New York
Hospital—Cornell
  Medical Center
Westchester Division
White Plains, NY

H. M. Wiesniewski, MD, PhD
Institute for Basic Research in
  Developmental Disabilities
Staten Island, NY

J. Wegiel
Institute for Basic Research in
  Developmental Disabilities
Staten Island, NY

Preface

Alzheimer's disease is a chronic neurodegenerative disorder heterogeneous in etiology and possibly clinical presentation. It is estimated there are millions of Americans suffering from this disorder and the number is growing significantly each year. Despite its recognition, there is a widespread perception by experts in the field that the majority of Alzheimer's disease patients remain underdiagnosed and are never treated. Ongoing research into etiology and pharmacotherapeutics gives us potential for treatments which improve symptoms, prevent the onset or slow the progression of the illness. We also have drugs at our disposal to treat associated psychiatric problems, depression, paranoia, agitation, and other behavior problems. Alzheimer's disease is a disease not just of patients, but of families and caregiver distress has been emerging as a major problem associated with depression, physical illness and ultimately inability to provide care.

The major focus of this book, *Advances in the Diagnosis and Treatment of Alzheimer's Disease*, is to describe the recent research findings regarding the epidemiology, genetics, diagnostic methods, and various pharmacological and nonpharmacological management strategies. We are delighted to have several of the most noted experts in the field as authors of various chapters. They not only reviewed the recent research findings but in several instances have described their experience and provide practical advice for clinicians.

The most important task for the clinician is to recognize the illness, make a comprehensive diagnosis, prescribe appropriate treatments (pharmacological and nonpharmacological), answer all the questions of family members regarding day-to-day management, and research findings in various aspects of the illness. Family members desire to satisfy themselves that they have provided the best treatment available in the world to their loved ones.

Our review of the field showed that none of the publications met the needs of clinicians. Therefore we embarked upon this volume to review and discuss the *Advances in Diagnosis and Treatment of Alzheimer's Disease*. For the convenience of the readers, we have divided this volume into three main sections:

1. "General Issues," which includes the highlights of what is known about the epidemiology, etiology, pathogenesis, biochemical deficits and genetics of Alzheimer's disease.
2. The section on "Diagnostic Updates" includes chapters on neurological and psychiatric evaluation, neuropsychological evaluation, neuroimaging techniques to diagnose Alzheimer's disease, and biological tests to develop the diagnosis.
3. The section on "Treatment Updates" includes the diagnosis and management of depression, paranoid delusions, agitation and other behavioral problems, cholinergic drug therapies, noncholinergic drug therapies, care providers, stress, psychopathology and its treatment, community management of Alzheimer's disease, ethical issues, and the future direction for clinical practice and research.

We have attempted to provide a balance between the scientific knowledge, and practical management strategies in the context of an overall humanistic approach to this devastating illness. We believe this to be a comprehensive volume that can be used by psychiatrists, neurologists, family practitioners, internists, neuropsychologists and other professionals in their clinical practice. We hope that the reader will judge this to be a successful effort.

Vinod Kumar, MD, MRC, Psych., DPM
Carl Eisdorfer, MD, PhD

PART ONE

General Issues

CHAPTER 1

Epidemiology of Alzheimer's Disease

Jasenka Demirovic

Dementia is the most common disease of the aging brain and can be defined broadly as a "syndrome of global loss of cognitive function, especially memory, sufficient to impair social or occupational function" (Larson, Kukull, & Katzman, 1992). Dementia is a frequent finding among elderly persons (65 years of age and above) and represents a growing public health problem as the population ages. A World Health Organization (WHO) report estimated that, by the year 2000, there will be more than 423 million elderly people worldwide (1991). It also has been estimated that the proportion of older adults in the U.S. population will increase from 11% in 1980 to 21% in 2030 (Gliford,1988). Furthermore, the subgroup of persons 85 years of age and above is growing six times faster than the rest of the U.S. population (Committee on a National Agenda on Aging, 1991; Schneider & Gurainick, 1990).

This work was supported in part by the National Institute on Aging Grant RO1AG09461 to the South Florida Program on Aging and Health ("The Epidemiology of Alzheimer's Disease in Three Ethnic Groups").

The U.S. National Health Interview Survey showed that 23% of elderly persons are unable to perform at least one of the major activities of daily living, such as bathing, dressing, or grooming, and that about half of those older than 80 are dependent on self-care (National Center for Health Statistics, 1985). In the United States, dementia is the leading cause of institutionalization (von Vostrand, 1977). Weiler (1987) showed that dementia would be the fourth or fifth leading cause of death in the United States if it were cited on the death certificates of persons for whom dementia was the underlying cause of death. Many disorders cause dementia. In the United States and Western Europe, Alzheimer's disease (AD) is by far the most frequent cause, accounting for up to two-thirds of all dementia cases (Tatemichi, Sacktor, & Mayeux, 1994). AD was first described as a discrete disease in a 51-year-old woman (Alzheimer, 1907). Until the mid-1970s, the term "Alzheimer's disease" was used only for progressive dementia coming on in late midlife but preceding the usual senile age. Meanwhile, it was shown that old people who were dying of progressive senile dementia had cerebral lesions identical to those found in persons who had died from AD. The term "senile dementia of Alzheimer's type" is frequently used today to designate such cases. Evans (1990) estimated that the number of elderly people with AD in the United States will increase from 2.88 million in 1980 to more than 10.3 million in 2050. All these facts demonstrate the public health importance of AD. Numerous epidemiologic and clinical studies have been conducted to estimate the prevalence and incidence of AD in various populations, as well as to identify risk factors. This chapter summarizes briefly their major findings and points to future research needs.

PREVALENCE STUDIES

Although there are more than 90 reports on the prevalence of dementia worldwide, the prevalence of AD is not known precisely. A cross-national comparison of the occurrence of AD and vascular dementia showed a predominance of AD in North America and Europe, whereas in Russia, Japan, and China, vascular dementia is more common (Jorm, 1991a). An exception is the study in Shanghai, China (Zhang et al., 1990), where AD accounted for 65% of all cases of dementia.The first published meta-analysis of the prevalence of AD and vascular dementia, which included 47 studies conducted from 1946 to 1985, showed a great variety (by a factor 7) of prevalence rates (Jorm, Korton, & Henderson, 1987). These studies also varied greatly in design and in clinical or diagnostic differentiation between AD and other forms of dementia.

In general, higher prevalence rates were reported for urban than for rural populations, for studies in which cases of mild dementia were not enumerated, and for studies in which the total population was investigated. In a recent review of studies published since Jorm's 1987 article, Rockwood and Stadnyk (1994) summarize results of prevalence studies among elderly people, using the following criteria:

1. a sample representative of the population under study;
2. an assessment by a physician using the Diagnostic Statistical Manual of Mental Disorders (DSM-III) (American Psychiatric Association, 1980) or equivalent criteria for assessing dementia; or
3. an assessment using the National Institute of Neurologic and Communicative Disorders and Stroke and the Alzheimer's Disease and Related Disorders Association (NINCDS-ADRDA) criteria (McKhann et al., 1984), DSM-III-R (American Psychiatric Association, 1987) or equivalent criteria for assessing AD.

A total of 18 studies met inclusion criteria, of which 3 were from North America, 8 from Europe, and 7 from Asia. Table 1.1 shows estimates of the prevalence of dementia in general and AD in particular. The rates of dementia varied from 2.2% to 8.4% (ages 65 + years), 10.5% to 16.0%

TABLE 1.1 Range of Reported Prevalence Rates of Dementia and Alzheimer's Disease Worldwide (in percentages)

Age Group	All Dementias (%)	Alzheimer's Disease (%)
65–74	2.2–8.4	1.6–15.3
75–84	10.5–16.0	4.1– 7.9
85 +	15.2–38.9	7.1–47.2

Note: Included studies met the following criteria: a sample representative of the population under study; an assessment by a physician using DSM-III or equivalent criteria for assessment of dementia, or NINCDS-ADRDA, DSM-III-R, or equivalent criteria for assessment of Alzheimer's disease. From "The Prevalence of Dementia in the Elderly: A Review," by K. Rockwood and K. Stadnyk, 1994, Canadian Journal of Psychiatry, 39, pp. 253–257. Copyright 1994 by the Canadian Journal of Psychiatry. Reprinted with permission.

(ages 75 + years), and 15.2% to 38.9% (ages 85 + years). Mild dementia accounted for 50% to 65% of all dementia cases. The rates of moderate and severe dementia showed a wide range of variation across geographic areas, with the highest rates among older adults of North America, followed by European and Asian populations. Table 1.1 shows the prevalence rates of AD, based on data from seven studies. The rates varied from 1.6% in Asia to 15.3% in North America (ages 65 + years) and from 7.1% in Asia to 47.2% in North America (ages 85 + years). Of interest to the U.S. population are results of a community study initiated in 1982 in East Boston, Massachusetts (Evans et al., 1989). From a group of 3,623 persons ages 65 or older (none of whom resided in institutions), and who had a brief memory test in their homes, a sample was selected for extensive neurologic, psychologic, and laboratory evaluations. The prevalence rate of clinically diagnosed AD increased greatly with advancing age, from 3% in those 65–74 years of age to 19% in those 75–84 years of age, and up to 47% among those 85 years of age or older. The prevalence rates of AD found in this study were higher than those previously reported. Prevalence studies of AD vary greatly in sampling and screening methods and in case ascertainment. It has been suggested that up to 76% of this variation in rates could be accounted for by methodological differences (Corrada, Brookmeyer, & Kawas, 1995). The prevalence rates also are affected by the survival rate and migration. Thus, incidence studies are more appropriate for comparing populations.

INCIDENCE STUDIES

The first study on the incidence of AD and of vascular dementia was carried out in Lundby, Sweden (Rorsman, Hagnell, & Lanke, 1986). The study population was first examined in 1947 and followed for 25 years. The lifetime risk for developing dementia found in this study was approximately 35% for women and 25% for men. Several other European studies reported incidence rates of AD and of dementia similar to those found in the Lundby study (Katzman & Kawas, 1994). The U.S. Baltimore Longitudinal Study of Aging, initiated in 1958, showed a significant increase in risk for developing primary degenerative dementia (presumably AD) between the ages of 75 and 85; the estimated incidence rate of AD among men age 80 was 3.2% (Sluss, Gruenberg, & Kramer, 1981). The U.S. Bronx Aging Study, a prospective study of a cohort of old persons, began in 1980 and included 488 nondemented subjects 75 to 84 years old who were volunteers in the study (Aronson et al., 1991). A 1.3% annual incidence rate of dementia was found among those 75 to 79 years old, 3.5% among those 80 to 84 years old, and 6.0% among those 85 years old and above. In another well designed, large scale cohort study, in Framingham, Massachusetts, the 5-year incidence rate of AD doubled with successive 5-year age groups, from 3.5 per 1,000 at ages 65 to 69, to 72.8 per 1,000 at ages 85 to 89 (Bachman et al., 1993). In the population-based East Boston study (Hebert et al., 1995), the estimated age-specific annual incidence rates of AD were substantially higher than those of previous investigations (see Fig. 1.1).

It has been suggested that methodological issues may account for these high rates, such as an emphasis on psychometric tests for diagnosis of

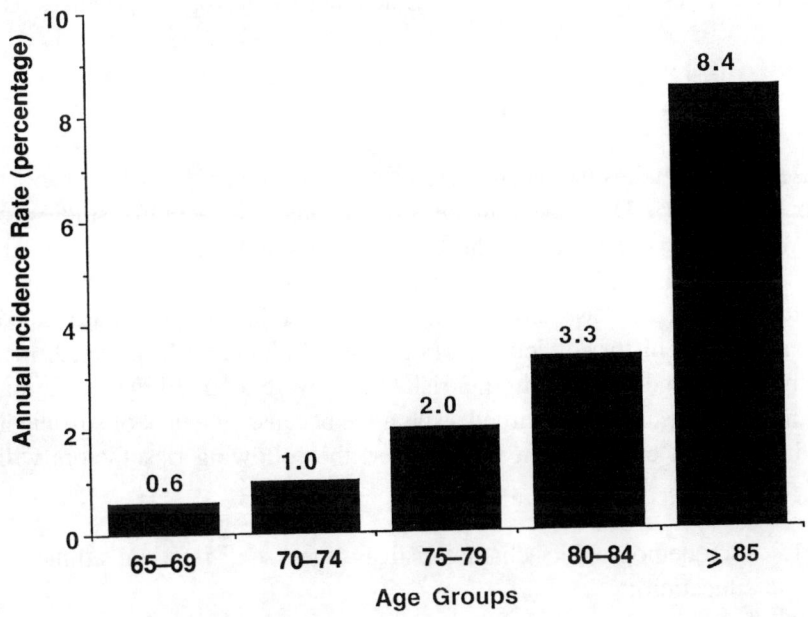

FIGURE 1.1 Annual incidence rates of Alzheimer's disease by age group. The East Boston study.

From "Age Specific Incidence of Alzheimer's Disease in a Community Population," by L. E. Hebert et al., 1995, *Journal of the American Medical Association, 293,* pp. 1354–1359. Copyright 1995 by the *Journal of the American Medical Association.* Reprinted with permission.

AD in a sample with low levels of education. This further points to the necessity of conducting comparative studies of the incidence of AD within and between countries using the same methods. Six ongoing studies of AD included the European Concerted Action on Epidemiology of Dementia (EURODEM) are:

1. PAQUID, France;
2. the Italian Longitudinal Study of Aging;
3. the Rotterdam Elderly Study, The Netherlands;
4. the Zaragosa study, Spain;
5. the Multicenter Study of Cognitive Functioning and Aging, United Kingdom; and
6. the Alpha study, Liverpool, United Kingdom.

These studies have adopted a core protocol that allows comparison of incidence rates and risk factor levels across their European populations.

RISK FACTORS

Case-control studies have generated most of the current knowledge about risk factors for AD. A meta-analysis of 11 major case-control studies (6 of which were conducted in the United States and the others in Japan, Australia, Finland, Italy, and The Netherlands) revealed that the only factors consistently associated with excess risk for AD were advanced age and family history of dementia (van Duijn, Stijnen, & Hofman, 1991a). Although a large number of other risk factors were reported in association with AD, these are still regarded as putative because of a lack of sufficient and consistent evidence. In this chapter, the following risk factors will be discussed:

1. sociodemographic characteristics (age, sex, race or ethnicity, education);
2. family history of dementia, Down's syndrome, and Parkinson's disease, parental age;
3. genetic factors, medical history of head trauma, hypothyroidism, depression, and epilepsy;
4. lifestyle factors (cigarette smoking, alcohol consumption, diet); and
5. environmental exposures (aluminum, lead, solvents).

Sociodemographic Characteristics

Age

Age is a well-established risk factor for AD: between ages 65 and 85, the prevalence rate of AD doubles every 5 years (Jorm, 1987). A direct and significant association between the age and AD incidence is demonstrated by the East Boston study data shown in Figure 1.1: the incidence rate of AD among persons ages 85 and older is approximately 14 times greater than the rate among persons ages 65 to 69 (Hebert et al., 1995).

Sex

AD occurs more frequently in women, contrary to vascular dementia, which affects men more often than women. A meta-analysis of 47 studies (Jorm, 1987) showed this excess prevalence of AD among women, and this was confirmed by other studies (Bachman et al., 1992; Rocca et al., 1991a). In the Framingham study, for cohort members 75 years of age and older, the female to male ratio of the AD prevalence rate was 2.8 (Bachman et al., 1992). Heyman et al., 1991, found a significantly higher prevalence rate of dementia for black women (19.9%) than for black men (8.9%). Women have a greater life expectancy than men, and the survival advantage of women may account for some of the difference. However, Rocca et al., 1991a, found greater age-specific prevalence rates of AD in women than in men. Similar findings were reported from the incidence studies of AD (Aronson et al., 1990; Katzman et al., 1989; Kokmen, Chandra, & Schonberg, 1988; Molsa et al., 1982). In the Framingham study, age-specific incidence rates of AD were generally higher among women than among men (see Fig. 1.2), but the difference was not statistically significant (Bachman et al., 1993). The authors suggested that the limited sample size did not have the power to detect a difference in incidence between men and women. Several mechanisms are considered in explaining the role of sex in the occurrence of AD. Gonadal hormones affect synapse formation and neurite growth; therefore, they may play a role in the development of dementia (Gould, Wooley, Frankfurt, & McEwen, 1990; Matsumoto, 1991). Estrogen deprivation in postmenopausal women may contribute to the development of AD (Aronson et al., 1990; Paganini-Hill & Henderson, 1994), but this hypothesis needs further

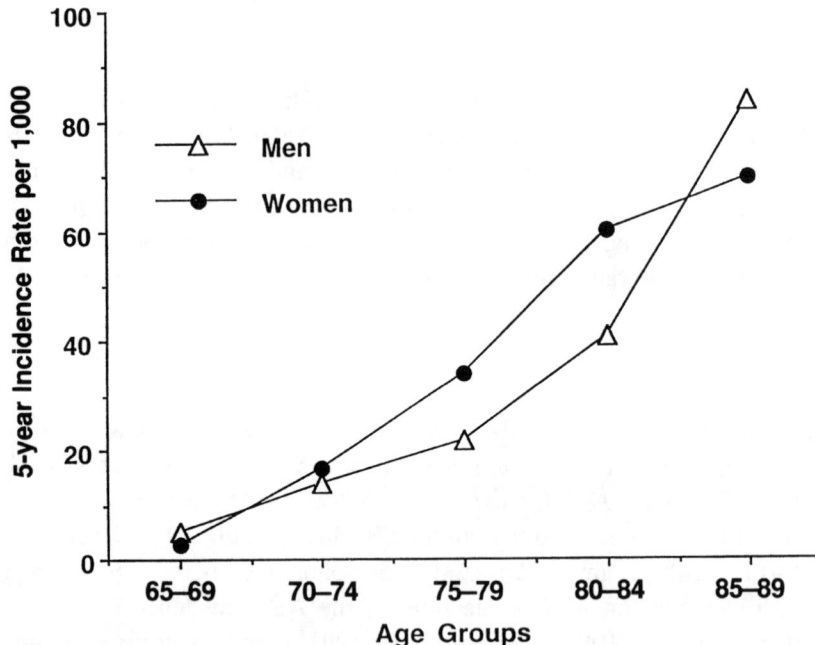

FIGURE 1.2 Age- and sex-specific incidence rates of Alzheimer's disease. The Framingham study.

From "Incidence of Dementia and Probable Alzheimer's Disease in a General Population," by D. L. Bachman et al., *Neurology, 43*, pp. 515–519. Copyright 1993 by *Neurology*. Reprinted with permission.

investigation. Studies examining the association between estrogen replacement therapy (ETR) and cognitive function and dementia have provided conflicting results (Barret-Connor & Kritz-Silverstein, 1993; Brenner et al., 1994; Paganini-Hill & Henderson, 1994; Szklo et al., 1996). In a review of future therapeutic developments of estrogen use, Fillit (1995) suggested that several clinical questions need to be answered regarding the role of ERT in the cognitive and affective dysfunctions associated with menopause and senile dementia. These are:

1. Does long-term ERT prevent cognitive decline in late life if initiated at the time of menopause?
2. Can ERT improve cognition and affective function in postmenopausal women with AD, and does ERT prevent the progression of AD in these patients?

3. Should ERT be used for a menopausal woman whose sole complaint is cognitive or affective dysfunction?
4. Do the vascular effects of ERT play a role in the treatment or prevention of both AD and vascular dementia?

It also has been hypothesized that the sex difference in the occurrence of AD could be related to a relative lack of education among women (Katzman & Kawas, 1994). Furthermore, men have more cardiovascular risk factors and, therefore, may be more likely classified as having vascular or mixed dementia than AD (Rocca, 1994). Further research is needed to determine whether the female sex itself is an independent risk factor for AD.

Race/Ethnicity

Information is scarce on race- or ethnic-specific prevalence and incidence rates of dementia in general and AD in particular. In a study among community residents in North Carolina, Heyman et al., 1991, found a significantly higher prevalence of dementia among blacks (16.0%) than among whites (3.0%). In this study, blacks were more likely than whites to have a history of hypertension, stroke, and other chronic diseases that might contribute to the development of dementia. The rate of institutionalization was higher among whites than among blacks. Ogunniyi, Osuntokun, Lekwauwa, and Falope (1992) and Osuntokun, Ogunniyi, Lekwauwa, and Oyediran (1991) reported that AD is absent in Nigerians. It also was reported that AD is rare among Cree Indians compared to Caucasians (Hendrie et al., 1993). Several large, population-based studies in the United States, in Indianapolis (Hendrie et al., 1995), Honolulu (White et al., 1994), and Miami (Prineas et al., 1995), are expected to provide new information about the prevalence and incidence rates of AD and other dementias among African, Japanese, and Cuban Americans.

Education

Numerous cross-sectional studies have found an inverse association between AD and educational attainment (Bonaiuto et al., 1990; Dartigues et al., 1991; Fratiglioni et al., 1991; Korczyn, Kahana, & Galper, 1991; Rocca et al., 1990; Sulkava et al., 1985; Zhang et al., 1990). In a study in Shanghai, China (Zhang et al., 1990), where approximately 27% of the study participants had never been to school and were illiterate, and 63% had 6 years or less of schooling, the age-adjusted relative risk for developing dementia was two times higher for those with no education compared with those who had attended middle or elementary school. Similar findings (with various strengths of association) have been reported from studies in Italy (Bonaiuto et al.; Rocca et al., 1990), France (Dartigues et al., 1991), Sweden (Fratiglioni et al., 1991), Finland (Sulkava et al., 1985), and Israel (Korczyn et al., 1991). In a Rochester, Minnesota, study (Beard, Kokmen, Offord, & Kurland, 1992), no association was found between education and the risk for developing dementia. Most participants in this study were well educated. One recent study in New York City suggested that increased educational and occupational attainment may reduce the incidence of AD (Stern et al., 1994).

Several explanations have been offered for the inverse association between education and dementia. The relationship may be causal (Friedland, 1993), and education may protect against clinical manifestations of dementia by increasing "brain reserve" and delaying clinical symptoms of dementia by up to 5 years and reducing prevalence overall (Katzman, 1993; Mortimer, 1988; Gurland, 1981; Satz, 1993; Stern et al., 1994), or it may be that individuals with lower educational levels perform worse on the psychometric tests that are used to diagnose dementia (Kittner et al., 1986). The concept of "brain reserve" is supported by a recent finding that cognitive decline in AD is predicted by neocortical synaptic density (Katzman, 1993). Education is postulated to increase "brain reserve" by increasing neocortical synaptic density (Katzman, 1993). This hypothesis needs confirmation by quantitative follow-up studies to include biological markers of synaptic density and change over time. Other issues that need clarification include potential confounders concerning the relationship between education and cognition, such as nutritional and other socioeconomic deprivations during childhood, as well as modification of the educational process by cognitive activities in later life (Katzman, 1993).

Family History/Genetic Factors

Familial aggregation of AD was found in numerous studies. Family history of *dementia* is, in addition to age, the only well-established risk for AD. van Duijn et al. (1991a) found a 3.5 times greater risk for AD in those with at least one first-degree relative with dementia than in those without a family history. The risk is stronger in the earlier age of onset in the proband. It has been suggested that familial aggregation of AD is due to an autosomal dominant inheritance (van Duijn et al., 1991a), but other authors suggest more complex mechanisms (Hirst, Yee, & Sadovnick, 1994). A significant positive association of family history of *Down's syndrome* with AD was also found: patients with a positive family history of Down's syndrome had a 2.7 greater risk of AD compared with those without a family history (van Duijn et al., 1991a). The risk was enhanced in those who also had a positive family history of dementia. A family history of *Parkinson's disease* was associated with a 2.4 times higher risk of AD compared with those without a family history (van Duijn et al., 1991a). It has been hypothesized that AD and Parkinson's disease have a common etiology because they share common clinical, pathologic, and biochemical features. *Late maternal age* at birth (40 and above) was associated with an increased risk of AD in 4 of the 11 major case-control studies, and 3 of these studies suggested that a very early maternal age (15 to 19 years) also may be a risk factor for AD (Rocca et al., 1991b). Explanations for this association included chromosomal and other mechanisms, such as suggestions that late or early maternal age at birth may influence psychological and cognitive developments of a child so as to make him or her predisposed to AD in later life (Rocca et al., 1991b).

Genetic Factors

Genetic defects on *chromosomes 14, 19, and 21* have been linked to AD, suggesting a genetic heterogeneity of AD (Schellenberg et al., 1993; van Duijn et al., 1994). There is now a considerable body of evidence that the *e4 allele of apolipoprotein E* (Apo E-e4) is associated with an increased risk of familial and sporadic forms of late-onset AD in both white and nonwhite populations (Brousseau et al., 1994; Hendrie et al., 1995; Saunders et al., 1993). Approximately 2–3% of the United States population is homozygous for the Apo E-e4 (Edelberg & Wei, 1996). It has been shown that the prevalence of Apo E-e4 varies by population according to the prevalence of AD; it is increased in the Finnish, Sudanese, and Aborigines, and decreased in the Chinese and Japanese (Edelberg & Wei, 1996). Because competing risks of heart disease and death, also related to Apo E-e4, may account for the Apo E-e4 association with AD, population-based prospective studies are needed to clarify these issues. Hofman et al. (1997) suggested an interaction between apolipoprotein E and atherosclerosis to the effect that the increase in the prevalence of AD with atherosclerosis is pronounced in those with the Apo E-e4 genotype. This cross-sectional association also needs further clarification in prospective epidemiologic studies.

Medical History

Head Trauma

Head trauma was associated positively with AD in most case-control studies (Amaducci et al., 1986; Broe et al., 1990; Chandra, Kokmen, Schoenberg, & Beard, 1989; Chandra, Philpose, Bell, Lazaroff, & Schoenberg, 1987; Graves et al., 1990a; Heyman et al., 1984; Kondo & Yamashita, 1990; Mortimer, French, Hutton, & Schuman, 1985; Shalat, Seltzer, Pidcack, & Baker, Jr., 1987), but not in all (Ferini-Strambi, Smirne, Garancini, Pinto, & Franceshi, 1990; Soininen & Heinonen, 1982). Although a majority of case-control studies, as well as one prospective study (Paschalis et al., 1990) showed no statistically significant positive association, one population-based case-control study found a significant increase in the risk for developing AD associated with the head trauma that occurred within 10 years prior to the onset of AD (van Duijn et al., 1992). This finding was consistent with an earlier report (Graves et al., 1990a) of a greater risk of AD the shorter the period between head trauma and the onset of AD. Pooling of data from case-control studies of the relationship between head trauma and loss of consciousness showed a significant positive association with AD (van Duijn et al., 1992). A small elevation of risk for developing AD associated with head trauma also was found in a follow-up study based on a review of medical records (Chandra et al., 1989). Several reports showed an increased risk of falls and head trauma in AD patients compared with subjects without dementia (Buchner & Larson, 1987; Friedland et al., 1988; Morris, Rubin, Morris, & Mandel, 1987), suggesting that head trauma may be a consequence of early stage dementia rather than an etiologic factor (van Duijn et al., 1992). Two explanations for the association of head trauma with AD have been suggested: (1) head trauma may play a role in the pathogenesis of AD; and (2) head trauma may be a consequence of an early stage of AD (van Duijn et al., 1992). The findings of neurofibrillary tangles and diffuse cortical plaques (indistinguishable from those seen in AD) in patients with dementia pugilistica (the dementia found in boxers who have had repeated head trauma) supported the etiologic role of head trauma in AD (Merz, 1989; Roberts, 1988). It has been hypothesized that head trauma causes changes in the blood-brain barrier affecting immunological protection of brain tissue and entry of toxins and viruses that produce damage years later (Heyman et al., 1984; Merz, 1989). It has been further suggested that head trauma may also cause rupture of small brain vessels, already damaged by amyloid, leading to onset of manifest AD shortly after the trauma (Merz). In a recent population-based case-control study, Mayeux et al. (1993) found an increased risk of AD associated with head trauma and loss of consciousness: the association was stronger for head injuries that occurred after age 70. The authors suggested that, although it is regarded as a putative risk factor for AD, the association of head trauma with AD is consonant with current concepts on the role of amyloid in AD, and that the temporal relationship between head injury and AD warrants future investigation.

Hypothyroidism

In 1984, Heyman et al. reported a positive association of AD with a history of hypothyroidism. This finding was not confirmed by several other studies (Broe et al., 1990; Chandra et al., 1987; French et al., 1985; Graves et al., 1990b; Kokmen et al., 1991; Shalat et al., 1987). A meta-analysis of nine case-control studies showed a positive and significant association (Breteler et al., 1991). Yoshimasu et al. (1991) found an increased risk of AD associated with myxedema, although the association was not statistically significant. The mechanism by which hypothyroidism may affect cognition is not fully explained. The thyroid hormone may play a role, either through effects on maturation of the nervous system and on neuritic outgrowth (Benjamin, Cambray-Deakin, & Burgoyne, 1988; Hargreaves, Yusta, Aranda, Avila, & Pascual, 1988), or through its functional relationship with other hormones and trophic factors of importance in neurodegenerative disorders (Hefti, Hartikka, & Knusel, 1989).

Depression

A significant positive association of history of depression with late onset AD was found in a meta-analysis of six case-control studies in which data on history of medically treated depression were collected (Jorm et al., 1991). The episodes of depression occurred more than 10 years before the onset of AD, as well as during the decade of onset of AD. This and other (Speck et al., 1995) reports suggested that depression may be not only a prodromal feature of AD but also an etiologic factor. It also was suggested that antidepressant drugs may play a role in this association because of their anticholinergic effects (Jorm et al., 1991b). Another explanation included disruption of the neurotransmitter system found in depression and in early onset AD (Rossor, Iversen, Reynolds, Mountjoy, & Roth, 1984).

Epilepsy

Epilepsy also was found to be associated with AD. Epileptic seizures may be among the first symptoms of AD, preceding by 10 years onset of clinically diagnosed AD. Although case-control studies included in the EURODEM analysis showed a consistent association of a history of epilepsy with AD, the association failed to reach statistical significance (Breteler et al., 1991).

An inverse association of AD with several other medical conditions and treatments (osteoarthritis, headaches, including migraine, blood transfusion, and nonsteroid anti-inflammatory drug use), was found in the EURODEM pooled analysis of case-control studies (Breteler et al., 1991). These associations, however, need further investigation in prospective epidemiologic studies.

Lifestyle Factors

Cigarette Smoking

Case-control epidemiologic studies have yielded inconsistent results on the relationship between cigarette smoking and cognitive impairment (Ferini-Strambi et al., 1990; Grossberg, Nakra, Woodward, & Russel, 1989; Joya, Pardo, & Landono, 1990; Shalat et al., 1987; van Duijn & Hofman, 1991b). A meta-analysis of eight case-control studies showed a significant inverse association between the lifetime prevalence of cigarette smoking and AD (Graves et al., 1991). This finding was not confirmed by one cohort study conducted in the United States (Hebert et al., 1992), but another population-based study among older adults in France showed that current and past smokers had about a 50% lower risk of cognitive impairment than did adults who never smoked (Letennuer et al., 1994). The suggested mechanism by which cigarette smoking affects the risk of AD has been linked to nicotinic binding site density in the cerebral cortex. Experimental studies have shown that nicotine increases the number of nicotinic cholinergic recognition sites in the cortex (Schwartz & Kaellar, 1985). A reduced density of nicotinic binding sites has been found in autopsy brains of AD patients (Nordberg et al., 1989; Whitehouse, Martino, Antuono, & Loewenstein, 1986). Similar findings were reported for Parkinson's disease (Perry et al., 1987). This similarity has strengthened further the hypothesis that cigarette smoking may be protective against both AD and Parkinson's disease. The association of cigarette smoking with cognitive impairment and AD remains controversial and needs further clarification by prospective population-based studies.

Alcohol Consumption

Alcohol consumption is associated with dementia in general and has been investigated in relation to AD (Freund & Ballinger, 1992). Although alcoholic dementia (a form of dementia found in alcoholics) has long been recognized, the association between AD and average weekly intake of alcohol failed to show a significant relationship in both case-control (Graves et al., 1991) and prospective studies (Hebert et al., 1992). However, one population-based case-control study in Sweden (Fratiglioni, Ahlbom, Vitanen, & Winblad, 1993), which used modified DSM-III-R criteria for diagnosis of AD, showed an excess risk of AD associated with alcohol intake. Terry, Hughes, and Larson (1990) also found accelerated cognitive decline in AD patients that was associated with alcohol consumption. Further population-based prospective studies are needed to assess more accurately the relationship between mild and moderate alcohol consumption and cognitive decline in general and AD in particular.

Diet

Studies of dietary intakes and risk of AD are scarce and most of them have been performed among institutionalized patients. Deficiencies of vitamin B^{12}, thiamine, folate, and niacin have been reported in association with AD (Litchford & Wakefield, 1987; Sandman, Adolfsson, Nygren, Hallmans, & Winblad, 1987). Population-based studies also showed a negative association between vitamin B^{12} and AD (Cole & Prchal, 1984;

Renvall, Spindler, Rampsell, & Paskavan, 1989). Free radicals have been implicated in the etiology of neurodegenerative disease, including AD (Jenner, 1994). Reports from animal studies warrant further investigations of this relationship to humans (Hsiao, Johannssdotir, & Yunis, 1994; Socci & Arendash, 1994). One recent cross-sectional, population-based study of 5,182 community participants in Rotterdam, The Netherlands, showed no association between cognitive function and intakes of vitamins C and E, and suggested that beta-carotene-rich foods may protect against cognitive impairment in older people (Warsama Jama et al., 1996). Another cross-sectional community study of 2,759 older people in South Florida showed that high dietary intakes of vitamin C and of beta-carotene were associated with better cognitive function (Prineas, Bean, Demirovic, & Rudolph, 1996). A recent report from the Zutphen Elderly Study (Kalmijin, Feskens, Launer, & Kromhout, 1997) suggested that high linoleic acid intake is positively associated with cognitive impairment in older people and that high fish consumption is inversely associated. None of the antioxidants examined in this study were protective against cognitive impairment. Few data are available on the relationship between antioxidants and incidence of AD, and this relationship needs further investigation.

Environmental Exposures

Aluminum

Aluminum accumulation in AD patients' brain lesions suggested a link between the disease and exposure. Epidemiologic evidence of the relationship between aluminum and AD is difficult to obtain because most people are abundantly exposed (Ganrot, 1986). One study by Graves et al. (1990a) showed a positive association between the use of aluminum containing antiperspirants and AD, whereas other studies failed to show a significant relationship (Broe et al., 1990; Crapper McLachlan, Kruck, Lakiw, & Krishnan, 1991; Heyman et al., 1984; Li et al., 1992). Ecologic studies have suggested that aluminum concentration in tap water is associated with a higher risk of AD (Flaten, 1990; Martyn et al., 1989). Because of the public health concerns about the potential risk of AD associated with aluminum in drinking water, a number of reports have addressed this issue, ranging from proposals for public policy to limit exposure by reducing the aluminum content in drinking water (Crapper McLachlan et al., 1991; Kraus & Forbes, 1992) to reports by those who do not support this view (Sherrard, 1991; Spink, 1992; Whalley, McGonigal, & Thomas, 1992; Wisniewski, Moretz, & Iqbal, 1986). The issue remains controversial. Occupational exposures to *lead and to solvents* also have been suggested as risk factors for dementia (Axelson, Hane, & Hogstedt, 1976; Hogstedt, Hane, Agrell, & Bodin, 1983), but a meta-analysis of several case-control studies showed no significant association of AD with either factor (Graves et al., 1990c). One recent report suggested an increased risk of AD for those with occupational *exposures to glues, pesticides, and fertilizers* (Canadian Study of Health and Aging Investigators, 1994).

COMMENT

Although much has been learned in recent years about the epidemiology of AD in different populations, many questions remain. For example, it is unknown whether the epidemiology of AD and other dementias in Latin America, Africa, and much of Asia is different from that seen in North America, Europe, China, and Japan. Moreover, because most of the current findings on risk factors for AD are derived from case-control studies, population-based prospective studies are needed for many putative risk factors. From a public health perspective, community studies of AD are important to provide information necessary for defining public health policy and for finding preventive measures. More people are surviving to old age. Those who develop dementia live longer after onset. Burdens are great for families and society as a whole. Only about one fifth of older adults with dementia are in nursing homes. Cases that reach hospitals or nursing homes represent only a subsample of all cases, and they may be different from those who remain in the community. As suggested in the "World Mental Health Situation Report: Dementia" (WHO, 1991), high priority areas for further epidemiologic research include:

1. the incidence rate of AD within and between countries using the same methods;
2. studies of special populations, such as those with reputedly low or high rates for dementias including AD; and
3. longitudinal studies of large community samples in order to examine the range of cognitive decline in late life and the risk factors that may influence accelerated cognitive and functional decline.

In conclusion, the problem is immense and it is growing. Research is greatly needed—from epidemiologic, clinical, laboratory, and experimental disciplines—to provide a basis for sound care and preventive policy.

REFERENCES

Alzheimer, A. (1907). Über eine eigenartige Erkrankung der Hirnrinde. *Allgemeine Zeitschrifs fir Psychiatric und Psychiatrische-Gerichts Medizin, 64,* 146–148.

Amaducci, L. A., Fratiglioni, L., Rocca, W. A., Fieschi, C., Livrea, P., Pedone, D., Bracco, L., Lippi, A., Gandolfo, C., Bino, G., Prencipe, M., Bonatti, M. L., Girotti, F., Carella, F., Tavolato, B., Ferla, S., Lenzi, G. L., Carolei, A., Gambi, A., Grigoletto, F., Schoenberg, B. S. (1986). Risk factors for clinically diagnosed Alzheimer's disease: A case-control study of an Italian population. *Neurology, 36,* 922–931.

American Psychiatric Association. (1980). *APA Diagnostic and Statistical Manual* (3rd ed.). Washington, DC: American Psychiatric Press.

American Psychiatric Association. (1987). *APA Diagnostic and Statistical Manual* (3rd ed. rev.). Washington, DC: American Psychiatric Press.

Aronson, M. K., Ooi, W. L., Geva, D. L., Masur, D., Blau, A., & Frishman, W. (1991). Age-dependent incidence, prevalence, and mortality in the old old. *Archives of Internal Medicine, 151,* 989–992.

Aronson, M. K., Ooi, W. L., Morgenstern, H., Hafner, A., Masur, D., Crystal, H., Frishman, W. H., Fisher, D., & Katzman, R. (1990). Women, myocardial infarction and dementia in the very old. *Neurology, 40,* 1102–1106.

Axelson, O., Hane, M., & Hogstedt, C. (1976). A case-reference study on neuropsychiatric disorders among workers exposed to solvents. *Scandinavian Journal of Work Environment Health, 2,* 14–20.

Bachman, D. L., Wolf, P. A., Linn, R., Knoefel, J. E., Cobb, J., Belanger, A., D'Agostino, R. B., & White, L. R. (1992). Prevalence of dementia and probable senile dementia of the Alzheimer type in the Framingham study. *Neurology, 42,* 115–119.

Bachman, D. L., Wolf, P. A., Linn, R. T., Knoefel, J. E., Cobb, J. L., Belanger, A. J., White, L. R., & D'Agostino, R. B. (1993). Incidence of dementia and probable Alzheimer's disease in a general population: The Framingham study. *Neurology, 43,* 515–519.

Barret-Connor, E., & Kritz-Silverstein, D. (1993). Estrogen replacement therapy and cognitive function in older women. *Journal of the American Medical Association, 269,* 2637–2641.

Beard, C. M., Kokmen, E., Offord, K. P., & Kurland, L. T. (1992). Lack of association between Alzheimer's disease and education, occupation, marital status, or living arrangements. *Neurology, 42,* 2063–2068.

Benjamin, S., Cambray-Deakin, M. A., & Burgoyne, R. D. (1988). Effect of hypothyroidism on the expression of three microtubule associated proteins (1A, 1B and 2) in developing rat cerebellum. *Neuroscience, 27,* 931–939.
Bonaiuto, S., Rocca, W. A., Lippi, A., Luciani, P., Turtu, F., Cavarzeran, F., Amaducci, L. (1990). Impact of education and occupation on prevalence of Alzheimer's disease (AD) and multi-infarct dementia (MID) in Appignano, Macerata Province, Italy. *Neurology, 40*(Suppl. 1), 346.
Brenner, D. E., Kukull, W. A., Stergachis, A., van Belle, G., Bowen, J. D., McCormick, W. C., Teri, L., & Larson, E. B. (1994). Postmenopausal estrogen replacement therapy and the risk of Alzheimer's disease: A population-based case-control study. *American Journal of Epidemiology, 140,* 262–267.
Breteler, M. M. B., van Duijn, C. M., Chandra, V., Fratiglioni, L., Graves, A. B., Heyman, A., Jorm, A. F., Kokmen, E., Kondo, K., Mortimer, J. A., Rocca, W. A., Shalat, S. L., Soininen, H., & Hofman, A., for the Eurodem Risk Factors Research Group. (1991). Medical history and the risk of Alzheimer's disease: A collaborative re-analysis of case-control studies. *International Journal of Epidemiology, 20*(Suppl. 2), S36–S42.
Broe, G. A., Henderson, A. S., Creasey, H., McCusker, E., Korten, A. E., Jorm, A. F., Longley, W., & Anthony, J. C. (1990). A case-control study of Alzheimer's disease in Australia. *Neurology, 40,* 1698–1707.
Brousseau, T., Legrain, S., Berr, C., Gourlet, V., Vidal, O., & Amouyel, P. (1994). Confirmation of the e4 allele of the apolipoprotein E gene as a risk factor for late-onset Alzheimer's disease. *Neurology, 44,* 342–344.
Buchner, D. M., & Larson, E. B. (1987). Falls and fractures in patients with Alzheimer-type dementia. *Journal of the American Medical Association, 257,* 1492–1495.
Canadian Study of Health and Aging Investigators. (1994). The Canadian Study of Health and Aging: Risk factors for Alzheimer's disease in Canada. *Neurology, 40,* 2073–2080.
Chandra, V., Kokmen, E., Schoenberg, B. S., & Beard, C. M. (1989). Head trauma with loss of consciousness as a risk factor for Alzheimer's disease. *Neurology, 39,* 1576–1578.
Chandra, V., Philipose, V., Bell, P. A., Lazaroff, A., & Schoenberg, B. S. (1987). Case-control study of late-onset "probable Alzheimer's disease." *Neurology, 37,* 1295–1300.
Cole, M. G., & Prchal, J. F. (1984). Low serum vitamin B_{12} in Alzheimer type dementia. *Age and Aging, 13,* 101–105.
Committee on a National Agenda on Aging. (1991). *Extending life, enhancing life. A national research agenda on aging.* Washington, DC: National Academy Press, Institute of Medicine.
Corrada, M., Brookmeyer R., & Kawas, C. (1995). Sources of variability in prevalence rates of Alzheimer's disease. *International Journal of Epidemiology, 24,* 1000–1005.

Crapper McLachlan, D. R., Kruck, T. P., Lukiw, W. J., & Krishnan, S. S. (1991). Would decreased aluminum ingestion reduce the incidence of Alzheimer's disease? *Canadian Medical Association Journal, 145,* 793–804.

Dartigues, J. F., Gagnon, M., Michel, P., Letenneur, L., Commenges, D., Barberger-Gateau, P., Auriacombe, S., Rigal, B., Bedry, R., Alperovitch, A., Orgogozo, J. M., Henry, P., Loiseau, P., Salamon, R., et Groupe d'Etude Paquid. (1991). Le programme de recherche paquid sur l'épidémiologie de la demence méthodes et résultats initiaux. *Révue Neurologie (Paris), 147,* 225–230.

Edelberg, H. K., & Wei, J. Y. (1996). The biology of Alzheimer's disease. *Mechanisms of Ageing and Development, 91,* 95–114.

Evans, D. (1990). Estimated prevalence of Alzheimer's disease in the United States. *Milbank Quarterly, 68,* 267–289.

Evans, D., Funkenstein, H., Albert, M., Scherr, P., Cook, N., Chown, M., Hebert, L., Hennekens, C., & Taylor, J. (1989). Prevalence of Alzheimer's disease in a community population of older persons. *Journal of the American Medical Association, 262,* 2551–2556.

Ferini-Strambi, L., Smirne, S., Garancini, P., Pinto, P., & Franceshi, M. (1990). Clinical and epidemiological aspects of Alzheimer's disease with presenile onset: A case-control study. *Neuroepidemiology, 9,* 39–49.

Fillit, H. (1995). Future therapeutic developments of estrogen use. *Journal of Clinical Pharmacology, 35*(Suppl. 9), 25S–28S.

Flaten, T. P. (1990). Geographical association between aluminum in drinking water and death rates with dementia (including Alzheimer's disease), Parkinson's disease and amyotrophic lateral sclerosis in Norway. *Environmental and Geochemical Health, 12,* 152–168.

Fratiglioni, L., Ahlbom, A., Viitanen, M., & Winblad, B. (1993). Risk factors for late-onset Alzheimer's disease: A population-based case-control study. *Annals of Neurology, 33,* 258–266.

Fratiglioni, L., Grut, M., Forsell, Y., Viitanen, M., Grafstrom, M., Holmen, K., Ericsson, K., Backman, L., Ahlbom, A., & Winblad, B. (1991). Prevalence of Alzheimer's disease and other dementias in an elderly urban population: Relationship with age, sex and education. *Neurology, 41,* 1886–1892.

French, L. R., Schuman, L. M., Mortimer, J. A., Hutton, J. T., Boatman, R. A., & Christians, B. (1985). A case-control study of dementia of the Alzheimer type. *American Journal of Epidemiology, 121,* 414–421.

Freund, G., & Ballinger, W. E. (1992). Alzheimer's disease and alcoholism. Possible interactions. *Alcohol, 9,* 233–240.

Friedland, R. P. (1993). Epidemiology, education, and the ecology of Alzheimer's disease. *Neurology, 43,* 246–249.

Friedland, R. P., Koss, E., Kumar, A., Gaine, S., Metzler, D., Haxby, J. V., & Moore, A. (1988). Motor vehicle crashes in dementia of the Alzheimer type. *Annals of Neurology, 24,* 782–786.

Ganrot, P. O. (1986). Metabolism and possible health effects of aluminum. *Environmental Health Perspective, 65,* 363–441.
Gliford, D. M. (Ed). (1988). *The aging population in the twenty-first century.* Washington, DC: National Academy Press.
Gould, E., Wooley, C. S., Frankfurt, M., & McEwen, B. S. (1990). Gonadal steroids regulate dendric spine density in hippocampal pyramidal cells in adulthood. *Journal of Neuroscience, 10,* 1286–1291.
Graves, A. B., van Duijn, C. M., Chandra, V., Fratiglioni, L., Heyman, A., & Jorm, A. F. (1991). Alcohol and tobacco consumption as risk factor for Alzheimer's disease: A collaborative re-analysis of case-control studies. *International Journal of Epidemiology, 20*(Suppl. 2), S48–S57.
Graves, A. B., White, E., Koepsell, T. D., Reifler, B. V., van Belle, G., & Larson, E. B. (1990c). The association between aluminum-containing products and Alzheimer's disease. *Journal of Clinical Epidemiology, 43,* 35–44.
Graves, A. B., White, E., Koepsell, T. D., Reifler, B. V., van Belle, G., Larson, E. B., & Raskind, M. (1990a). The association between head trauma and Alzheimer's disease. *American Journal of Epidemiology, 131,* 491–501.
Graves, A. B., White, E., Koepsell, T. D., Reifler, B. V., van Belle, G., Larson, E. B., & Raskind, M. (1990b). A case-control study of Alzheimer's disease. *Annals of Neurology, 28,* 766–774.
Grossberg, G. T., Nakra, R., Woodward, V., & Russel, T. (1989). Smoking as a risk factor for Alzheimer's disease. *Journal of the American Geriatric Society, 37,* 822.
Gurland, B. J. (1981). The borderlands of dementia: The influence of sociocultural characteristics on rates of dementia occurring in the senium. *Aging, 15,* 61–84.
Hargreaves, A., Yusta, B., Aranda, A., Avila, J., & Pascual, A. (1988). Triiodothyronine (T3) induces neurite formation and increases synthesis of a protein related to MAP1B in cultured cells of neuronal origin. *Developmental Brain Research, 38,* 141–148.
Hebert, L. E., Scherr, P. A., Beckett, L. A., Albert, M. S., Pilgrim, D. M., Chown, M. J., Funkenstein, H., & Evans, D. (1995). Age-specific incidence of Alzheimer's disease in a community population. *Journal of the American Medical Association, 273,* 1354–1359.
Hebert, L. E., Scherr, P. A., Beckett, L. A., Funkenstein, H. H., Albert, M. S., Chown, M. J., & Evans, D. A. (1992). Relation of smoking and alcohol consumption to incident Alzheimer's disease. *American Journal of Epidemiology, 135,* 347–355.
Hefti, F., Hartikka, J., & Knusel, B. (1989). Function of neurotrophic factors in the adult and aging brain and their possible use in the treatment of neurodegenerative diseases. *Neurobiology of Aging, 10,* 515–533.
Hendrie, H. C., Hall, K. S., Hui, S., Unverzagt, F. W., Yu, C. E., Lahiri, D. K., Sahota, A., Farlow, M., Musick, B., Class, C. A., Brashear, A., Burdine, V.

E., Osuntokun, B. O., Ogunniyi, A. O., Gureje, O., Baiyewu, O., & Schellenberg, G. D. (1995). Apolipoprotein E genotypes and Alzheimer's disease in a community study of elderly African Americans. *Annals of Neurology, 37,* 118-120.
Hendrie, H. C., Hall, K. S., Pillay, N., Rodgers, D., Prince, C., Norton, J., Brittain H., Nath, A., Blue, A., & Kaufert, J. (1993). Alzheimer's disease is rare in Cree. *International Journal of Psychogeriatrics, 5,* 5-14.
Heyman, A., Fillenbaum, G., Prosnitz, B., Raiford, K., Burchett, B., & Clark, C. (1991). Estimated prevalence of dementia among elderly black and white community residents. *Archives of Neurology, 48,* 594-598.
Heyman, A., Wilkinson, W. E., Stafford, J. A., Helms, M. J., Sigmon, A. H., & Weinberg, T. (1984). Alzheimer's disease: A study of epidemiological aspects. *Annals of Neurology, 15,* 335-341.
Hirst, C., Yee, I. M., & Sadovnick, A. D. (1994). Familial risks for Alzheimer's disease from a population-based series. *Genetic Epidemiology, 11,* 365-374.
Hofman, A., Ott, A., Breteler, M. B., Bots, M. L., Slooter, A. J., van Harskamp, F., van Duijn, C. N., van Broeckhoven, C., & Grobbee, D. E. (1997). Atherosclerosis, apolipoprotein E, and prevalence of dementia and Alzheimer's disease in the Rotterdam study. *Lancet, 349,* 151-154.
Hogstedt, C., Hane, M., Agrell, A., & Bodin, L. (1983). Neuropsychological test results and symptoms among workers with well defined long-term exposure to lead. *British Journal of Industrial Medicine, 40,* 99-105.
Hsiao, K. K., Johannssdotir, R., & Yunis, W. (1994). *Vitamin E delays onset of neurologic disorder in transgenic (TG) mice expressing human amyloid precursor protein (APP) variants.* Paper presented at the annual meeting of the Society for Neurosciences, Miami Beach, Florida.
Jenner, P. (1994). Oxidative damage in neurodegenerative disease. *Lancet, 344,* 769-772.
Jorm, A. F. (1991a). Cross-national comparisons of the occurrence of Alzheimer's and vascular dementias. *European Archives of Psychiatry and Clinical Neuroscience, 240,* 218-222.
Jorm, A. F., Korton, A. E., & Henderson, A. S. (1987). The prevalence of dementia: A quantitative integration of the literature. *Acta Psychiatrica Scandinavica, 76,* 465-479.
Jorm, A. F., van Duijn, C. M., Chandra, V., Fratiglioni, L., Graves, A. B., Heyman, A., Kokmen, E., Kondo, K., Mortimer, J. A., Rocca, W. A., Shalat, S. L., Soininen, H., & Hofman, A., for the EURODEM Risk Factors Research Group. (1991). Psychiatric history and related exposures as risk factors for Alzheimer's disease: A collaborative re-analysis of case-control studies. *International Journal of Epidemiology, 20*(Suppl. 2), S43-S47.
Joya, C. J., Pardo, C. A., & Londono, J. L. (1990). Risk factors in clinically diagnosed Alzheimer's disease: A case-control study in Colombia (South America). *Neurobiology of Aging, 11,* 296.

Kalmijn, S., Feskens, E. J. M., Launer, L. J., & Kromhout, D. (1997). Polyunsaturated fatty acids, antioxidants, and cognitive function in very old. *American Journal of Epidemiology, 145,* 33–41.
Katzman, R. (1993). Education and the prevalence of dementia and Alzheimer's disease. *Neurology, 43,* 13–20.
Katzman, R., Aronson, M., Fuld, P., Kawas, C., Brown, T., Morgenstern, H., Fishman, W., Gidez, L., Eder, H., & Ooi, W. L. (1989). Development of dementing illness in an 80-year-old volunteer cohort. *Annals of Neurology, 25,* 317–324.
Katzman, R., & Kawas, C. H. (1994). The epidemiology of dementia and Alzheimer's disease. In R. D. Terry, R. Katzman, & K. L. Bick (Eds.), *Alzheimer disease* (pp. 105–122). New York: Raven Press.
Kittner, S. J., White, L. R., Farmer, M. E., Wolz, M., Kaplan, E., Moes, E., Brody, J. A., & Feinleib, M. (1986). Methodological issues in screening for dementia: The problem of education adjustment. *Journal of Chronic Disease, 39,* 163–170.
Kokmen, E., Beard, C. M., Chandra, V., Offord, K. P., Schoenberg, B. S., & Ballard, D. J. (1991). Clinical risk factors for Alzheimer's disease: A population-based case-control study. *Neurology, 41,* 1393–1397.
Kokmen, E., Chandra, V., & Schonberg, B. S. (1988). Trends in incidence of dementing illness in Rochester, Minnesota, in three quinquennial periods, 1960–1974. *Neurology, 38,* 975–980.
Kondo, K., & Yamashita, I. (1990). A case-control study of Alzheimer's disease in Japan: Association with inactive psychosocial behaviors. In K. Hasegawa & A. Homma (Eds.), *Psychogeriatrics: Biomedical and social advances* (pp. 49–53). Amsterdam, The Netherlands: Excerpta Medica.
Korczyn, A. D., Kahana, E., & Galper, Y. (1991). Epidemiology of dementia in Ashkelon, Israel. *Neuroepidemiology, 10,* 100.
Kraus, A. S., & Forbes, W. F. (1992). Aluminum, fluoride and the prevention of Alzheimer's disease. *Canadian Journal of Public Health, 83,* 97–100.
Larson, E. B., Kukull, W. A., & Katzman, R. L. (1992). Cognitive impairment: Dementia and Alzheimer's disease. *Annual Review of Public Health, 13,* 431–449.
Letennuer, L., Dartigues, J. F., Commenges, D., Barberger-Gateau, P., Tessier, J. F., & Orgogozo, J. M. (1994). Tobacco consumption and cognitive impairment in elderly people. A population-based study. *Annals of Epidemiology, 4,* 449–454.
Li, G., Shen, Y. C., Li, Y. T., Chen, C. H., Zhau, Y. W., & Silverman, J. M. (1992). A case-control study of Alzheimer's disease in China. *Neurology, 42,* 1481–1488.
Litchford, M. D, & Wakefield, L. M. (1987). Nutrient intakes and energy expenditures of residents with senile dementia of the Alzheimer's type. *Journal of the American Dietetic Association, 87,* 211–213.

Martyn, C. N. (1992). The epidemiology of Alzheimer's disease in relation to aluminium. In *Aluminium in biology and medicine. Ciba Foundation Symposium, 169*, 69–86.

Martyn, C. N., Barker, D. J. P., Osmond, C., Harris, E. C., Edwardson, J. A., & Lacely, R. F. (1989). Geographical relation between Alzheimer's disease and aluminum in drinking water. *Lancet, 1*, 59–62.

Matsumoto, A. (1991). Synaptogenic action of sex steroids in [the] developing and adult neuroendocrine brain. *Psychoneuroendocrinology, 16*, 25–40.

Mayeux, R., Ottman, R., Tang, M. X., Noboa-Bauza, L., Marder, K., Gurland, B., & Stern, J. (1993). Genetic susceptibility and head injury as risk factors for Alzheimer's disease among community-dwelling elderly persons and their first-degree relatives. *Annals of Neurology, 33*, 494–501.

McKhann, G., Drachman, D., Folstein, M., Katzman, R., Price, D., & Stadlan, E. M. (1984). Clinical diagnosis of Alzheimer's disease (Report of the NINCDS-ADRDA work group under the auspices of the Department of Health and Human Services Task Force on Alzheimer's Disease). *Neurology, 34*, 939–944.

Merz, B. (1989). Is boxing a risk factor for Alzheimer's? *Journal of the American Medical Association, 261*, 2597–2598.

Molsa, P. K., Marttila, R. J., & Rinne, U. K. (1982). Epidemiology of dementia in a Finnish population. *Acta Neurologica Scandinavica, 65*, 541–552.

Morris, J. C., Rubin, E. H., Morris, E. J., & Mandel, S. A. (1987). Senile dementia of the Alzheimer's type: An important risk factor for serious falls. *Journal of Gerontology, 42*, 412–417.

Mortimer, J. A. (1988). Do psychosocial risk factors contribute to Alzheimer's disease? In A. S. Henderson & J. H. Henderson (Eds.), *Etiology of Dementia of Alzheimer's Type* (pp. 39–52). New York: John Wiley.

Mortimer, J. A., French, L. R., Hutton, J. T., & Schuman, L. M. (1985). Head injury as a risk factor for Alzheimer's disease. *Neurology, 35*, 264–267.

National Center for Health Statistics. (1985). National Health Interview Survey. Vital and Health Interview Survey. *Health Statistics* (Ser. 10, No. 150, DHHS Publication No. PHS 85-1587). Washington, DC: U.S. Government Printing Office.

Nordberg A., Nilsson-Hakansson, L., Adam, A., Hardy, J., Alafuzoff, I., Lai, Z., Herrera-Marschitz, M., & Winblad, B. (1989). The role of nicotinic receptors in the pathophysiology of Alzheimer's disease. In A. Nordberg, K. Fuxe, B. Holmsted, & A. Sundwall (Eds.), *Progress in Brain Research* (Vol. 79, pp. 353–362). Amsterdam, New York, Oxford: Elsevier.

Ogunniyi, A. O., Osuntokun, B. O., Lekwauwa, U. B., & Falope, Z. F. (1992). Rarity of dementia (by DSM-III-R) in an urban community in Nigeria. *East African Medical Journal, 69*, 64–68.

Osuntokun, B. O., Ogunniyi, A. O., Lekwauwa, G. U., & Oyediran, A. B. O. O. (1991). Epidemiology of age-related dementias in the third world and

aetiological clues of Alzheimer's disease. *Tropical and Geographical Medicine,* 345–531.
Paganini-Hill, A., & Henderson, V. W. (1994). Estrogen deficiency and risk of Alzheimer's disease in women. *American Journal of Epidemiology, 140,* 256–261.
Paschalis, C., Polychronopoulos, P., Lekka, N. P., Harrison, M. J. G., Papapetropoulos, T. (1990). The role of head injury, surgical anaesthesia and family history as aetiological factors in dementia of Alzheimer type: A prospective study. *Dementia, 1,* 52–55.
Perry, E. K., Perry, R. H., Smith, C. J., Dick, D. J., Candy, J. M., Edwardson, J. A., Fairbairn, A., & Blessed, G. (1987). Nicotinic receptor abnormalities in Alzheimer's and Parkinson's diseases. *Journal of Neurology Neurosurgery and Psychiatry, 50,* 806–809.
Prineas, R., Bean, J., Demirovic, J., & Rudolph, M. (1996). Aging, cognitive function and dietary antioxidants in an elderly multiethnic population: The South Florida Program on Aging and Health. *American Journal of Epidemiology, 143*(Suppl.), S64.
Prineas, R., Demirovic, J., Bean, J., Duara, R., Gomez-Marin, O., Loewenstein, D., Sevush, S., Stitt, F., & Szapocznik, J. (1995). The South Florida Program on Aging and Health. Assessing the prevalence of Alzheimer's disease in three ethnic groups. *Journal of the Florida Medical Association, 82,* 805–810.
Renvall, M. J., Spindler, A., Rampsell, J. W., & Paskavan, M. (1989). Nutritional status of free living Alzheimer's patients. *American Journal of Medical Science, 298,* 20–27.
Roberts, G. W. (1988). Immunocytochemistry of neurofibrillary tangles in dementia pugilistica and Alzheimer's disease: Evidence for common genesis. *Lancet, 2,* 1456–1458.
Rocca, W. A. (1994). Frequency, distribution, and risk factors for Alzheimer's disease. *Nursing Clinics of North America, 29,* 101–111.
Rocca, W. A., Bonaiuto, S., Lippi, A., Luciani, P., Turtu, F., Cavarzeran, F., & Amaducci, L. (1990). Prevalence of clinically diagnosed Alzheimer's disease and other dementing disorders: A door-to-door survey in Appignano, Macerata Province, Italy. *Neurology, 40,* 626–631.
Rocca, W. A., Hofman, A., Brayne, C., Breteler, M. M. B., Clarke, M., Copeland, J. R. M., Dartigues, J. F., Engedal, K., Hagnell, O., Heeren, T. J., Jonker, C., Lindsey, J., Lobo, A., Mann, A. H., Molsa, P. K., Morgan, K., O'Connor, D. W., da Silva Droux, A., Sulkava, R., Kay, D. W. K., Amaducci, L., for the EURODERM-Prevalence Research Group. (1991a). Frequency and distribution of Alzheimer's disease in Europe: A collaborative study of 1980–1990 prevalence findings. *Annals of Neurology, 30,* 381–390.
Rocca, W. A., van Duijn, C. M., Clayton, D., Chandra, V., Fratiglioni, L., Graves, A. B., Heyman, A., Jorm, A. F., Kokmen, E., Kondo, K., Mortimer,

J. A., Shalat, S. L., Soininen, H., & Hofman, A., for the EURODEM Risk Factors Research Group. (1991b). Maternal age and Alzheimer's disease: A collaborative re-analysis of case-control studies. *International Journal of Epidemiology, 20*(Suppl. 2), S21–S27.

Rockwood, K., & Stadnyk, K. (1994). The prevalence of dementia in the elderly: A review. *Canadian Journal of Psychiatry, 39*, 253–257.

Rorsman, B., Hagnell, O., & Lanke, J. (1986). Prevalence and incidence of senile and multi-infarct dementia in the Lundby study: A comparison between the time periods 1947–1957 and 1957–1972. *Neuropsychobiology, 15*, 122–129.

Rossor, M. N., Iversen, L. L., Reynolds, G. P., Mountjoy, C. R., & Roth, M. (1984). Neurochemical characteristics of early and late onset types of Alzheimer's disease. *British Medical Journal, 288*, 961–964.

Sandman, P. O., Adolfsson, R., Nygren, C., Hallmans, G., & Winblad, B. (1987). Nutritional status and dietary intake in institutionalized patients with Alzheimer's disease and multiinfarct dementia. *Journal of the American Geriatric Society, 35*, 31–38.

Satz, P. (1993). Brain reserve capacity on symptom onset after brain injury: A formulation and review of evidence for threshold theory. *Neuropsychology, 7*, 273–295.

Saunders, A. M., Strittmatter, W. J., Schmechel, D., George-Hyslop, P. H., Pericak-Vance, M. A., Joo, S. H., Rosi, B. L., Gussela, J. F., Crapper MacLachlan, D. R., & Alberts, M. J. (1993). Association of apolipoprotein E allele epsilon 4 with late-onset familial and sporadic Alzheimer's disease. *Neurology, 44*, 2420–2421.

Schellenberg, G. D., Bird, T. D., Wijsman, E. M., Orr, H. T., Anderson, L., Nemens, E., White, J. A., Bonnycastle, L., Weber, J. L., & Alonso, M. E. (1992). Genetic linkage evidence for a familial Alzheimer's disease locus on chromosome 14. *Science, 258*, 668–671.

Schneider, E. L., & Gurainick, J. M. (1990). The aging of America. Impact on health care costs. *Journal of the American Medical Association, 263*, 2335–2340.

Schwartz, R. D., & Kaellar, K. J. (1985). In vivo regulation of (3H) acetylcholine recognition sites in brain by nicotinic cholinergic drugs. *Journal of Neurochemistry, 45*, 427–433.

Shalat, S. L., Seltzer, B., Pidcock, C., & Baker, E. L., Jr. (1987). Risk factors for Alzheimer's disease: A case-control study. *Neurology, 37*, 1630–1633.

Sherrard, D. J. (1991). Aluminum—Much ado about something. *New England Journal of Medicine, 324*, 558–559.

Sluss, T. K., Gruenberg, E. M., & Kramer, M. (1981). The use of longitudinal studies in the investigation of risk factors for senile dementia—Alzheimer's type. In J. A. Mortimer & L. M. Schuman (Eds.), *The Epidemiology of Dementia* (pp. 132–154). London: Oxford University Press.

Socci, D. J., & Arendash, G. W. (1994). *Chronic antioxidant treatment improves the cognitive function of aged rats.* Paper presented at the Annual Meeting of the Society for Neurosciences, Miami Beach, Florida.

Soininen, H., & Heinonen, O. P. (1982). Clinical and etiological aspects of senile dementia. *European Neurology, 21,* 401–410.

Speck, C. E., Kukull, W. A., Brenner, D. E., Bowen, J. D., McCormick, W. C., Teri, L., Pfanschmidt, M. L., Thompson, J. D., & Larson, E. B. (1995). History of depression as a risk factor for Alzheimer's disease. *Epidemiology, 6,* 366–369.

Spink, D. (1992). Aluminum and Alzheimer's disease. *Canadian Medical Association Journal, 146,* 431.

Stern, Y., Gurland, B., Tatemichi, T. K., Tang, M. X., Wilder, D., & Mayeux, R. (1994). Influence of education and occupation on the incidence of Alzheimer's disease. *Journal of the American Medical Association, 271,* 1004–1010.

Sulkava, R., Wikstrom, J., Aromaa, Raitasalo, R., Lehtinen, V., Lahtela, K., & Palo, J. (1985). Prevalence of severe dementia in Finland. *Neurology, 35,* 1025–1029.

Szklo, M., Cerhan, J., Diez-Roux, A. V., Chambless, L., Cooper, L., Folsom, A. R., Fried, L. P., Knopman, D., & Nieto, J. F. (1996). Estrogen replacement therapy and cognitive functioning in the Atherosclerosis Risk in Communities (ARIC) Study. *American Journal of Epidemiology, 144,* 1048–1057.

Tatemichi, T. K., Sacktor, N., & Mayeux, R. (1994). Dementia associated with cerebrovascular disease, other degenerative diseases, and metabolic disorders. In R. D. Terry, R. Katzman, & K. L. Bick (Eds.), *Alzheimer Disease.* New York: Raven Press.

Terry, L., Hughes, G. P., & Larson, E. B. (1990). Cognitive deterioration in Alzheimer's disease: Behavioral and health factors. *Journal of Gerontology, 45,* P58–P63.

van Duijn, C. M., Hendriks, L., Farrer, L. A., Backhovens, H., Cruts, M., Wehert, A., Hofman, A., & van Brockhoven, C. (1994). A population-based study of familial Alzheimer's disease: Linkage to chromosome 14, 19, and 21. *American Journal of Human Genetics, 55,* 714–727.

van Duijn, C. M., Stijnen, T., & Hofman, A. (1991a). Risk factors for Alzheimer's disease: Overview of the EURODERM collaborative re-analysis of case-control studies. *International Journal of Epidemiology, 20*(Suppl. 2), S4–S11.

van Duijn, C., & Hoffman, A. (1991b). Relation between nicotine intake and Alzheimer's disease. *British Medical Journal, 302,* 1491–1494.

van Duijn, C., Tanja, T. A., Haaxma, R., Schulte, W., Saan, R. J., Lameris, A. J., Antonides-Hendriks, G., & Hofman, A. (1992). Head trauma and the risk of Alzheimer's disease. *American Journal of Epidemiology, 135,* 775–782.

von Vostrand, J. (1977). The National Nursing Home Survey: 1977 Summary for the United States. *National Center for Health Statistics* (Ser. 13, No.

43, DHEW Publication No. 43 [PHS] 79-1794). Washington, DC: U.S. Government Printing Office.

Warsama Jama, J., Launer, L. J., Witteman, J. C. M., den Breeijen, J. H., Breteler, M. M. B., Groobbee, D. E., & Hofman, A. (1996). Dietary antioxidants and cognitive function in a population-based sample of older persons. *American Journal of Epidemiology, 144,* 275–280.

Weiler, P. (1987). The public health impact of Alzheimer's disease. *American Journal of Public Health, 77,* 1157–1158.

Whalley, L. J., McGonigal, G., & Thomas, B. (1992). Aluminium and dementia. *Lancet, 339,* 1235–1236.

White, L. R., Ross, G. W., Petrovitch, H., Masaki, K., Chiu, D., & Teng, E. (1994). Estimation of the sensitivity of a dementia screening test in a population-based study. *Neurobiology of Aging, 15*(Suppl. 1), S42.

Whitehouse, P. J., Martino, A. M., Antuono, & Loewenstein, P. R. (1986). Nicotinic acetylcholine binding sites in Alzheimer's disease. *Brain Research, 371,* 146–151.

Wisniewski, H. M., Moretz, R. C., & Iqbal, K. (1986). No evidence for aluminum in etiology and pathogenesis of Alzheimer's disease. *Neurobiology of Aging, 7,* 532–535.

World Health Organization. (1991). *Eighth Report on the World Health Situation* (Publication No. EB89/10), Geneva, Switzerland: Author.

Yoshimasu, F., Kokmen, E., Hay, I. D., Beard, C. M., Offord, K. P., & Kurland, L. T. (1991). The association between Alzheimer's disease and thyroid disease in Rochester, Minnesota. *Neurology, 41,* 1745–1747.

Zhang, M. Y., Katzman, R., Salmon, D., Jin, H., Cai, G. J., Wang, Z. Y., Qu, G. Y., Grant, I., Yu, E., & Levy, P. (1990). The prevalence of dementia and Alzheimer's disease in Shanghai, China: Impact of age, gender and education. *Annals of Neurology, 27,* 428–437.

CHAPTER 2

Etiology and Neuropathogenesis of Alzheimer's Disease

H. M. Wisniewski
T. Pirttilä
J. Wegiel

Alzheimer's disease (AD) is a neurodegenerative disorder characterized by accumulation of fibrillar amyloid-β (Aβ) protein in plaques in brain parenchyma and in the walls of leptomeningeal and parenchymal vessels, neurofibrillary changes in neurons and their processes, and extensive progressive synaptic and neuronal loss. β-amyloidosis and neurofibrillary changes are such consistent features that postmortem diagnosis of AD is based on semiquantitative assessment of plaques and tangles (Khachaturian, 1985).

The etiology of Alzheimer's disease is complex. The well-established risk factors for AD include aging, genetics, and some environmental

---

This grant was supported in part by funds from the New York State Office of Mental Retardation and Developmental Disabilities, grants from the National Institutes of Health, National Institute on Aging, Nos. PO1 AG 04220 and PO1 AG 11531, and the fund for the Center for Trace Element Studies and Environmental Toxicology.

factors. A combination of pathological events in genetically vulnerable individuals may initiate and facilitate development of AD neuropathology.

At least four different genetic loci that cause AD or confer susceptibility to the disease have been identified. Mutations in the gene encoding amyloid-β precursor protein (βAPP) on chromosome 21 segregate with rare forms of early-onset familial AD (causing 2%–3% of familial AD) or inherited forms of cerebrovascular amyloidosis (Baringa, 1995). However, 70%–80% of cases of familial early-onset AD (and 5%–10% of all AD) are linked to a gene locus on chromosome 14 (Baringa, 1995). The first genetic linkage reported for late-onset AD was to chromosome 19 (Pericak-Vance et al., 1991). Later on, investigators showed that the apolipoprotein E (apo E) polymorphism is associated with late-onset AD (Saunders et al., 1993). Three common alleles of human apo E gene on chromosome 19 produce three isoforms: apo E2, apo E3, and apo E4. A number of studies have shown that the apo E4 allele increases the risk for the development of late-onset AD and lowers the average age of onset of AD (Corder et al., 1993). However, the association between the apo E4 allele, especially apo E ∈4 heterozygosity, and an increased risk of AD is weaker in African Americans than in whites or Hispanics (Maestre et al., 1995). Also, the presence of the apo E4 allele does not correlate with the development of AD pathology in patients with Down's syndrome (DS) (Wisniewski, Morelli, et al., 1995). These findings indicate that other modifier genes or environmental factors are important in AD.

Aβ accumulates in the neuropil in two different forms: (1) diffuse or benign plaques that contain nonfibrillar Aβ, and (2) neuritic or malignant plaques consisting of fibrillar Aβ, and abnormal neurites and activated glial cells (Wisniewski & Wegiel, 1995b). Recent data indicate that different types of Aβ deposits appear to have different cellular origins. Specifically, nonfibrillar plaques appear to be produced by neurons, whereas microglia, perivascular cells, and smooth muscle cells appear to produce fibrillar amyloid. Also, evidence is accumulating that additional factors, such as some components of basement membrane or extracellular matrix, and Aβ carrier proteins, affect fibrillization of Aβ in the areas of amyloid formation. The intermediary processes causing cell damage related to amyloidosis include neurotoxicity of fibrillar Aβ, oxidative injury, and immune activation associated with the plaques.

Amyloid plaques do not show reliable regional specificity, whereas neurofibrillary tangles (NFTs), neuronal loss, and the atrophy of brain structures exhibit a consistent and characteristic region-specific, lamina-specific, and cell-type-specific pattern. Neurofibrillary pathology is the major contributor to neuronal loss in AD, and the gradual cognitive deterioration is correlated by the concomitant progress of neurofibrillary changes. Recent data suggest that β-amyloidosis and NFT pathology may be caused by different factors or may be triggered independently by a common factor (Silverman et al., 1993).

AMYLOID-β PRECURSOR PROTEIN

The core protein of amyloid plaques is a 4-kDa peptide, amyloid-β protein (Aβ) that is derived from a much larger precursor protein (βAPP). Several isoforms of βAPP are generated by alternative splicing of mRNA transcribed from a single gene on chromosome 21 (Ashall & Goate, 1994). βAPP is synthesized as an integral membrane molecule. Aβ is secreted as a product of proteolytic cleavage of βAPP. There are at least two secretory pathways for βAPP. The vast majority of βAPP is cleaved at the Lys16/Leu17 bond of Aβ by α-secretase, which is not amyloidogenic. Some βAPP is cleaved at the β-secretase site, which is prior to the amyloid sequence. This leaves a C-terminal βAPP fragment that can be processed further, by γ-secretase, to release Aβ.

SOLUBLE AND FIBRILLAR AMYLOID-β

The presence of soluble Aβ (sAβ) in cerebrospinal fluid (CSF) and tissue culture supernatants (Seubert et al., 1992) indicates that Aβ-protein may exist in a nonfibrillar form. Immunohistochemical studies revealed diffuse thioflavine S- and Congo red-negative foci of Aβ without any evidence of neuropil pathology or reactive glia (Tagliavini, Giaccone, Frangione, & Bugiani, 1988). They are usually called diffuse, preamyloid, or benign plaques (Wisniewski & Wegiel, 1995b). Fibrillar β-peptide is the main component of vascular amyloid deposits and neuritic plaques. The latter are complex lesions that contain abnormal neurites, activated microglia, and astrocytes. It appears that fibrillar amyloid deposits cause neuronal degeneration. Therefore, fibrillar amyloid plaques are also called malignant plaques (Wisniewski & Wegiel, 1995b). They are most prominent in association cortices and limbic structures.

Aβ in amyloid plaques and vascular amyloid is formed of different monomers, 40- and 42-amino acid peptides (Miller et al., 1993), which suggests that different cells and different processing mechanisms may be engaged. Immunocytochemical and biochemical studies revealed that the Aβ1-42 or 17-42 peptide is present in diffuse plaques (Gowing et al., 1994; Kida, Wisniewski, & Wisniewski, 1995; Tamaoka et al., 1995), whereas both Aβ42 and Aβ40 are found in the fibrillized plaques (Iwatsubo, Mann, Odaka, Susuki, & Ihara, 1995). Therefore, different types of Aβ deposits appear to have a different cellular origin. Neurons and microglia have been postulated to be responsible for the production of amyloid in the neuropil (Busciglio, Gabuzda, Matsudaira, & Yankner, 1993). Diffuse plaques are of neuronal (Probst, Langui, Ipsen, Robakis, & Ulrich, 1991) or vascular (Pluta et al., 1994) origin. However, there is no consensus about what happens next to diffuse plaques. According to some investigators, they progress and become neuritic fibrillized plaques (Probst et al., 1991). Our recent studies showed, however, that diffuse plaques appeared in very young individuals with DS (15 years of age) and that the number of these plaques increased with age. On the other hand, the numbers of fibrillized, thioflavine-S-positive, neuritic plaques were small even in the oldest group (61 to 70 years of age). Furthermore, the cerebellar diffuse plaques are often found in AD but do not progress into fibrillized neuritic plaques. Our studies of old dogs demonstrated the presence of many diffuse plaques, none of which developed into thioflavine-S-positive plaques. Also, the brains of mice transgenic for βAPP contain diffuse plaques—not malignant neuritic plaques—when the expression of transgene is limited to neurons (Kotula & Wisniewski, 1995). However, when the transgene is expressed in neuronal and nonneuronal cells, thioflavine S-positive and Congo red-positive neuritic plaques appear to develop in addition to diffuse plaques. Taken together, these data suggest that only a small proportion of human diffuse plaques progress into fibrillized neuritic plaques.

As mentioned previously, we hypothesized that diffuse and neuritic plaques may have separate origins. We have shown that microglia produce Aβ that fibrillizes readily, and newly formed amyloid fibrils appear in the deep cytoplasmic membrane infoldings and channels of microglial cells (Wisniewski, Vorbrodt, Wegiel, Morys, & Lossinsky, 1990). We have also demonstrated that perivascular cells of capillaries and smooth muscle cells (SMCs) of the leptomeningeal vessels are responsible for amyloid formation in amyloid angiopathy (Wisniewski & Wegiel, 1993,

1994). The deposit of β-protein in vascular wall in vivo occurs mainly as amyloid fibrils located in the basement membrane. The cells engaged in the formation of vascular amyloid appear to be smooth muscle cells of the tunica media (Wisniewski & Wegiel, 1996). Cultured SMCs produce β-protein and accumulate it intracellularly as fibrillar and nonfibrillar deposits (Wisniewski, Frackowiak, et al., 1995).

The microinjection of soluble Aβ into the brain of experimental animals does not induce neuronal degeneration (Winkler et al., 1994). The presence of many diffuse plaques in brains from elderly nondemented individuals (Tagliavini et al., 1988), and the lack of neuritic pathology in association with diffuse Aβ deposits, indicates that the mere presence of Aβ deposits is insufficient to induce cytopathology. Many different laboratories have shown that aggregation or fibrillization of Aβ is necessary for neurotoxicity (Selkoe, 1995). Recently, we showed that Alzheimer-type functional impairment in DS appears to be related to the appearance of and the increase in the number of neuritic fibrillized, thioflavine-positive, and tau-1-positive plaques.

Why does Aβ fibrillize at a given site but remain in a nonfibrillar form in other places? The stab-wound experiments and studies of transgenic mice show that overexpression of βAPP alone does not lead to amyloid formation, nor does the presence of soluble Aβ-protein (Fukuchi et al., 1994). Test tube studies of synthetic β-peptides showed that fibril formation is influenced by β-peptide concentration, pH, length of β-peptide, and interaction with other proteins (Selkoe, 1995). Investigators have proposed a kinetic model for amyloid formation (Schubert, 1994). The first step is a slow formation of the amyloid nucleus followed by a rapid deposition of aggregated Aβ into the nucleus, which leads to fibril growth. Recent data indicate that Aβ-42/43 may be the seed for the aggregation of Aβ40 in the brain (Tamaoka et al., 1994). Iwatsubo et al. (1995) showed that young DS brains contained mainly Aβ42/43-positive, Aβ40-negative diffuse plaques, whereas the proportion of Aβ40-positive plaques increased in old DS brains. Also, diffuse plaques in the cerebellum of AD patients are composed mainly of Aβ1-42/43 and Aβ17-42 (Tamaoka et al., 1995).

Current data indicate that additional factors promoting fibrillization of Aβ are operative in the area of amyloid formation. For years, it has been known that other proteins are associated with amyloid deposits; the most common are amyloid component P (AP), apo E, and glycosaminoglycans. Soluble Aβ in cerebrospinal fluid forms complexes with apo E and apo

J. Binding of β-peptide with carriers, or with chaperon proteins, including transthyretin (Schwarzman et al., 1994) and apolipoproteins E, J, and A1, is now considered a physiological mechanism for mediating solubility, transport, and clearance of β-peptide.

Apo E is involved in transport and cellular uptake of lipid complexes via the low-density lipoprotein receptor (LDL-R) and the LDL-R-related protein receptor (LRP) (Mahley, 1988). Both of these receptors are expressed in the human brain (Rebeck, Harr, Strickland, & Hyman, 1995). Apo E binds to Aβ (Strittmatter et al., 1993) and is present in β-amyloid plaques, dystrophic neurites, and NFTs (Namba, Tomonaga, Kawasaki, Otomo, & Ikeda, 1991). It has been suggested that LRP-mediated uptake of apo E/Aβ complexes may be a mechanism of Aβ clearance from the neuropil (Rebeck et al., 1995). Intracellular Aβ deposits in cultured SMCs also contained apo E (Mazur-Kolecka, Frackowiak, & Wisniewski, 1995). Exogenous apo E may sequester the β-peptide produced by SMCs and mediate internalization of the apo E/Aβ complex via LDL receptors.

Some components of the basement membrane and extracellular matrix may be necessary for the initial steps in amyloid formation (Leveugle & Fillit, 1994). The highly sulfated proteoglycans of the extracellular matrix promote aggregation of β-peptide (Snow et al., 1994). On the other hand, sulfated proteoglycans interact with a number of molecules, including apo E (Ji et al., 1993). Immobilization of apo E by matrix components may prevent the cellular uptake of the apo E/Aβ complexes and decrease the intracellular accumulation of β-peptide. The altered equilibrium of apolipoproteins, transthyretin, and matrix components appears to create a cell microenvironment for amyloids to form and to participate in β-peptide transport and clearance.

NEUROFIBRILLARY TANGLES

NFTs are the major contributors to neuronal death and dementia in AD. They are formed of paired helical filaments (PHFs) that contain abnormally and overphosphorylated tau-protein (Grundke-Iqbal et al., 1986). The abnormal phosphorylation of tau precedes the formation of NFTs, suggesting that an abnormality in the regulation of the protein phosphorylation-dephosphorylation system is one of the early events in Alzheimer cytoskeletal pathology.

Tau is a phosphoprotein, with two to four phosphates per mole in a normal adult brain (Smith & Anderton, 1994). In cells, its role is to stabilize microtubules, which are essential for neurite outgrowth. Hyperphosphorylated tau self-associates via its microtubule-binding domain (Smith & Anderton, 1994). The normal cytoskeleton of microtubules and neurofilaments is reduced in neurons with PHFs. Such neurons will have a failure of axoplasmic transport and other functions, which depend upon an intact cytoskeleton. The accumulation of PHFs in cell cytoplasm causes neuronal death associated with synaptic loss and deterioration in function.

STAGING OF NEUROFIBRILLARY CHANGES

Amyloid plaques do not show reliable regional specificity; however, NFTs, neuronal loss, and the atrophy of brain structures exhibit a consistent and characteristic region-specific, lamina-specific, and cell-type pattern. Much of the neuronal loss in AD is related to the development of NFTs that are detectable many years before death (Ohm, Muller, Braak, & Bohl, 1995). The gradual cognitive deterioration is correlated with the concomitant progression of NFT formation. We have shown that AD patients resistant to neurofibrillary pathology do not develop dementia even though they may have many neuritic plaques in their brains (Barcikowska, Wisniewski, Bancher, & Grundke-Iqbal, 1989).

Neurofibrillary changes start in the allocortex—the transentorhinal and entorhinal cortex (transentorhinal stages). However, patients in this stage do not exhibit obvious cognitive decline (preclinical phase). Mild to moderate impairment of cognition and personality changes are seen when the transentorhinal and entorhinal cortex are severely affected, and mild changes affect sector CA1 in the cornu ammonis and subcortical nuclei (amygdala, anterodorsal thalamic nucleus, magnocellular nuclei of the basal forebrain, and tuberomammillary nucleus; limbic stages). Further progression in previously affected structures and spread of the neurofibrillary changes and neuronal loss into the association areas of the isocortex as well as the dentate gyrus and substantia nigra characterize the late and end stages of AD (isocortical stages). In these stages, substantial loss of cortical neurons with corresponding shrinkage of the gyri, widening of the sulci, and loss of the brain weight is seen (Braak, Braak, & Bohl, 1993). Neuronal loss in the hippocampal formation appears to be a major component of the memory impairment observed in AD (Hyman, Van Hoesen, Damasio, & Barnes, 1985). The total number of neurons decreases by 84% and 78% in the pyramidal layer of the cornu ammonis and subiculum, respectively. Moreover, the number of neurons in the granular layer of the dentate gyrus decreases by 43%. Volumetric loss of the cornu ammonis, subicular complex, and entorhinal cortex correlates with the stage and duration of AD (Bobinski et al., 1995). Atrophy of the hippocampal formation progresses linearly, even in the end stage of AD, when clinical symptoms of dementia are out of range of psychometric and mental status tests (Bobinski et al., 1996).

In addition to region-specific development of NFTs, there appears to be neuron-specific susceptibility to the neurofibrillary changes. It is puzzling that one neuron is affected by NFT pathology, whereas the nearby neuron remains intact even though they both are under the same influence of time and microenvironment. The reasons for the different vulnerability of the neurons are not clear. However, there are at least seven allelic forms of tau (Goedert, Spillantini, Jakes, Rutherford, & Crowther, 1989), and it is possible that some of them form PHF more readily than the others. Another explanation may be related to differences in mitochondrial pathology. Mitochondria in neurons divide and thus acquire the same problems as any dividing cell. Therefore, mitochondrial activity may be affected in some but not all neurons. Insufficiency of mitochondrial activity may then influence tau phosphorylation.

Despite the lengthy debate, the relationship between the development of β-amyloidosis and neurofibrillary pathology remains unresolved. On the basis of data pertaining to the topographic relationship between plaques and tangles, we hypothesize that β-amyloidosis and NFT pathology may be caused by different factors or be triggered by a common factor rather than be developed in the form of a cascade (i.e., amyloid causing NFT formation, or vice versa).

NEUROTOXICITY OF AMYLOID

The symptoms of dementia in AD are a consequence of NFT formation and synaptic and neuronal loss. There are two basic pathways to cell death—necrosis and apoptosis—both of which have characteristic morphological features. Necrosis has been suggested to reflect cellular degeneration as the result of an insult that causes acute loss of cellular regulation and function, such as traumatic or ischemic injury (Kerr & Harmon, 1991). On the other hand, apoptosis is considered to be a programmed cellular death that may be triggered by various signals, including toxins, loss of neurotrophic support, and oxidative damage, or via a homeostatic cellular signaling pathway.

Apoptosis may be a mechanism of cell loss in AD (Cotman & Anderson, 1995). In vitro studies showed that Aβ, by itself, induces neurons to undergo apoptosis (Loo et al., 1993). On the other hand, Aβ may compromise calcium homeostasis of cultured neurons and enhance their vulnerability to other insults such as excitotoxic or peroxidative damage, hypoxia, or hypoglycemia. Calcium appears to play an important role in apoptosis and has been linked to the regulation of cellular signaling pathways associated with apoptosis. Recent studies showed that increases in intracellular Ca^{2+} in cultured cells can replicate some of the biochemical features of AD: alterations in the phosphorylation of tau-microtubule-associated protein and increased production of Aβ peptide (Mattson et al., 1993).

Many studies have found evidence of oxidative stress in AD brains (Bowling & Beal, 1995; Smith, Sayre, Monnier, & Perry, 1995). Free radicals have been suggested to contribute to β-amyloidosis and tissue injury in AD (Friedlich & Butcher, 1994). Recent data indicate that Aβ itself may generate free radicals and cause oxidative damage to neurons (Harris, 1995).

Test tube studies and tissue culture studies have increased our knowledge considerably of βPP secretion, processing, and metabolism. However, one should remember that nonfibrillar β-protein in vivo does not structurally affect neurites. The fibrillogenesis of Aβ seems to result from interactive pathological processes that are highly dependent on the local microenvironment. Therefore, it is unlikely that tissue culture data on the toxicity of sAβ are applicable to the living brain.

INFLAMMATORY RESPONSE IN AD

Various elements of the immune system, including features associated with both the innate and adaptive immune mechanisms, are associated with the principal lesions characterizing AD. Microglia and astrocytes are components of neuritic, fibrillar plaques and extracellular NFTs but are lacking in most diffuse plaques. The expression of microglial activation markers such as Class II major histocompatibility antigens, Fc-receptors, receptors belonging to the leucocyte adhesion family (β-2 integrins), and the vitronectin receptors is enhanced in AD brains (McGeer, Rogers, & McGeer, 1994). Moreover, microglia associated with amyloid plaques show intensive staining for many interleukins (ILs) such as IL-1∝, IL-1β, and IL-6, and tumor necrosis factor (TNF) (Eikelenboom, Zhan, van Gool, & Allsop, 1994).

Immunocytochemical studies showed that a number of complement factors of the classical complement pathway and their inhibitors are localized in diffuse and neuritic plaques in the neocortex and the cerebellum in patients with AD and DS. Although many acute phase proteins (∝1-antitrypsin, AT; ∝1-antichymotrypsin, ACT; ∝2-macroglobulin, MG; C-reactive protein, CRP; and amyloid P component, AP) are found in neuritic plaques, only some of them such as AP and ACT are also present in diffuse plaques (Eikelenboom et al., 1994).

Inflammatory proteins in amyloid deposits may be derived from blood through the abnormal blood-brain barrier resulting from amyloid angiopathy. mRNA of AP and CRP have not been found in the brain (Kalaria, 1993). However, current evidence suggests that the mRNAs of many complement factors, acute phase proteins, and cytokines are expressed in brain tissue and appear to be produced mainly by glial cells. Some complement factors or inhibitors, and their mRNAs, including C1, C3, C4, CD59, and clusterin, seem to be unregulated in AD (McGeer, Rogers, & McGeer, 1994). Also, the levels of some cytokines, for example, IL-1β and IL-6, in AD brains are elevated, compared to those in controls (Cacabelos et al., 1994; Wood et al., 1993).

Inflammatory response may contribute to several crucial events in the pathogenetic cascade of AD. It may

1. modify the secretion and processing of βAPP;
2. modify Aβ deposition or fibrillization;
3. cause tissue damage via the activation of classical complement pathway or release of potentially toxic products such as proteases, nitric oxide, and free radicals from activated microglia; and
4. induce an abortive regenerative response in AD brains.

Activated microglia and astrocytes secrete neurotoxic factors such as eicosanoids, free radicals, and nitric oxide, as well as interleukins, proteases, and protease inhibitors (Eikelenboom et al., 1994; Lipton & Gendelman, 1995). IL-1, IL-6, and some growth factors were shown to stimulate βAPP mRNA and induce increased production and altered processing of βAPP in neuronal or endothelial cultures (Del Bo, Angeretti, Lucca, Grazia De Simoni, & Forloni, 1995; Forloni, Demichelli, Giorgi, Bendotti, &

Angeretti, 1992; Ohyagi & Tabira, 1993; Vasilakos et al., 1994). In turn, Aβ stimulates glial cells in culture to produce cytokines such as IL-1, TNF-∝, and basic fibroblast growth factor (Araujo & Cotman, 1992; Meda et al., 1995). Coculture experiments demonstrated that activation of microglia with Aβ leads to the production of reactive nitrogen intermediates and neuronal cell injury in vitro (Meda et al., 1995).

Some acute phase proteins may act as pathological chaperon proteins. ACT binds to Aβ and accelerates Aβ fibrillogenesis (Ma, Yee, Brewer, Das, & Potter, 1994). Also, AP enhances the resistance of amyloid fibrils to proteolytic cleavage and may therefore contribute to their persistence (Tennent, Lovat, & Pepys, 1995).

The complement system seems to be involved intrinsically in cerebral amyloidosis. The pattern of complement fragments in AD brains indicates activation of the classical complement pathway (Kalaria, 1993; McGeer et al., 1994). Lack of immunoglobulins in neuritic plaques suggests an antibody-independent mechanism. Aβ avidly binds C1q, and this binding activates complement in vitro (Jiang, Burdick, Glabe, Cotman, & Tenner, 1994). The attachment of C1q to aggregated Aβ in the brain may trigger the activation of the complement cascade, the establishment of the membrane attack complex (MAC), and a lytic assault on the surrounding tissue. The association of the MAC with dystrophic neurites and neurofibrillary tangles suggests that the MAC is directed against neurons (Kalaria).

Many protease inhibitors have potential neurite growth-promoting activity, and they may be released from astrocytes in response to neuronal degeneration (Kalaria, 1993). Investigators have demonstrated signs of a regenerative process in AD brains that may involve a complex network of proteases, cytokines, growth-promoting factors, protease inhibitors, integrins, and adhesion molecules (Eikelenboom et al., 1994).

In conclusion, the present data point to the operation of a low-grade chronic inflammatory response that shares some features with a chronic granulomatous-type lesion and contributes to the progression of the disease and cell death. Activated microglia appear to be the main immunocompetent cells contributing to the response.

RISK FACTORS FOR AD

The cause of AD is unknown. AD can be considered a disease with multiple risk factors (polyetiology) (Khachaturian, 1986; Wisniewski & Wegiel, 1995c).

There are allele-specific interactions between apo E and Aβ that may contribute to the increased risk of AD in the presence of apo E4 (Strittmatter et al., 1993). Apo E4 accelerates fibrillization and stabilizes amyloid in vitro (Ma et al., 1994). In the brains of patients with the apo E4/4 genotype, amyloid plaque density is more than 50% greater than that in the brains of patients with the apo E3/3 genotype (Rebeck, Reiter, Strickland, & Hyman, 1993). Recently, it also has been suggested that apo E may be involved in the development of neurofibrillary pathology in AD (Strittmatter et al., 1994). Apo E3 binds to the microtubule-binding domain of tau in vitro, whereas apo E4 shows no such binding (Strittmatter et al., 1994). The presence of apo E3 may decrease tau phosphorylation and self-assembly into PHFs.

Sherrington et al. (1995) recently identified the gene on chromosome 14 that is associated with most familial early-onset AD. Thirty-five missense mutations in this gene cosegregated with the disease. The function of the gene's product, called S182 protein, remains to be shown. The general topology of S182 protein suggests that it is an integral membrane protein, such as a receptor, a channel protein, or a structural membrane protein. Its amino acids bear similarity to those of a membrane protein known as SPE-4 from nematode worm, *Caenorhabditis elegans*, sperm. SPE-4 is needed in the transport and storage of soluble and membrane-bound polypeptides Presenilen (S182) protein could be involved in the docking of other membrane-bound proteins such as βPP or in the axonal transport and fusion budding of membrane-bound vesicles during protein transport. The mutations of the protein may result in aberrant transport and processing of βPP or abnormal interactions with cytoskeletal proteins such as the microtubule-associated protein, tau.

Changes in mitochondrial activity and oxidative damage in the brain are a well-documented consequence of aging (Bowling & Beal, 1995). Amyloid-related cytotoxic events may precipitate the disease on a background of compromised cells with age. The pathogenetic effects of βAPP mutations are thought to include increased formation of Aβ from mutant βAPP (Citron et al., 1994), greater propensity of mutant Aβ to aggregate into amyloid fibrils (Clements, Walsh, Williams, & Allsop, 1993), and increased formation from βAPP of longer, more amyloidogenetic forms of Aβ (Suzuki et al., 1994).

FROM NEUROPATHOLOGY TO THERAPY

Loss of synapses, neurofibrillary pathology, and neuronal death leads to multisystem neurotransmitter failure and dementia in AD. Until recently, the main pharmacological approach in AD has been to achieve a symptomatic improvement of cognitive functions by treatment of neurotransmitter deficiency, most often the cholinergic deficit. Advances in neuropathology, molecular biology, and biochemistry have increased the understanding of the processes that lead to AD. It is now understood that a combination of pathological processes interacts in AD brains, and targeting each one of them may affect the progression of the disease.

The new strategies for treatment of AD include development of drugs that intervene in:

1. the specific pathogenetic processes such as amyloidogenesis or NFT formation;
2. secondary events such as oxidative injury or inflammatory response that contribute to the progression of the disease; and
3. the final pathways to cell death such as apoptosis or intracellular Ca^{2+} regulatory mechanisms.

The most promising approaches to slow down amyloid formation include the use of pharmacological agents that divert βAPP molecules from amyloidogenic to nonamyloidogenic proteolytic processing pathways or intervene with proteins promoting fibrillization of Aβ. Another therapeutic approach could be to modulate some intermediate steps in AD pathology. Although oxidative stress is well established in AD (see Bowling & Beal, 1995; Smith et al., 1995), and antioxidants protect cells against Aβ toxicity (Goodman, Steiner, & Mattson, 1994), the role of antioxidants and compounds that improve mitochondrial function in AD patients has not been widely studied. Recent data showed that some anti-inflammatory drugs may be beneficial in the treatment of AD (Rich et al., 1995), but more extensive clinical trials are needed to determine whether manipulation of inflammatory response can slow the progression of AD.

REFERENCES

Araujo, D. M., & Cotman, C. W. (1992). Beta-amyloid stimulates glial cells in vitro to produce growth factors that accumulate in senile plaques in Alzheimer's disease. *Brain Research, 569,* 141–145.

Ashall, F., & Goate, A. M. (1994). Role of the β-amyloid precursor protein in Alzheimer's disease. *Trends in Biochemical Science, 19,* 42–46.

Barcikowska, M., Wisniewski, H. M., Bancher, C., & Grundke-Iqbal, I. (1989). About the presence of paired helical filaments in dystrophic neurites participating in the plaque formation. *Acta Neuropathologica, 78,* 225–231.
Barinaga, M. (1995). New Alzheimer's gene found. *Science, 268,* 1845–1846.
Bobinski, M., Wegiel, J., Wisniewski, H. M., Tarnawski, M., Reisberg, B., Mlodzik, M., de Leon, M. J., & Miller, D. S. (1995). Atrophy of hippocampal formation subdivisions correlates with stage and duration of Alzheimer disease. *Dementia, 6,* 205–210.
Bobinski, M., Wegiel, J., Wisniewski, H. M., Tarnawski, M., Reisberg, B., de Leon, M. J., & Miller, D. C. (1996). Neurofibrillary pathology—correlation with hippocampal formation atrophy in Alzheimer disease. *Neurobiology of Aging, 17,* 909–919.
Bowling, A. C., & Beal, M. F. (1995). Bioenergetic and oxidative stress in neurodegenerative disease. *Life Science, 56,* 1151–1171.
Braak, H., Braak, E., & Bohl, J. (1993). Staging of Alzheimer-related cortical destruction. *European Neurology, 33,* 403–408.
Busciglio, J., Gabuzda, D. H., Matssudaira, P., & Yankner, B. A. (1993). Generation of β-amyloid in the secretory pathway in neuronal and nonneuronal cells. *Proceedings of the National Academy of Sciences, USA, 90,* 2092–2096.
Cacabelos, R., Alvarez, X. A., Fernandez-Novoa, L., Franco, A., Mangues, R., Pellicer, A., & Nishimura, T. (1994). Brain interleukin-1β in Alzheimer's disease and vascular dementia. Methods Find Exp *Clinical Pharmacology, 16,* 141–151.
Citron, M., Vigo-Pelfrey, C., Teplow, D. B., Miller, C., Schenk, D., Johnston, J., Winblad, B., Venizelos, N., Lannfelt, L., & Selkoe, D. J. (1994). Excessive production of amyloid β-protein by peripheral cells of symptomatic and presymptomatic patients carrying the Swedish familial Alzheimer disease mutation. *Proceedings of the National Academy of Sciences, USA, 91,* 11993–11997.
Clements, A., Walsh, D. M., Williams, C. H., & Allsop, D. (1993). Effects of the mutations Glu[22] to Gln and Ala[21] to Gly on the aggregation of a synthetic fragment of the Alzheimer's amyloid β/A4 peptide. *Neuroscience Letter, 161,* 17–20.
Corder, E. H., Saunders, A. M., Strittmatter, W. J., Schmechel, D. E., Gaskell, P. C., Small, G. W., Roses, A. D., Haines, J. L., & Pericak-Vance, M. A. (1993). Gene dose of apolipoprotein E type 4 allele and the risk of Alzheimer's disease in late onset families. *Science, 261,* 921–923.
Cork, L. C., Masters, C., Beyreuther, K., & Price, D. L. (1990). Development of senile plaques. Relationships of neuronal abnormalities and amyloid deposits. *American Journal of Pathology, 137,* 1383–1392.
Cotman, C. W., & Anderson, A. J. (1995). A potential role for apoptosis in neurodegeneration and Alzheimer's disease. *Molecular Neurobiology, 10,* 19–45.

Etiology and Neuropathogenesis of AD 45

Del Bo, R., Angeretti, N., Lucca, E., Grazia De Simoni, M., & Forloni, G. (1995). Reciprocal control of inflammatory cytokines, IL-1 and IL-6, and β-amyloid production in cultures. *Neuroscience Letter, 188,* 70–74.

Eikelenboom, P., Zhan, S. S., van Gool, W. A., & Allsop, D. (1994). Inflammatory mechanisms in Alzheimer's disease. *Trends in Pharmacologic Science, 15,* 447–450.

Forloni, G., Demichelli, F., Giorgi, S., Bendotti, C., & Angeretti, N. (1992). Expression of amyloid precursor protein mRNAs in endothelial, neuronal and glial cells: Modulation by interleukin-1. *Molecular Brain Research, 16,* 128–134.

Frackowiak, J., Mazur-Kolecka, B., Wisniewski, H. M., Potempska, A., Carroll, R. T., Emmerling, M. R., & Kim, K. S. (1995). Secretion and accumulation of Alzheimer's β-protein by cultured vascular smooth muscle cells from old and young dogs. *Brain Research, 676,* 225–230.

Friedlich, A. L., & Butcher, L. L. (1994). Involvement of free oxygen radicals in β-amyloidosis: An hypothesis. *Neurobiology of Aging, 15,* 443–455.

Fukuchi, K. I., Ogburn, C. E., Smith, A. C., Kunkel, D. D., Furlong, C. E., Deeb, S. S., Nochlin, D., Sumi, S. M., & Martin, G. M. (1994). Transgenic animal models of Alzheimer's disease. *Annals of the New York Academy of Science, 695,* 217–223.

Ghiso, J., Matsubara, E., Koudinow, A., Choi-Miura, N. H., Tomita, M., Wisniewski, T., & Frangione, B. (1993). The cerebrospinal fluid soluble form of Alzheimer's amyloid beta is complexed to SP-40,40 (apolipoprotein J), an inhibitor of the complement membrane-attack complex. *Biochemical Journal, 293,* 27–30.

Goedert, M., Spillantini, M. G., Jakes, R., Rutherford, D., & Crowther, R. A. (1989). Multiple isoforms of human microtubule-associated protein tau: Sequences and localization in neurofibrillary tangles of Alzheimer's disease. *Neuron, 3,* 519–526.

Goldman, J. E., & Yen, S. H. (1986). Cytoskeletal protein abnormalities in neurodegenerative diseases. *Annals of Neurology, 19,* 209–223.

Goodman, Y., Steiner, S. M., & Mattson, M. P. (1994). Nordihydroguaiaretic acid protects hippocampal neurons against amyloid β-peptide toxicity, and attenuates free radical and calcium accumulation. *Brain Research, 654,* 171–176.

Gowing, E., Roher, A. E., Woods, A. S., Cotter, R. J., Chaney, M., Little, S. P., & Ball, M. J. (1994). Chemical characterization of Aβ17-42 peptide, a component of diffuse amyloid deposits of Alzheimer disease. *Journal of Biological Chemistry, 269,* 10987–10990.

Gray, E. G., Paula Barbosa, M., & Roher, A. (1987). Alzheimer's disease: Paired helical filaments and cytomembranes. *Neuropathology Applied to Neurobiology, 13,* 91–110.

Grundke-Iqbal, I., Iqbal, K., Tung, Y. C., Quinlan, M., Wisniewski, H. M., & Binder, L. I. (1986). Abnormal phosphorylation of the microtubule associated protein tau in Alzheimer cytoskeletal pathology. *Proceedings of the National Academy of Sciences, USA, 83,* 4913–4917.

Harris, M. E., Hensley, K., Butterfield, D. A., Leedle, R. A., & Carney, J. M. (1995). Direct evidence of oxidative injury produced by the Alzheimer's β-amyloid peptide (1-40) in cultured hippocampal neurons. *Experimental Neurology, 131,* 193–202.

Hyman, B. T., Van Hoesen, G. W., Damasio, A. R., & Barnes, C. L. (1985). Alzheimer's disease: Cell-specific pathology isolates the hippocampal formation. *Science, 225,* 1168–1170.

Iwatsubo, T., Mann, D. M. A., Odaka, A., Suzuki, N., & Ihara, Y. (1995). Amyloid β protein (Aβ) deposition: Aβ42(43) precedes Aβ40 in Down syndrome. *Annals of Neurology, 37,* 294–299.

Ji, Z., Brecht, W. J., Miranda, R. D., Hussain, M. M., Innerarity, T. L., & Mahley, R. W. (1993). Role of heparan sulfate proteoglycans in the binding and uptake of apolipoprotein E-enriched remnant lipoproteins by cultured cells. *Journal of Biological Chemistry, 268,* 10160–10167.

Jiang, H., Burdick, D., Glabe, C. G., Cotman, C. W., & Tenner, A. J. (1994). β-amyloid activates complement by binding to a specific region of the collagen-like doamin of the C1q A chain. *Journal of Immunology, 152,* 5050–5059.

Kalaria, R. N. (1993). The immunopathology of Alzheimer's disease and some related disorders. *Brain Pathology, 3,* 333–347.

Kang, J., Lemaire, H. G., Unterbeck, A., Salbaum, J. M., Masters, C. L., Grzescik, K. H., Multhaup, G., Beyreuther, K., & Muller-Hill, B. (1987). The precursor of Alzheimer's disease amyloid A4 protein resembles a cell-surface receptor. *Nature, 325,* 733–736.

Kerr, J. F. R., & Harmon, B. V. (1991). Definition and incidence of apoptosis: An historical perspective. In L. D. Tomei & F. O. Cope (Eds.), *Apoptosis: The Molecular Basis of Cell Death* (Vol. 3, pp. 5–29). Cold Spring Harbor, NY: Cold Spring Harbor Laboratory.

Khachaturian, Z. S. (1986). Aluminium toxicity among other views on the etiology of Alzheimer disease. *Neurobiology of Aging, 7,* 537–539.

Khachaturian, Z. S. (1985). Diagnosis of Alzheimer's disease. *Archives of Neurology, 42,* 1097–1105.

Kida, E., Wisniewski, K. E., & Wisniewski, H. M. (1995). Early amyloid-β deposits show different immunoreactivity to the amino- and carboxy-terminal regions of β-peptide in Alzheimer's disease and Down's syndrome brain. *Neuroscience Letter, 193,* 1–4.

Kotula, L., & Wisnieswski, H. M. (1995). New hopes arise with the transgenic model for Alzheimer's disease. *Neurobiology of Aging, 16,* 701–703.

Koudinow, A., Matsubara, E., Frangione, B., & Ghiso, J. (1994). The soluble form of Alzheimer's amyloid beta protein is complexed to high density lipoprotein 3 and very high density lipoprotein in normal human plasma. *Biochemical and Biophysical Research Communication, 205,* 1164–1171.

Lehtimäki, T., Pirttilä, T., Mehta, P. D., Wisniewski, H. M., Frey, H., & Nikkari, T. (1995). Apolipoprotein E (apo E) polymorphism and its influence on apo E concentrations in the cerebrospinal fluid in Finnish patients with Alzheimer's disease. *Human Genetics, 95,* 39–42.

Leveugle, B., & Fillit, H. (1994). Proteoglycans and the acute-phase response in Alzheimer's disease brain. *Molecular Neurobiology, 9,* 25–32.

Levy, E., Carman, M. D., Fernandez-Madrid, I. J., Power, M. D., Lieberburg, I., Van Duinen, S. G., Bots, GThA, Luyendijk, W., & Frangione, B. (1990). Mutation of the Alzheimer's disease amyloid gene in hereditary cerebral hemorrhage, Dutch type. *Science, 248,* 1124–1126.

Lipton, S. A., & Gendelman, H. E. (1995). Dementia associated with the acquired immunodeficiency syndrome. *New England Journal of Medicine, 332,* 934–940.

Loo, D. T., Copani, A. G., Pike, C. J., Whittemore, E. R., Walencewicz, A. J., & Cotman, C. W. (1993). Apoptosis is induced by beta-amyloid in cultured central nervous system neurons. *Proceedings of the National Academy of Sciences, USA, 90,* 7951–7955.

Ma, J., Yee, A., Brewer, B., Jr., Das, S., & Potter, H. (1994). Amyloid-associated proteins ∝1-antichymotrypsin and apolipoprotein E promote assembly of Alzheimer β-protein into filaments. *Nature, 372,* 92–94.

Maestre, G., Ottman, R., Stern, Y., Gurland, B., Chun, M., Tang, M. X., Shelanski, M., Tycko, B., & Mayeux, R. (1995). Apolipoprotein E and Alzheimer's disease: Ethnic variation in genotypic risks. *Annals of Neurology, 37,* 254–259.

Mahley, R. W. (1988). Apolipoprotein E: Cholesterol transport protein with expanding role in cell biology. *Science, 240,* 622–630.

Mattson, M. P., Barger, S. W., Cheng, B., Lieberburg, I., Smith, S. V., & Rydel, R. E. (1993). Beta-amyloid precursor protein metabolites and loss of neuronal Ca2+ homeostasis in Alzheimer's disease. *Trends in Neuroscience, 16,* 409–414.

Mazur-Kolecka, B., Frackowiak, J., & Wisniewski, H. M. (1995). Apolipoproteins E3 and E4 induce, and transthyretin prevents accumulation of the Alzheimer's β-amyloid peptide in cultured vascular smooth muscle cells. *Brain Research, 698,* 217–222.

McGeer, P. L., Rogers, J., & McGeer, E. G. (1994). Neuroimmune mechanisms in Alzheimer disease pathogenesis. *Alzheimer Disease Associated Disorders, 8,* 149–158.

Meda, L., Cassatella, M. A., Szendrel, G. I., Otvos, L., Jr., Baron, P., Villalba, M., Ferrari, D., & Rossi, F. (1995). Activation of microglial cells by β-amyloid protein and interferon-γ. *Nature, 374,* 647–650.

Mehta, P. D., Kim, K. S., & Wisniewski, H. M. (1991). ELISA as a laboratory test to aid the diagnosis of Alzheimer's disease. *Techniques in Diagnostic Pathology, 2,* 99–112.

Miller, D. L., Papayannopoulos, I. A., Styles, J., Bobin, S. A., Lin, Y. Y., Biemann, K., & Iqbal, K. (1993). Peptide compositions of the cerebrovascular and senile plaque core amyloid deposits of Alzheimer's disease. *Archives of Biochemistry and Biophysics, 301,* 41–52.

Namba, Y., Tomonaga, M., Kawasaki, H., Otomo, E., & Ikeda, K. (1991). Apolipoprotein E immunoreactivity in cerebral amyloid deposits and neurofibrillary tangles in Alzheimer's disease and kuru plaque amyloid in Creutzfeldt-Jakob disease. *Brain Research, 541,* 163–166.

Ohm, T. G., Muller, H., Braak, H., & Bohl, J. (1995). Close-meshed prevalence rates of different stages as a tool to uncover the rate of Alzheimer's disease-related neurofibrillary changes. *Neuroscience, 64,* 209–217.

Ohyagi, Y., & Tabira, T. (1993). Effect of growth factors and cytokines on expression of amyloid β protein precursor mRNAs in cultured neural cells. *Molecular Brain Research, 18,* 127–132.

Pericak-Vance, M. A., Bebout, J. L., Gaskell, P. C., Yamaoka, L. H., Hung, W. Y., Alberts, M. J., Walker, A. P., Bartlett, R. J., Haynes, C. A., Welsh, K. A., Earl, N. L., Heyman, A., Clark, C. M., & Roses, A. D. (1991). Linkage studies in familial Alzheimer disease: Evidence for chromosome 19 linkage. *American Journal of Human Genetics, 48,* 1034–1050.

Pluta, R., Kida, E., Lossinsky, A. S., Golabek, A. A., Mossakowski, M. J., & Wisniewski, H. M. (1994). Complete cerebral ischemia with short-term survival in rats induced by cardiac arrest. Part 1. Extracellular accumulation of Alzheimer's β-amyloid protein precursor in the brain. *Brain Research, 649,* 323–328.

Probst, A., Langui, D., Ipsen, S., Robakis, N., & Ulrich, J. (1991). Deposition of β/A4 protein along neuronal plasma membranes in diffuse senile plaques. *Acta Neuropathologica, 83,* 21–29.

Rebeck, G. W., Harr, S. D., Strickland, D. K., & Hyman, B. T. (1995). Multiple, diverse senile plaque-associated proteins are ligands of an apolipoprotein E receptor, the ∝2-macroglobulin receptor/low-density-lipoprotein receptor-related protein. *Annals of Neurology, 37,* 211–217.

Rebeck, G. W., Reiter, J. S., Strickland, D. K., & Hyman, B. T. (1993). Apolipoprotein E in sporadic Alzheimer's disease: Allelic variation and receptor interactions. *Neuron, 11,* 575–580.

Rich, J. B., Rasmusson, D. X., Folstein, M. F., Carson, K. A., Kawas, C., & Brandt, J. (1995). Nonsteroidal anti-inflammatory drugs in Alzheimer's disease. *Neurology, 45,* 51–55.

Sandhu, F. A., Salim, M., & Zain, S. B. (1991). Expression of the human β-amyloid protein of Alzheimer's disease specifically in the brains of transgenic mice. *Journal of Biological Chemistry, 266,* 21331–21334.
Saunders, A. M., Strittmatter, W. J., Schmechel, D., St. George-Hyslop, P. H., Pericak-Vance, M. A., Joo, S. H., Rosi, B. L., Gusella, J. F., Crapper-MacLachlan, D. R., Alberts, M. J., Hulette, C., Crain, B., Goldgaber, D., & Roses, A. D. (1993). Association of apolipoprotein E allele ε4 with late-onset familial and sporadic Alzheimer's disease. *Neurology, 43,* 1467–1472.
Schubert, D. (1994). Structural properties of amyloid beta protein and its precursor. In *The structure and function of Alzheimer's amyloid beta proteins* (chap. 2, pp. 11–35). Austin, TX: R. G. Landes.
Schwarzman, A. L., Gregori, L., Vitek, M. P., Lyubski, S., Strittmatter, W. J., Enghilde, J. J., Bhasin, R., Silverman, J., Weigraber, K. H., Coyle, P. K., Zagorski, M. G., Talafous, J., Eisenberg, M., Saunders, A. M., Roses, A. D., & Goldgaber, D. (1994). Transthyretin sequesters amyloid β protein and prevents amyloid formation. *Proceedings of the National Academy of Sciences, USA, 91,* 8368–8372.
Selkoe, D. J. (1995). Deciphering Alzheimer's disease: Molecular genetics and cell biology yield major clues. *Journal of the National Institutes of Health Research, 7,* 57–64.
Seubert, P., Vigo-Pelfrey, C., Esch, F., Lee, M., Dovey, H., Davis, D., Shinha, S., Schlossmacher, M., Whaley, J., Swindlehurst, C., McCormack, R., Wolfert, R., Selkoe, D., Lieberburg, I., & Schenk, D. (1992). Isolation and quantitation of soluble Alzheimer's β-peptide from biological fluids. *Nature, 359,* 325–327.
Sherrington, R., Rogaev, E. I., Liang, Y., Rogaeva, E. A., Levesque, G., Ikeda, M., Chi, H., Lin, C., Li, G., Holman, K., Tsuda, T., Mar, L., Foncin, J. F., Bruni, A. C., Montesi, M. P., Sorbi, S., Rainero, I., Pinessi, L., Nee, L., Chumakov, I., Pollen, D., Brookes, A., Sanseau, P., Polinsky, R. J., Wasco, W., Da Silva, H. A. R., Haines, J. L., Pericak-Vance, M. A., Tanzi, R. E., Roses, A. D., Fraser, P. E., Rommens, J. M., & St. George-Hyslop, H. (1995). Cloning of a gene bearing missense mutations in early-onset familial Alzheimer's disease. *Nature, 375,* 754–760.
Silverman, W., Popovitch, E., Schupf, N., Zigman, W. B., Rabe, A., Sersen, E., & Wisniewski, H. M. (1993). Alzheimer neuropathology in mentally retarded adults: Statistical independence of regional amyloid plaque and neurofibrillary tangle densities. *Acta Neuropathologica, 85,* 260–266.
Smith, C., & Anderton, B. H. (1994). The molecular pathology of Alzheimer's disease: Are we any closer to understanding the neurodegenerative process? *Neuropathology Applied to Neurobiology, 20,* 322–338.
Smith, M. A., Sayre, L. M., Monnier, V. M., & Perry, G. (1995). Radical AGEing in Alzheimer's disease. *Trends in Neuroscience, 18,* 172–176.

Snow, A. D., Sekiguchi, R., Nochlin, D., Fraser, P., Kimata, K., Mizutani, A., Arai, M., Schreier, W. A., & Morgan, D. G. (1994). An important role of heparan sulfate proteoglycan (Perlecan) in a model system for the deposition and persistence of fibrillar Aβ-amyloid in rat brain. *Neuron, 12,* 219–234.

Strittmatter, W. J., Saunders, A. M., Goedert, M., Weisgraber, K. H., Dong, L. M., Jakes, R., Huang, D. Y., Pericak-Vance, M., Schmechel, D., & Roses, A. D. (1994). Isoform-specific interactions of apolipoprotein E with microtubule-associated protein tau: Implications for Alzheimer disease. *Proceedings of the National Academy of Sciences, USA, 91,* 11183–11186.

Strittmatter, W. J., Weisgraber, K. H., Huang, D. Y., Dong, L. M., Salvesen, G. S., Pericak-Vance, M., Schmechel, D., Saunders, A. M., Goldgaber, D., & Roses, A. D. (1993). Binding of human apolipoprotein E to synthetic amyloid β peptide: Isoform-specific effects and implications for late-onset Alzheimer disease. *Proceedings of the National Academy of Sciences, USA, 90,* 8098–8102.

Suzuki, N., Cheung, T. T., Cai, X. D., Odaka, A., Otvos, L., Jr., Eckman, C., Golde, T. E., & Younkin, S. G. (1994). An increased percentage of long amyloid β protein secreted by familial amyloid β protein precursor (βAPP$_{717}$) mutants. *Science, 264,* 1336–1340.

Tagliavini, F., Giaccone, G., Frangione, B., & Bugiani, O. (1988). Pre-amyloid deposits in the cerebral cortex of patients with Alzheimer's disease and nondemented individuals. *Neuroscience Letter, 93,* 191–196.

Tamaoka, A., Kondo, T., Okada, A., Sahara, N., Sawamura, N., Ozawa, K., Suzuki, N., Shoji, S., & Mori, H. (1994). Biochemical evidence for the longtail form (Aβ1-42/43) of amyloid β protein as a seed molecule in cerebral deposits of Alzheimer's disease. *Biochemical and Biophysical Research Communication, 205,* 834–842.

Tamaoka, A., Sawamura, N., Odaka, A., Suzuki, N., Mizusawa, H., Shoji, S., & Mori, H. (1995). Amyloid β protein 1-42/43 (Aβ 1-42/43) in cerebellar diffuse plaques: Enzyme-linked immunosorbent assay and immunocytochemical study. *Brain Research, 679,* 151–156.

Tennent, G. A., Lovat, L. B., & Pepys, M. B. (1995). Serum amyloid P component prevents proteolysis of the amyloid fibrils of Alzheimer disease and systemic amyloidosis. *Proceedings of the National Academy of Science, USA, 92,* 4299–4303.

Vasilakos, J. P., Carroll, R. T., Emmerling, M. R., Doyle, P. D., Davis, R. E., Kim, K. S., & Shivers, B. D. (1994). Interleukin-1β dissociates β-amyloid precursor protein and β-amyloid peptide secretion. *Federation of European Biochemical Societies Letter, 354,* 289–292.

Wegiel, J., & Wisniewski, H. M. (1990). The complex of microglia cells and amyloid star in three-dimensional reconstruction. *Acta Neuropathologica, 81,* 116–124.

Wegiel, J., Wisniewski, H. M., Dziewiatkowski, J., Tarnawski, M., Dziewiatkowska, A., Soltysiak, Z., & Kim, K. S. (1995). Fibrillar and non-fibrillar amyloid in the brain of aged dogs. In K. Iqbal, J. Mortimer, B. Winblad, & H. M. Wisniewski (Eds.), *Research advances in Alzheimer's disease and related disorders* (pp. 703–706). Chichester, England: John Wiley.

Winkler, J., Connor, D. J., Frautschy, S. A., Behl, C., Waite, J. J., Cole, G. M., & Thal, L. J. (1994). Lack of long-term effects after β-amyloid protein injections in rat brain. *Neurobiology and Aging, 15*, 601–607.

Wisniewski, H. M., Frackowiak, J., & Mazur-Kolecka, B. (1995). In vitro production of β-amyloid in smooth muscle cells isolated from amyloid angiopathy-affected vessels. *Neuroscience Letter, 183*, 120–123.

Wisniewski, H. M., Frackowiak, J., Zoltowska, A., & Kim, K. S. (1994). Vascular β-amyloid in Alzheimer's disease angiopathy is produced by proliferating and degenerating smooth muscle cells. *Amyloid International Journal of Clinical Experimentation and Investment, 1*, 8–16.

Wisniewski, H. M., Narang, H. K., & Terry, R. D. (1976). Neurofibrillary tangles of paired helical filaments. *Journal of Neurological Science, 27*, 173–181.

Wisniewski, H. M., Vorbrodt, A. W., Wegiel, J., Morys, J., & Lossinsky, A. S. (1990). Ultrastructure of the cells forming amyloid fibers in Alzheimer disease and scrapie. *American Journal of Medical Genetics*, (Supplement 7), 287–297.

Wisniewski, H. M., & Wegiel, J. (1993). Migration of perivascular cells into the neuropil and their involvement in β-amyloid plaque formation. *Acta Neuropathologica, 85*, 586–595.

Wisniewski, H. M., & Wegiel, J. (1994). β-amyloid formation by myocytes of leptomeningeal vessels. *Acta Neuropathologica, 87*, 233–241.

Wisniewski, H. M., & Wegiel, J. (1995a). Alzheimer's disease and the pathogenesis of β and paired helical filaments (tau) protein fibrillization. In K. Iqbal, J. A. Mortimer, B. Winblad, & H. M. Wisniewski (Eds.), *Research advances in Alzheimer's disease and related disorders* (pp. 569–575). Chichester, England: John Wiley.

Wisniewski, H. M., & Wegiel, J. (1995b). Commentary—Do neurofibrillary tangles initiate plaque formation, or is it β-amyloidosis that leads to NFT pathology? *Neurobiology of Aging, 16*, 341–343.

Wisniewski, H. M., Wegiel, J., & Popovitch, E. R. (1994). Age-associated development of diffuse and thioflavine-S-positive plaques in Down syndrome. *Developmental Brain Dysfunction, 7*, 330–339.

Wisniewski, H. M., Wegiel, J., Wang, K. C., Kujawa, M., & Lach, B. (1989). Ultrastructural studies of the cells forming amyloid fibers in classical plaques. *Canadian Journal of Neurological Science, 16*, 535–542.

Wisniewski, T., Morelli, L., Wegiel, J., Levy, E., Wisniewski, H. M., & Frangione, B. (1995). The influence of apolipoprotein E isotypes on Alzheimer's disease pathology in 40 cases of Down's syndrome. *Annals of Neurology, 37,* 136–138.

Wood, J. A., Wood, P. L., Ryan, R., Graff-Radford, N. R., Pilapil, C., Robitaille, Y., & Quirion, R. (1993). Cytokine indices in Alzheimer's temporal cortex: No changes in mature IL-1β or IL-1RA but increases in the associated acute phase proteins IL-6, ∝2-macroglobulin and C-reactive protein. *Brain Research, 629,* 245–252.

CHAPTER 3

Neurobiological Systems Disrupted by Alzheimer's Disease and Molecular Biological Theories of Vulnerability

J. Wesson Ashford
Mark Mattson
Vinod Kumar

Alzheimer's disease (AD) is a neuropathological process that devastates progressively and relentlessly the brains of its victims. The AD pathology produces progressively severe deficits in cognition, behavior, and activities of daily living over a time course of deterioration averaging 8 years (Ashford, Shan, Butler, Rajasekar, & Schmitt, 1995).

This work was supported in part by the National Institute on Aging Grant AGO5144 for Drs. Ashford and Mattson, and Grant NS30583 from the Alzheimer's Association and the Metropolitan Life Foundation for Dr. Mattson.
We are indebted to Sandy Tipton for stenographic assistance.

Most of the studies of AD pathology have examined the composition and distribution of the neurofibrillary tangles and senile plaques first described by Alois Alzheimer in 1907. However, Alzheimer's first comments on this disease referred to the psychosocial disruptions that he found in his patients. To solve this disease, the psychosocial clinical problems and the neurobiological system dysfunctions must be defined to the point that they indicate what neuromolecular mechanisms are attacked by the AD process.

The AD process has no direct effects on most functions of the body and is restricted in its attack on the brain. Investigations into the biology of AD have not yet revealed the basis of this process. Clearly, the most important factor associated with the development of AD is age, with AD changes appearing in many individuals at a young age and developing in a majority of individuals as age progresses past 60 years (Ohm, Muller, Braak, & Bohl, 1995). Studies of family constellations, DNA polymorphisms, and genetic mechanisms have revealed that genetic factors play a significant role in predisposing some individuals to AD (the genetic aspects of AD are discussed in chapter 4 of this volume). Certain environmental factors, including a possible contribution by aluminum (Bertholf, 1987; Lovell, Ehmann, & Markerbery, 1993; Forbes, Gentleman, & Maxwell, 1995), also may influence the onset of the disease. However, a major concern is understanding which neuronal systems in the brain are affected by the AD process and how their unique physiological processes may predispose them to allow the development of this disease. The affected neurobiological systems seem to be those that underlie learning, and the AD process appears to attack mechanisms for storing new information from molecular biological machinery to specific neurotransmitter systems to macroscopic anatomical structures of the cerebrum (Ashford & Jarvik, 1985; see Table 3.1). Through more understanding of the attack of the AD process, it is hoped that approaches can be developed to prevent or slow the development of AD.

PSYCHOSOCIAL SYSTEMS AFFECTED BY AD

In the study of AD, the first principle is that investigations of pathology must be linked to clinical dysfunctions. In AD, there is a progressive development of complex psychological and social symptoms. However, it is important to decipher these complex changes into simple psychological precepts that can be related meaningfully to the underlying organic disease.

TABLE 3.1 Biopsychosocial Systems Affected by AD (Mnemonic Function at Each Level Is Attacked by AD)

Social systems
    dysfunction in instrumental behaviors (early AD)
        (remembering a grocery list or phone number)
    dysfunction in personal care (late AD)
        (remembering how to dress or bathe)

Psychological systems
    primary loss of ability to learn new information including inability to know of this deficit
    secondary loss of previously learned information
    later loss of learned perceptual and motor skills (aphasia, agnosia, apraxia)

Cortical systems
    - entorhinal cortex (memory network) (early AD)
    - hippocampus (archicortex) - locational memory
    - amygdala (paleocortex) - emotional memory
    - temporal-parietal cortex (neocortex) (middle AD) sensory analysis and perception storage
    - frontal cortex - executive function (mid-late AD)
    - primary cortex - primary sensory/motor analysis (late)

Cortical neurotransmitter systems
    - glutamate (information storage mediation)
    - gaba-somatostatin (unknown mnemonic function)

Subcortical neurochemical systems projecting to cortex
    - nucleus basalis of meynert - acetylcholine
        (memory; classical conditioning)
    - rostral raphe nuclei - serotonin
        (sensitization conditioning)
    - locus coeruleus - norepinephrine
        (reward-related conditioning)

Neuronal systems (primarily cortical)
    - microtubule-associated protein - tau
        (process growth for establishing new synapses)
        neurofibrillary tangles, neuritic plaques
    - amyloid preprotein (APP)
        (possible involvement in formation of new synapses)
    - β-amyloid in senile plaques, amyloid angiopathy

Although the psychological and social difficulties of the AD patients seem diverse, there may be a common thread in the signs and symptoms that is the failure of memory (Ashford, Kolm, Colliver, Bekian, & Hsu, 1989a; Carlesino & Oscar-Berman, 1992), and, more specifically, the disruption of the fundamental mechanism for storing new information.

In most cases, the first reported symptoms of AD patients are failures of memory for recent events. Tests of the most mildly affected patients indicate that the earliest difficulties involve the storage of new information into memory, that is, learning (Ashford et al., 1989a; 1995; Welsh, Butters, Hughes, Mohs, & Heyman, 1991; Fillenbaum, Wilkinson, Welsh, & Mohs, 1994). Even various psychiatric symptoms found in AD patients (Cohen et al., 1993) can be linked to the failure of learning mechanisms. For example, claims of "stolen keys" usually turn out to be keys that were placed consciously, but the placement was not retained. "Unfaithful spouses" are in fact spouses whose whereabouts the night before is not available for recall, although they were within the patient's view the entire time. Thus, the primary symptoms of AD seem to relate to difficulties with the neural mechanism for storing new information.

As AD progresses into moderate phases, patients begin to lose the ability to recall information that had been learned prior to the onset of the disease. Neurological signs and symptoms such as aphasia, agnosia, and apraxia, which develop insidiously during the middle course of the disease, bear no resemblance to the failures seen after such critical brain injuries as stroke, but rather relate to the associative failure to recall a word, the purpose of an object, or how to perform a specific task. Consequently, the middle phase psychosocial symptoms of AD point to a disruption of neural connections related to the long-term storage of memory mechanisms.

As AD progresses into later phases, a host of diverse symptoms develop, including disruption of activities of daily living. Yet, with careful consideration, each of the symptoms can be traced to failures of cortical information retention.

The logical leap in making the connection between memory mechanisms and such diverse symptoms as inability to shop, bathe, or toilette lies in understanding that information is stored in the brain in a distributed fashion (Ashford & Fuster, 1985; Fuster, 1995). As new information is stored, it is placed (Lewandowsky & Murdock, 1989) on top of the information that is already in place (Fuster, 1995; Ungerleider, 1995). If the mechanism for storing the new information disrupts neuronal structure, then slowly, old information and habits will be lost as well. Consequently, the psychosocial symptoms and their progression point to a neuropathological process that attacks the mechanism for learning or storing information. This brain mechanism that is so vulnerable to the AD process is presumed to be neuroplasticity (Ashford & Jarvik, 1985; Di Patre, 1991; Geddes & Cotman, 1991; Larner, 1995; Woolf & Butcher, 1990).

NEUROBIOLOGIC SYSTEMS AFFECTED BY ALZHEIMER PATHOLOGY

AD is known as a neurodegenerative disorder. The major signs of the disorder are dystrophic neurites, neurofibrillary tangles (NFTs), and neuritic amyloid plaques (NAPs). The dystrophic neurites and the NFTs are composed of paired helical filaments (PHFs), which are primarily abnormally phosphorylated microtubule associate protein-tau (Trojanowski & Lee, 1995). The PHFs clog the dendrites of the neurons and coalesce to form the NFTs in the neuronal cell bodies. They appear to reside indefinitely in situ after the neuron has died. NAPs are complex structures that contain a core of beta-amyloid (Aβ) and activated microglia (Itagaki et al., 1989; Streit & Kincaid-Colton, 1995), with reactive astrocytes (Sadowski, Morys, Barcikowska, & Narkiewicz, 1995) and invading neurites (Geddes, Anderson, & Cotman, 1986), which contain PHFs. The distribution of these changes is not random, preferentially occurring in particular regions of the cortex (Brun & Englund, 1981) and subcortical nucleii projecting to those cortical regions (German, White, & Sparkman, 1987). The process disrupts memory presumably by causing loss of synapses and the death of neurons.

Telencephalic Systems Affected by AD

Alzheimer pathology is concentrated in the structures of the temporal lobe, particularly the amygdala, the hippocampus, and the entorhinal cortex (Hyman, Van Hoesen, Damasio, & Barnes, 1984). The AD process makes its initial appearance in the transitional entorhinal cortex, then spreads to the entorhinal cortex, then selective regions of the hippocampus (Braak & Braak, 1995). At a later stage, about the time that there is a transition from mild memory loss to significant functional impairment, pathology begins to develop in the convexity of the temporal lobe (Bancher, Braak,

Fischer, & Jellinger, 1993). In some cases, dementia develops without significant pathology in the medial temporal lobe structures, but still in association with the lateral distribution. Development of pathology in the neocortex also follows a progression, with successive appearances of disease in the parietal cortex and the frontal cortex, and late in the primary cortical regions. Even the occipital cortex, containing the primary and secondary visual cortical regions, shows a gradient of pathological involvement, increasing from the primary visual area 17 to areas 18 and then to 19 (Lewis, Campbell, Terry, & Morrison, 1987). However, considerable variation occurs among individual cases. Alzheimer pathology can disproportionately affect one side of the brain or one lobe more in one case than in another.

The degree of clinically relevant AD pathology in specific regions of the cortex is indicated most clearly by the concentration of neurofibrillary tangles (Arriagada, Growdon, Hedley-Whyte, & Hyman, 1992; Hyman, 1994; Nagy et al., 1995), whereas plaques, diffuse or neuritic types, are less clearly associated with the severity of the pathology (Braak & Braak, 1995). However, the cortical change most closely associated with cognitive dysfunction is the loss of synapses (Davies, Mann, Sumpter, & Yates, 1987), occurring in the temporal (Scheff & Price, 1993), frontal (Scheff, DeKosky, & Price, 1990; DeKosky et al., 1992), and parietal regions (Terry et al., 1991). Nevertheless, it is not clear whether this association is based on the critical role of these cortical regions in functions that are most clearly measured by cognitive testing in the middle phases of the disease, rather than directly reflecting the global advance of the disease process.

In another analysis, atrophy of the hippocampal formation subdivisions corresponds closely to the stage (Bobinski et al., 1995) and the duration (Jobst et al., 1994) of AD. Since dementia symptoms are highly dependent on premorbid factors such as education and occupational attainment (Stern et al., 1994), and probably other factors, including variation in pathology between cases and in presentation, variability can be expected in the relationship between pathology and function. In the clarification of these relationships, it is important to analyze the time course of development of the pathological factors (Ashford et al., 1995).

The sequence of appearance of Alzheimer pathology in macroscopic structures is generally consistent with the concept that the principal target of the underlying process of Alzheimer pathology is a neuroplastic mechanism. The hippocampus has been long associated with memory formation

(Grady et al., 1995), and the amygdala also plays an important role in learning (Mishkin, 1982). However, why the entorhinal cortex would be the primary site of attack of the Alzheimer process is unclear. Part of the explanation could be that this region is the critical pathway connecting the neocortex to the hippocampus (Rosene & Van Hoesen, 1987) for consolidation of information into long-term memory. An important concept in this regard is that information is processed in the neocortex, whereas connections with the medial temporal lobe (in particular, the hippocampus and amygdala) serve to coordinate the encoding of that information in the neocortex (Coburn, Ashford, & Fuster, 1990; Ungerleider, 1995). Thus processed information is not actually transferred from associative cortical regions to the medial temporal lobe, but reciprocal connections with the medial temporal lobe through the entorhinal cortex serve to initiate and foster the consolidation of information bearing connections in those regions of the convexity of the brain.

Accordingly, the transitional region of the entorhinal cortex serves as the critical bridge between the medial and lateral structures during memory consolidation. The major burden of this role potentially explains why the AD process makes its initial appearance in this site. The evolutionary association of the olfactory system with the cortex, especially the medial temporal regions involved in memory, may further explain this vulnerability (see the discussion that follows). As AD progresses and information storage continues to be attempted in broadly distributed cortical regions, those regions that are burdened with relatively more storage requirements can be supposed to be affected earlier in the disease course than areas that have lower storage demands.

An important recent development in research is brain imaging. New techniques are being used to define and track the macroscopic development of AD pathology in the brains of living patients. As noted previously, atrophy of the hippocampus (Bobinski et al., 1995; Jobst et al., 1994) accompanies the progression of AD. Loss of metabolism in the temporal-parietal cortex also develops with respect to disease severity (Kuhl et al., 1985). Further, metabolic losses can be traced over time from the temporal to the parietal to the frontal regions (Jagust, 1994). Metabolic loss could be related to a variety of factors including local loss of neurons to loss of activation by projecting fibers.

However, the most parsimonious explanation of loss of local metabolic activity is loss of synapses. Synapse quantity is an indicator of the volume of the neuropil of a cortical region, and maintenance of membrane polarization of axonal and dendritic fibers in the neuropil is the major metabolic demand in the cortex. Loss of neuropil substance will result in a loss of metabolic activity and a resulting loss of blood flow. Although it does not directly reflect metabolism, the pattern of loss of cerebral blood flow in AD patients resembles the loss of glucose metabolism (Jagust, 1994) and does appear similar to the reported distribution of AD pathology in the brain (see Fig. 3.1). Both metabolism and blood flow changes can be quantified over time in the living patient. It is now important to link the temporal relationships of the development of pathology in the living patients with the concentration or rate of development of particular components of the cellular pathology, such as neurofibrillary tangles or senile plaques. The development of special ligands applicable for use in living patients for these primary, pathologic, microscopic structures would help to trace the time course of their appearance.

Neurotransmitter Systems Affected by AD

In recent years, researchers have found that several neurotransmitter systems are selectively disrupted in the brain of Alzheimer patients (see Fig. 3.2). The initial discovery of a lack of choline acetyltransferase (ChAT), an indicator of acetylcholine (ACh) activity, was followed by reports that several other neurotransmitters were deficient in the Alzheimer brain. However, the only systems that have been found to be consistently disrupted are ACh, serotonin, norepinephrine, glutamate, somatostatin (which colocalizes with GABA and represents a subpopulation of the GABA inhibitory neurons), neuropeptide-Y, and vasopressin. No other neurotransmitter systems are consistently reported to be significantly diminished in AD, including dopamine, GABA (as a whole), aspartate, and substance-P. In fact, the disruption is so selective that a particular neurotransmitter can be affected when it belongs to one neural system, but not when its neuronal cell bodies belong to a different system or even to a different cortical projection. The general pattern of disruption of the neurotransmitter systems also provides support for the notion that memory mechanisms are selectively attacked by the AD process. Neurotransmitter disruption also may be reflected to some extent by changes found in the cerebrospinal fluid. See Table 3.2 for a synopsis of measures of neurotransmitter losses in AD.

Neurotransmitter receptors are affected by the disease, but not necessarily in direct relation to the disruption of the neurotransmitters. A loss of

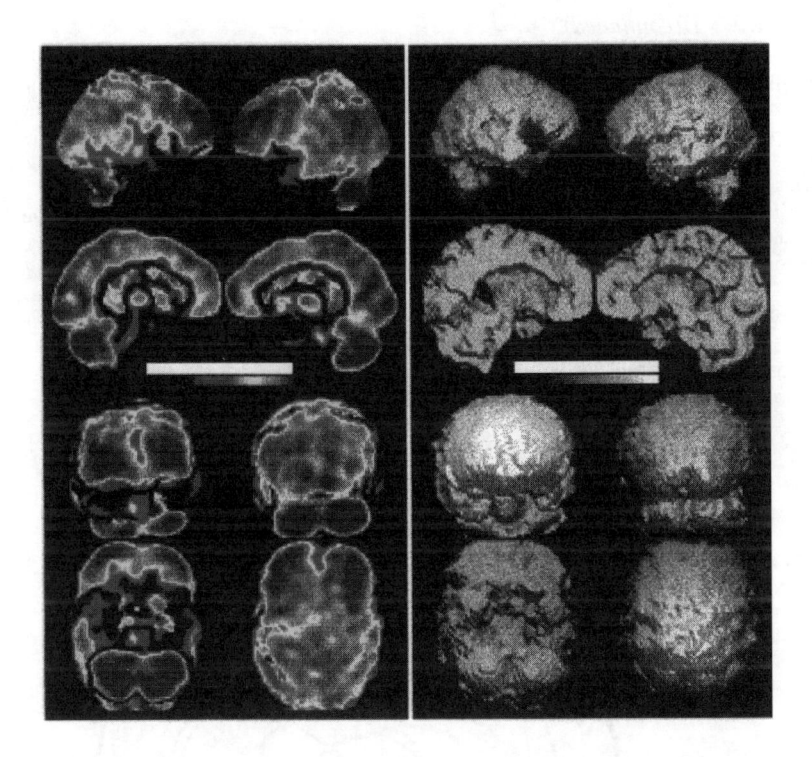

FIGURE 3.1   Cerebral blood flow in severe AD.

These images of cerebral blood flow were produced from SPECT (Single Photon Emission Computed Tomography) of a 75-year-old male with severe Alzheimer's disease (Mini-Mental State Score = 0). He was still able to walk and state his name (testing performed by Cathy Cool, R.N., M.S.N., VA Medical Center, Lexington). The SPECT images were obtained with Neurolite (ECD - ethylene cysteine dimer), which was injected intravenously. The patient was scanned after 30 minutes of resting in a dimly lit room. Scanning was performed with a three-headed Picker Prism camera for 20 minutes (horizontal detectors every 2 mm, 120 angles of acquisition; full-width, half-maximum resolution of 6.7 mm at 10 cm for the technetium tracer). Image data were back projected into a three-dimensional array with voxels 2 mm on a side. (The data array was provided by Dr. Wei-Jen Shih, VA Medical Center, Lexington.) The external surface images were constructed by directing lateral rays toward the brain, thresholding out nonbrain structures and seeking local maxima across three voxels. The anterior and posterior aspects of the left and right side views were justified with the anterior and posterior images so that these two images (only) did not show tangential diminution of cerebral blood flow activity. (Three-dimensional analysis and imaging program by J. W. Ashford.)

The color images on the left show blood flow with red being normal relative to the cerebellum and purple representing severe diminishment of flow. The black and white images on the right are three-dimensionally shaded reconstructions indicating the locations of the cerebral blood flow pixels. The top images represent the left and right lateral views. The bottom row shows the inferior and superior views.

FIGURE 3.1 *(continued)*

The medial and inferior aspects of the anterior temporal lobe show the most diminution of blood flow, with less decline spreading out over the lateral temporal and parietal lobes. A unique finding in this demonstration is the severe involvement of the entire limbic lobe, including the cingulate and basal frontal cortex. By contrast, aged matched normals show only slight decrease of flow in the limbic structures. Three-dimensional display characterizes the distribution of blood flow more clearly than cross-sectional images using SPECT or PET (Burdette et al., 1995).

Further, the distribution of the blood flow decline demonstrated here clearly corresponds to the distribution of pathology seen at autopsy ("Regional Pattern of Degeneration in Alzheimer's Disease: Neuronal Loss and Histopathological Grading," by A. Brun and E. Englund, 1981, *Histopathology, 5,* pp. 549–564. Copyright 1981 by *Histopathology*.), approximating a Braak stage of five ("Staging of Alzheimer's Disease-Related Neurofibrillary Changes," by H. Braak and E. Braak, 1995, *Neurobiology of Aging, 16,* pp. 271–284. Copyright 1995 by *Neurobiology of Aging*.). This approach provides a means to study Alzheimer pathology in the living patient.

Calibration bars are 128 mm wide and 5 mm high.

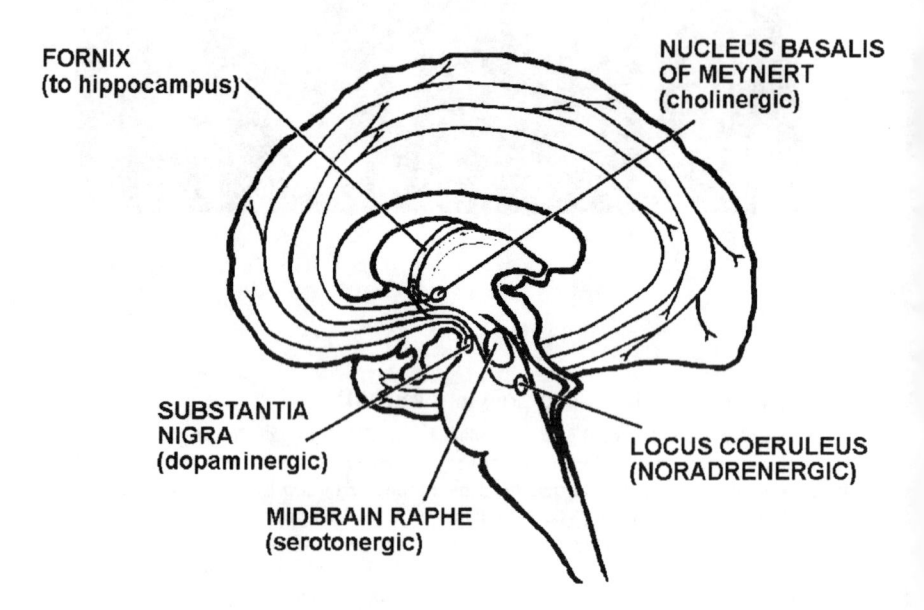

FIGURE 3.2   Neurotransmitter systems projecting from subcortical regions to the cortex.

Note. These systems project from subcortical regions throughout the cortex. They are: scattered neurons of the nucleus basalis of Meynert in the lateral hypothalamus; the serotonergic system of the midbrain raphe; and the noradrenergic neurons in the rostral locus coeruleus of the pons. These systems are all affected by AD. The dopamine system, which extends medial to the substantia nigra, projects to the frontal cortex but is generally unaffected by AD.

TABLE 3.2 Neurotransmitter Losses in AD: Concentrations from AD Brain as Percentage of Control

	Temporal	Frontal	Hippocampus	r^*
ChAT	40	50	50	$.6(a)^{**}, .4(p)^{***}$
Serotonin	30	10	20	$.5(a)$
	(51)	(65)		
Norepinephrine	50	60	60	$.2(a)$
	(48)	(67)		
Glutamate	(72)	(n.s.)	20	
Somatostatin	30	50	40	$.3(a), .5(p)$
	(61)	(n.s.)		
Neuropeptide-Y	30	50	40	
Vasopressin	(n.s.)	(n.s.)	70	

Note. Values for temporal and frontal cortex and hippocampus are from autopsy studies.

Values in parentheses and *r* values are from "Cortical Pyramidal Neuron Loss May Cause Glutamatergic Hypoactivity and Cognitive Impairment in Alzheimer's Disease," by Francis et al., *Journal of Neurochemistry, 60,* pp. 1589–1604. Copyright 1993 by the *Journal of Neurochemistry.* Reprinted with permission.

Other values are from "Changes in the Brain Catecholamines in Patients with Dementia of Alzheimer Types," by R. Adolfsson, C. G. Gottfries, B. E. Roos, and B. Winblad, 1979, *British Journal of Psychiatry, 135,* pp. 216–223. Copyright 1993 by the *British Journal of Psychiatry.* Reprinted with permission.

"Neurotransmitter Changes in Early- and Late-Onset Alzheimer-type Dementia," by H. Arai, Y. Ichimiya, K. Kosaka, T. Moroji, and R. Iizuka, 1992, *Progress in Neuro-Psychopharmacology and Biological Psychiatry, 16,* pp. 883–890. Copyright 1992 by *Progress in Neuro-Psychopharmacology and Biological Psychiatry.* Reprinted with permission.

"Neuropeptide Y Immunoreactivity Is Reduced in Cerebral Cortex in Alzheimer's Disease," by Beal et al., 1986a; *Annals of Neurology, 20,* pp. 282–288. Copyright 1986a by the *Annals of Neurology.* Reprinted with permission.

"Widespread Reduction of Somatostatin-like Immunoreactivity in the Cerebral Cortex in Alzheimer's Disease," by Beal et al., 1986b, *Annals of Neurology, 20,* pp. 489–495. Copyright 1986b by the *Annals of Neurology.* Reprinted with permission.

"Biochemical Changes in Dementia Disorders of Alzheimer Type (ADISDAT)," by Gottfries et al., 1983, *Neurobiology of Aging, 4,* pp. 261–271. Copyright 1983 by *Neurobiology of Aging.* Reprinted with permission.

"Vasopressin in Alzheimer's Disease: A Study of Postmortem Brain Concentrations," by M. F. Mazurek, F. Beal, E. D. Bird, and J. B. Martin, *Annals of Neurology, 20,* pp. 665–670. Copyright 1986 by the *Annals of Neurology.* Reprinted with permission.

"Excitatory Amino Acid-Releasing and Cholinergic Neurons in Alzheimer's Disease," by A. M. Palmer, A. W. Procter, G. C. Stratmann, & D. M. Bowen, 1986, *Neuroscience Letters, 66,* pp. 199–204. Copyright 1986 by *Neuroscience Letters.* Reprinted with permission.

"Presynaptic Serotonergic Dysfunction in Patients with Alzheimer's Disease," by Palmer et al., 1987, *Journal of Neurochemistry, 48,* pp. 8–15. Copyright 1987 by the *Journal of Neurochemistry.* Reprinted with permission.

(continued)

TABLE 3.2 *(continued)*
"Neurotransmitters and CNS Disease: Dementia," by M. N. Rossor, 1982, *Lancet,* __, pp. 1200–1204.
Copyright 1982 by *Lancet*. Reprinted with permission.
Only significant changes are listed. n.s. = not significant.
r^* = correlation with dementia severity; a^{**} = antemortem; p^{***} = postmortem.

a particular receptor may reflect loss of presynaptic activity, but there may be postsynaptic supersensitivity to compensate for the presynaptic loss. Loss in the postsynaptic neuron could reflect additional pathology in the local system. Certain neurotransmitter receptors seem to function as calcium channel gates, such as certain glutamate and nicotinic cholinergic receptors. Pathologic activation of these receptors could allow entry of calcium into the cell and initiate pathological cascades leading to AD pathology. Thus the particular neurotransmitter receptors a neuron carries on its dendrites may be more relevant to the AD pathological process than the neurotransmitter it releases at its axonal terminals.

The Cholinergic System

Findings of neurotransmitter changes in the brains of AD patients began in 1976, when three separate laboratories in the United Kingdom (Davies & Maloney, 1976; Bowen, Smith, White, & Davison, 1976; Perry, Perry, Blessed, & Tomlinson, 1977) discovered independently that ChAT is decreased in brains affected by AD, confirming long-standing suspicions about a cholinergic deficit in this disease (Bigl, Arendt, & Biesold, 1990). Numerous additional studies have supported the relevance of this finding, including:

1. widespread confirmation of the finding;
2. demonstration of a significant relation between a decline in metabolism of ACh in the cortex and dementia (Francis et al., 1985);
3. a selective loss of ACh neurons in the nucleus basalis of Meynert in the basal forebrain (Whitehouse et al., 1982); and
4. anatomical demonstration of a relationship between ChAT loss in small cortical regions and loss of projecting acetylcholine nerve groups in the nucleus basalis (Mesulam, Mufson, Levey, & Wainer, 1983).

However, additional findings have modified the implications of the ChAT loss (Harrison, 1986).

1. ACh neuron loss is relatively restricted to the nucleus basalis, and little loss of ACh neurons is found among numerous other groups of ACh neurons (Woolf & Butcher, 1990).
2. There is a major loss of brain nicotinic receptors, which are in part likely to be postsynaptic (Sugaya, Giacobini, & Chiappinelli, 1990).
3. Muscarinic receptors in the cortex are variably affected (Whitehouse & Kellar, 1987).
4. Numerous neurotransmitter systems other than ACh also are selectively affected in AD.
5. Treatment of AD patients with cholinergic agents has met limited success (Ashford, Sherman, & Kumar, 1989b).

The resulting picture indicates that the group of cholinergic neurons in the basal forebrain that projects to the neocortical and medial temporal regions affected by AD is selectively damaged. Pharmacologic disruption of the ACh function produces a severe impairment of learning (Drachman, 1977). Selective poisoning of these neurons in animals, including primates, also disrupts learning (Aigner et al., 1987). Therefore, the role that the basal forebrain ACh neurons play in memory storage offers an explanation for their vulnerability to the AD process. The affected neurons project long axons to the cortex that ramify extensively within a small region. Numerous substances are transmitted anterogradely in the axon (Steward & Banker, 1992), and other substances, including nerve growth factor (NGF), are transmitted retrogradely. Any of these substances, or aberrant byproducts of these substances, could put these long, fine fibers at particular risk for clogging, particularly at branch points and at the terminal ramifications. Disruption of axons in AD prevents retrograde transport of NGF, which is critical for sustaining the cholinergic neuron cell bodies (Scott, Mufson, Weingartner, Skau, & Crutcher, 1995). However, the mRNA for NGF is not decreased in the cortex of AD patients (Jette, Cole, & Fahnestock, 1994), thus supporting the premise that it is not lack of NGF that initiates Alzheimer pathology (Woolf & Butcher, 1990).

Other Cortically Projecting Neurotransmitter Systems

Two other cortically projecting neurotransmitter systems are selectively disrupted by the AD process in a manner similar to the ACh system, the norepinephrine neurons of the locus coeruleus and the serotonin neurons of the dorsal and central raphe nuclei. Although the specific functions of these neurons are not known, there are substantial conjectures that norepinephrine neurons mediate reward-related conditioning that pertains to cortical learning (Gratton & Wise, 1988), and that the serotonin neurons of these nuclei direct sensitization conditioning involving cortical functions (Bailey & Kandel, 1995; Jacobs & Azmitia, 1992). Accordingly, there are three cortically projecting neurotransmitter systems that are affected in AD, and each of these systems plays a significant role in the learning of new information. That role may explain the vulnerability of each system to the AD process.

Cortical Neurotransmitter Systems

In the cortex, the preponderance of neurons use the neurotransmitters glutamate and GABA. The glutamate neurons, which are the pyramidal cells, are devastated in regions of the brain affected by AD (Francis, Sims, Proctor, & Bowen, 1993). Glutamate is now known as a transmitter that can initiate and regulate process growth in postsynaptic neurons (Brewer & Cotman, 1989; Mattson, Dou, & Kater, 1988) and, consequently, seems to be a critical factor in learning and memory. Glutamate can open NMDA receptor channels, which allow Ca^{++} into the neuron, and Ca^{++} can initiate several learning-related changes in the neuron, but also can cause toxic changes. Some forms of mammalian associative conditioning may depend on interactions between ACh and glutamate in neocortical neurons, including classical conditioning (Woody & Gruen, 1993). The role of glutamate in memory offers an explanation why this group of neurons is affected by the AD process.

The role of GABA is inhibitory, and it is the GABA neurons that colocalize with the neuropeptide somatostatin, which are affected in regions of the brain attacked by the AD process (Bissette & Myers, 1992). However, the role of somatostatin in brain functioning is unclear, just as is the reason why this group of neurons is affected in AD.

Olfactory vs. Connectivity vs. Plasticity Theories of AD

The selective distribution of AD pathology in the brain, particularly, its apparent systematic spread from the entorhinal transitional area (Braak & Braak, 1995), suggests that some mechanism exists whereby the AD pathology can be transmitted from one group of neurons to another. An early observation in this regard suggested that memory dysfunction was due to the loss of connections between the entorhinal cortex and the hippocampus (Hyman et al., 1984), but this change does not account for the development of similar pathology in other regions of the brain. Another theory suggests that the AD process is transmitted directly from one neuron to another (De La Coste & White, 1993), but this theory does not explain why some of the most widely connected systems, including the thalamus, the cerebellum, and the primary cortical regions, are relatively spared by the AD process.

An important line of speculation has invoked the relation between the preferential distribution of AD pathology and the olfactory system (Ellison, 1995; Pearson, Esiri, Hiorns, Wilcock, & Powell, 1985), noting that many of the regions affected by Alzheimer pathology relate to ancient projections of the olfactory bulb to the "rhinencephalic cortex" (Brodal, 1969). One speculation suggested that the nasal epithelium may be infected by a substance that is transmitted to specific regions of the brain, then by certain connections to other regions (Roberts, 1986). This latter theory is not supported by the pathology (Davies, Brooks, & Lewis, 1993) or by the symptomatology that indicates that there is more impairment in olfactory recognition than detection (Serby, Larson, & Kalkstein, 1991). However, failure of the olfactory function, including recollection of odors, occurs early in the disease with patients' inability to detect most scents occurring in the middle phase (Serby et al.). Further, the olfactory bulb is affected profoundly in AD (Struble & Clark, 1992). Also, specific AD-related pathological changes occur in olfactory neurons (Talamo et al., 1989; Wolozin, Lesch, Lebovics, & Sunderland, 1993). Further, the losses in the olfactory function in AD patients, particularly olfactory memory, correlate highly with loss of volume (Kesslak, Nalcioglu, & Cotman, 1991) and metabolism (Buchsbaum et al., 1991) in the medial temporal lobe olfactory regions.

The olfactory system has played a major role in the development of the cortex (Nauta & Karten, 1970), particularly those regions now associated with learning and memory (Haberly, 1990; Stäubli, Le, & Lynch, 1995). Olfactory sensation involves a large number of receptors in the olfactory epithelium (Axel, 1995). The olfactory neurons transmit information to the olfactory bulb for a type of analysis, parallel distributed processing, which is similar to the analysis conducted on information distributed by the cortex (Kauer, 1991). Several neurotransmitters are used for this processing, including glutamate (Trombley & Shepherd, 1993; Kaba, Hayashi, Higuchi, & Nakanishi, 1994). The mechanism of olfactory memory, requiring a distributed representation of information, is actually the most similar to the mechanism thought to be at play in the storage of information in the neocortical association cortex.

Therefore, some important mechanism in the olfactory system associated with learning may explain the vulnerability of the brain to AD. The entorhinal transition cortex, which is first attacked by the AD process, sits in an evolutionary crossroads from the olfactory system to the archicortex (hippocampus), paleocortex (amygdala), and neocortex (Haberly, 1990). This position, with an abundance of plastic connections to numerous regions of the brain (Rosene & VanHoesen, 1987), may explain its vulnerability to the AD process. Thus the relationship between olfaction and AD is consistent with the hypothesis that a plastic mechanism is associated with the vulnerability to AD pathology (Ashford & Jarvik, 1985; Di Patre, 1991), and offers an evolutionary line of investigation to understand that mechanism.

NEUROMOLECULAR MECHANISMS AFFECTED BY AD

There is a clear genetic basis for some forms of AD with mutations in specific genes causing the disease (see Mullan & Crawford, 1993, for a review; see also Matsuyama, chap. 4 of this volume). Several familial forms of AD arise from mutations in the β-amyloid precursor protein (βAPP) gene, which is located on chromosome 21. The fact that essentially all persons with Down's syndrome (trisomy 21) develop AD pathology emphasizes the importance of chromosome 21 and the βAPP gene in the pathogenesis of AD. Other inherited forms of AD have been linked to mutations on chromosomes 1, 14, and 19. In addition, a "predisposition factor" was identified recently, namely, dosage of the apolipoprotein E4 allele (Saunders et al., 1993). Although some forms of AD have a genetic basis, the majority of cases are sporadic (i.e., not linked to specific mutations), and the cause(s) of most cases of AD are therefore unknown. The selective vulnerability of brain regions and neuronal populations in AD and the pattern of progression of the neurodegenerative process provide an explanation for the symptoms of the disease and clues to the cellular and molecular basis of the neurodegenerative process. Specific groups of neurons in the entorhinal cortex (Layer 2 cells) and hippocampus (CA1 pyramidal neurons) are among the first to degenerate (Braak & Braak, 1995). Other brain regions heavily involved in AD pathology include superior and middle temporal gyri, inferior parietal cortex, and multiple association cortices, whereas relatively nonvulnerable regions include the cerebellum and primary sensory and motor cortices.

Several hypotheses have been suggested to account for the neurodegenerative process in AD. Several of the most prominent hypotheses concerning vulnerability at the cellular level are probably correct and provide collectively an integrated view of the molecular and cellular bases of the neurodegenerative process in AD (see Fig. 3.3).

The Amyloid Hypothesis

Investigations of the molecular and cellular biology of βAPP have yielded information vital to our current understanding of the pathogenesis of AD (see Selkoe, 1993; Mattson et al., 1993a, for review). A hallmark histopathological feature of the AD brain is the accumulation of amyloid plaques, which are often associated with degenerating neurons. The plaques are comprised of amyloid β-peptide (Aβ), a 40-42 amino acid fragment of the βAPP-amyloid precursor protein (βAPP). βAPP is widely expressed in the brain, with both neurons and astrocytes being major cellular sources. βAPP can be enzymatically processed in two major ways, one of which involves a cleavage within the Aβ sequence liberating secreted forms of βAPP (sAPP) from the cell surface and precluding release of amyloidogenic Aβ. The other cleavage results in release of Aβ, which is normally produced in low amounts and circulates at nanomolar concentrations in CSF (cerebrospinal fluid) and blood.

A striking characteristic of Aβ is its ability to aggregate rapidly and form fibrils with β-sheet structure. Mutations in βAPP that cause some forms of AD may alter processing of βAPP such that increased amounts of Aβ are produced, or these mutations may cause Aβ to aggregate more readily. A causal role for Aβ in the neurodegenerative process in AD is suggested from experimental studies showing that Aβ can be neurotoxic and can increase neuronal vulnerability to excitotoxicity and energy deprivation (see Mattson et al., 1993a, for review). Specific mechanisms whereby Aβ damages neurons have been elucidated. Aβ itself can generate free radicals by a mechanism involving interaction of specific amino acids with molecular oxygen (Hensley et al., 1994); these peptide-derived radicals may play a central role in the covalent cross-linking of the peptide. Aβ accumulates at the plasma membrane, where it induces free radical production and lipid peroxidation (Goodman & Mattson, 1994; Mattson

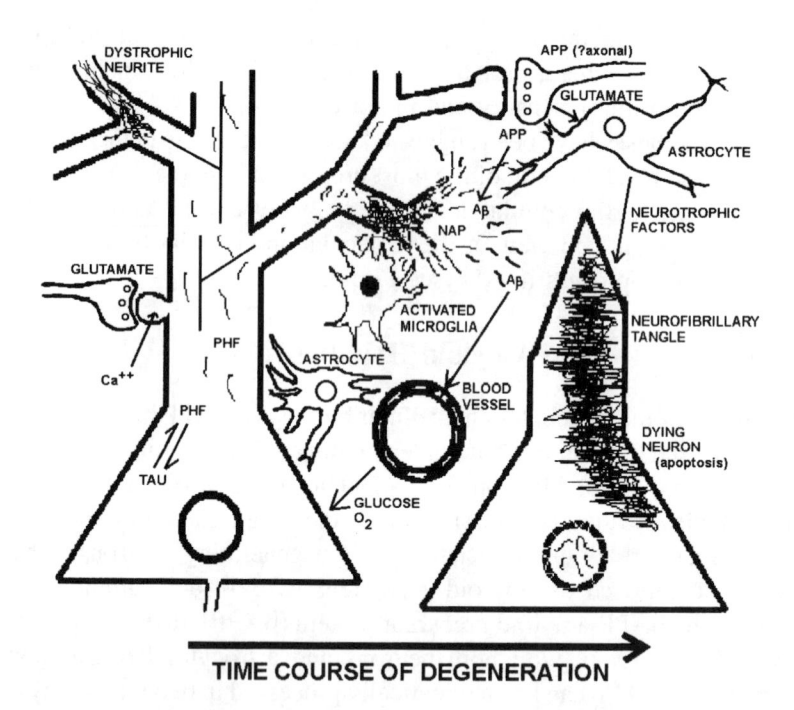

FIGURE 3.3   Model of neuromolecular progression of AD.

Note. In this model, glutamate activation of dendritic spines of highly plastic neurons causes entry of Ca^{++}, which plays a role in the induction of excess phosphorylation of tau and allows transformation of tau into PHFs. The PHFs accumulate in dendritic segments at some distance from the soma to form dystrophic neurites. These PHF deposits clog the dendrites, especially at branch points. With disruption of dendritic flow, portions of the dendrite distal to the soma lose their integrity, releasing their contents, including normal tau and PHFs, into extracellular space. APP may be axonally transported to terminal fields. If APP is abnormally released, it may be aberrantly transformed into $A\beta$, which can accumulate in the neuritic plaque (NAP). In the region of the dendrite break, extracellular PHF and $A\beta$ form amyloid cores that are surrounded by activated microglia. Under normal circumstances, astrocytes can keep Ca^{++} concentrations at nontoxic levels, absorb glutamate, and provide neurotrophic factors to axons and dendrites. When the Alzheimer state develops, excess neurotrophic activity may stimulate excess APP production, which may be transformed into $A\beta$, which can cause additional toxicity before being transported to blood vessel walls. As PHF production increases, due to the stress on the neuron, and accumulates, a neurofibrillary tangle is formed in the cell soma. As a late event, the cell becomes apoptotic and dies.

et al., 1993a). Lipid peroxidation results in dysfunction of membrane ion-motive ATPases (sodium and calcium pumps), resulting in disruption of ion homeostasis, membrane depolarization, and elevation of intracellular calcium levels (Mark, Hensley, Butterfield, & Mattson, 1995). Both calcium and free radicals contribute to damage of proteins, lipids, and DNA and to eventual cell death. Lower subtoxic levels of Aβ can severely disrupt signal transduction mechanisms and render neurons vulnerable to metabolic perturbations.

The role of Aβ in AD has been questioned because this substance is a frequent concomitant of aging, but its concentration has not been related to the severity of Alzheimer dementia or pathology (Arriagada et al., 1992), and in rare cases, AD has been diagnosed histopathologically in the absence of Aβ. Consequently, Aβ may be considered a major factor in the initiation of AD, but not a sufficient factor for pathogenesis (Selkoe, 1994). The stress of Aβ may be manifested significantly on those cells that have the greatest memory-related metabolic demands. The toxicity of this normally present substance may exert its deleterious effect over long periods of time and serve as a factor that induces neurofibrillary change and the consequent loss of cell processes and synapses. Curiously, Aβ levels are decreased in the CSF of AD patients (Motter et al., 1995; van Gool, Kuiper, Walstra, Wolters, & Bolhuis, 1995).

The Tau Hypothesis

The microtubule associated protein tau seems to play a central role in AD (Trojanowski & Lee, 1995). This protein becomes aberrantly phosphorylated early in the pathologic process in dystrophic neurites, which then serves to form the backbone for the PHFs, which turn into NFTs in the neuronal cell bodies. Why this aberrant phosphorylation occurs is unknown, but the critical problem could be a failure of dephosphorylation. Formations of the PHFs normal flow through axons and dendrites, and complete obstruction would eliminate all parts of the process distal to the cell body from the obstruction. The most vulnerable location for an obstruction would be at a dendritic or axonal branch point. Those parts of the cell process distal to the obstruction would become extravasated material, which could induce the formation of amyloid and plaques, with local attempts to regrow from the neuritic stump serving to produce the abnormal neurites in these structures (Geddes et al., 1985, 1986; Geddes & Cotman, 1991). In support of the concept of neuronal process breakage with extravasation of intracellular contents, several recent studies have found an elevation of tau in the CSF of AD patients (Arai et al., 1995; Hock, Golombowski, Naser, & Müller-Spahn, 1995; Mori et al., 1995;

Tato, Frank, & Hernanz, 1995; Vigo-Pelfrey et al., 1995; Jensen, Basun, & Lannfelt, 1995).

The Apolipoprotein E Hypothesis

Apolipoprotein E alleles have been shown to have a relationship with AD. The mechanism of interaction between this protein and AD pathology is not yet clear, but at least three mechanisms are possible. This protein could support peripheral vascular pathology, which instigates AD. Alternatively, the Apo E could work as a chaperon protein for amyloid or tau, with inadequate removal from normal turnover leading to the development of the AD pathology.

The Immune Hypothesis

The immune system also appears to be intimately involved in pathological processes occurring in the brain in AD. Several studies have found an elevation of immunoglobulins in serum (Cohen & Eisdorfer, 1980; Kumar, Cohen, & Eisdorfer, 1988) and CSF (McRae-Degueurce et al., 1987) of AD patients. Infiltration of microglia in the vicinity of amyloid plaques (Sadowski, 1995), and the recent reports of reduced incidence of AD in patients receiving chronic treatment with anti-inflammatory drugs, further supports a central role for an immune response in AD (Breitner et al., 1995). It is unclear if this response could initiate or exacerbate the pathology.

The Metabolic Hypothesis

A well-documented alteration in the brain of AD patients is reduced glucose metabolism (Burdette, Minoshima, Borght, Tran, & Kuhl, 1996; Hoyer, Oesterreich, & Wagner, 1988; Kuhl et al., 1987; Small, La Rue, Komo, Kaplan, & Mandelkern, 1995). Five possible causes of the reduced glucose uptake into brain cells are:

1. vascular alterations resulting in hypoperfusion;
2. decreased glucose uptake across the blood-brain barrier;
3. impaired glucose transport within neurons themselves;
4. a defect in energy metabolism (Beal, 1995); and

5. decreased demand for glucose due to diminished neuron surface membrane associated with loss of cell processes.

Reduced energy availability (possible Causes 1–4) would place neurons at risk because ATP (adenosine-triphosphate) is required to maintain ion homeostasis. Accordingly, reduced glucose availability to neurons would increase their vulnerability to glutamate excitotoxicity and Aβ toxicity (see the next paragraph).

This hypothesis predicts that neurons that express high levels of glutamate receptors are exposed to high levels of Aβ, would be expected to be very vulnerable in AD patients, and that larger neurons with a higher metabolic demand also would be more vulnerable. In this regard, the metabolic hypothesis is supported by the fact that vulnerable neurons tend to be large and express high levels of glutamate receptors. Since neurons with high levels of glutamate receptors are likely to be more involved with information storage, and the production of new processes places a metabolic load on neurons, the metabolic hypothesis also supports the central role of neuroplasticity in the vulnerability to the AD process.

The Free "Radical" Hypothesis

Considerable data indicate that free radical injury plays a major role in the damage to neurons in AD. Levels of protein oxidation, DNA damage, and lipid peroxidation are increased in vulnerable regions of the AD brain such as the hippocampus.

The causes of radical accumulation in AD are likely multifold and may include: (1) reduced energy availability due to circulatory alterations (see discussion later in this chapter); (2) Aβ deposition; and (3) formation of advanced glycation end products (Yan et al., 1994; see Benzi & Moretti, 1995, for review). Aβ has been shown to induce lipid peroxidation and accumulation of cellular peroxides in cultured neurons, as well as in synaptosomes (Butterfield, Hensley, Harris, Mattson, & Carney, 1994; Goodman & Mattson, 1994; Hensley et al., 1994). Generation of free radicals in response to Aβ appears to be an early event in the neurodegenerative process that occurs prior to disruption of ion homeostasis. As described previously, disruption of ion homeostasis by Aβ results from free radical damage to ion-motive ATPases (Mark et al., 1995). Trace elements also are implicated as inducers of free radical production in AD. Levels of both aluminum and iron are increased in neurofibrillary tangles. Iron damages neurons by inducing hydroxyl radical production via the Fenton reaction. Although most iron in the brain is normally in a bound (innocuous) form, it is conceivable that increased levels of free iron occur in AD and contribute to the neurodegenerative process.

The "Calcium" Hypothesis

Prolonged elevation of $[Ca^{2+}]_i$ can damage and kill neurons (Mattson, 1992). Studies of acute neurodegenerative conditions (e.g., stroke and traumatic brain injury) and chronic neurodegenerative disorders, including AD, suggest that elevation of $[Ca^{2+}]_i$ is a final, common pathway in the neurodegenerative process. Conditions believed to occur in the AD brain result in elevation of neuronal $[Ca^{2+}]_i$ in experimental paradigms. For example, reduced energy availability (glucose deprivation and hypoxia) results in elevation of $[Ca^{2+}]_i$, which precedes cell degeneration in cultured neurons, and Aβ induces an elevation of rest $[Ca^{2+}]_i$ and potentiates $[Ca^{2+}]_i$ responses to glutamate (Mattson et al., 1993a).

Studies of postmortem tissue from AD patients and age-matched controls suggest altered calcium homeostasis in AD. For example, Ca^{2+}-ATPase activity was reduced in synaptosomes from vulnerable regions of AD brain and Aβ impaired Na^+/K^+-ATPase and Ca^{2+}-ATPase activities in hippocampal synaptosomes from neurologically normal individuals (see Mark et al., 1995). Differential expression of components of the $[Ca^{2+}]_i$-regulating systems in neurons may contribute to the pattern of selective neuronal vulnerability in AD. For example, neurons expressing the calcium-binding protein calbindin may be resistant to Ca^{2+}-mediated injury, whereas neurons expressing high levels of NMDA glutamate receptors (a voltage- and ligand-regulated calcium channel) may be particularly vulnerable. Prolonged elevation of $[Ca^{2+}]_i$ results in damage to proteins, lipids, and DNA. This damage is mediated largely by proteases and free radicals.

The "Excitotoxicity" Hypothesis

Many studies have shown that glutamate, the major excitatory neurotransmitter in the brain, is capable of damaging and killing neurons when energy levels are reduced or when neurons are exposed to Aβ. Exposure of cultured brain cells or adult rat brain to excitatory amino acids results in alterations in the neuronal cytoskeleton similar to those seen in AD (Mattson, 1990; Stein-Behrens, Mattson, Chang, Yeh, & Sapolsky, 1994). Epidemiological data also support the excitotoxic hypothesis. For example, domoic acid intoxication in a group of Canadians that ingested shellfish containing high concentrations of this excitotoxin resulted in memory loss and massive accumulation of neurofibrillary tangles (Zattore, 1990). A compelling aspect of the excitotoxicity hypothesis is its links with other hypotheses of AD. For example, glutamate induces accumulation of calcium and free radicals in neurons; metabolic impairment increases the vulnerability of neurons to excitotoxicity (Beal, 1995); and neurons vulnerable in AD patients bear high levels of glutamate receptors.

The Neurotrophic Factor Hypothesis

Many studies have shown that neurotrophic factors, endogenous proteins in the brain that promote neuron survival, can protect neurons against many insults relevant to AD, including glutamate, Aβ, and metabolic insults (see Mattson, Cheng, & Smith-Swintosky, 1993b, for review). Included among such neurotrophic factors are basic fibroblast growth factor, brain-derived neurotrophic factor, and transforming growth factor-β. As noted previously, NGF production is not diminished in the cortex of AD patients, but its lack of transport to the nucleus basalis of Meynert may be largely responsible for the death of cholinergic neurons in that structure.

The Steroid Hypothesis

Steroid hormones also might play a role in the pathogenesis of AD. The evidence is strongest for glucocorticoids and estrogens. Glucocorticoids, the "stress steroids," have been shown to increase neuronal vulnerability to a variety of insults, including excitotoxins and ischemic conditions (Smith-Swintosky et al., 1995; Stein-Behrens et al., 1994). Alterations in function of the neuroendocrine system controlling glucocorticoid production have been documented in AD patients. Postmenopausal women receiving estrogen replacement therapy (ERT) have a reduced risk of developing AD (Henderson, Paganini-Hill, Emanuel, Dunn, & Buckwalter, 1994). In addition, estrogens have been shown to have antioxidant activity and may protect neurons against free radical damage (Goodman, Bruce, Cheng, & Mattson, 1996).

The Vascular Hypothesis

Alterations in the vasculature also may contribute to AD. Aβ is deposited in blood vessels, and numerous studies have documented alterations in the cerebral microvasculature in AD. The recent link between apolipoprotein E4 allele dosage and age of onset of AD bolsters a role for vascular alterations in AD because the E4 allele also increases the risk for atherosclerosis. Small emboli may cause transient episodes of ischemia, which could initiate a local onset of AD pathology, particularly in regions of vascular vulnerability such as the medial temporal lobe.

The Peripheral Medical Factor Hypotheses

There has been a broad search for peripheral diseases and medical conditions that might be associated with AD. For the most part, AD patients are generally no less healthy than age-matched controls (McCormick et al., 1994), although poor health may accelerate cognitive decline (Teri, Hughes, & Larson, 1990). However, there are certain conditions that have weak associations with AD, such as head trauma, cardiovascular disease, thyroid disease, and menopause. Each of these conditions puts stress on the neurons of the brain.

In neural trauma, connections between neurons are sheared and neuroplastic mechanisms must be taxed to reestablish functional connectivity.

Hypoxic injury to the brain, which allows the survival of a significant portion of the neurons, will still severely tax the capacity of the surviving neurons to reestablish a functioning neural network.

The thyroid hormone itself plays a role in the normal development of neuronal processes, which are associated with neuroplastic mechanisms. Low thyroid levels may stress dendritic arbors. Excessive thyroid levels may stimulate aberrant sprouting (Woolf & Butcher, 1990).

Other conditions such as peripheral amyloid deposits (Joachim et al., 1989) or calcium metabolism irregularities (Landfield et al., 1991) are medically benign, but may indicate that the affected individual may have a central vulnerability. Serum from elderly individuals and AD patients has been shown to stimulate Alzheimer-like changes in hippocampal neurons in culture (Brewer & Ashford, 1992). This finding indicates that peripheral factors may play a causative role in AD pathology in the brain, including Apo E dysfunction, through induction of vascular changes, and immunologic factors that could be initiated through temporary breaks in the blood-brain barrier.

Multivalent Cation Toxicity Theories

There has been considerable speculation that aluminum or some other element may contribute to the development of AD. At this time, the evidence for a primary etiologic role for aluminum remains inconclusive (Forbes et al., 1994; Lovell et al., 1993). However, the affinity of the AD pathological changes for the divalent silver cations leaves open the possibility that similar ions such as aluminum could interfere with the metabolism of those proteins whose disconformation leads to the AD pathology (Bertholf, 1987; Shin, Lee, & Trojanowski, 1994; Trojanowski & Lee, 1995). Similarly, there is weak evidence for roles for divalent cations such as mercury, zinc, and iron. Iron and aluminum are free radical catalysts that may facilitate aggregration of Aβ into amyloids. The calcium hypothesis, the role of zinc in the hippocampus, and the affinity of the AD pathologic structures for silver continue to sustain interest in a possible role for multivalent cations in AD.

SUMMATION

It can be appreciated, even from this brief discussion of the cellular and molecular underpinnings of AD, that the different hypotheses of AD are integrative in nature (Beal, 1995). For example, the fact that energy deprivation destabilizes neuronal calcium homeostasis and renders neurons vulnerable to excitotoxic insults and Aβ links the calcium and metabolic hypotheses. The interactive, and often synergistic, effects of calcium and free-radical-generating systems make calcium a key component of the free radical hypothesis. The ability of neurotrophic factors to stabilize $[Ca^{2+}]_i$ and protect neurons against excitotoxicity, metabolic insults, and Aβ toxicity emphasizes the importance of $[Ca^{2+}]_i$-regulating systems in the mechanism of neurotrophic factor action.

The vascular and hormonal hypotheses also are closely tied to the other hypotheses described previously. Free radicals and calcium appear to be convergence points for the different hypotheses. There is an important need to ascertain changes in these neuromolecular systems, particularly those associated with neuroplasticity, with respect to the clinical progression of AD, to focus on the most relevant factors associated with the development of the disease. Clearly, fundamental knowledge of cellular and molecular mechanisms of neuronal degeneration in AD are providing a large number of preventative and therapeutic strategies for this devastating neurodegenerative disorder.

REFERENCES

Adolfsson, R., Gottfries, C. G., Roos, B. E. & Winblad, B. (1979). Changes in the brain catecholamines in patients with dementia of Alzheimer type. *British Journal of Psychiatry, 135,* 216–223.

Aigner, T. G., Mitchell, S. J., Aggleton, J. P., DeLong, M. R., Struble, R. G., Price, D. L., Wenk, G. L., & Mishkin, M. (1987). Effects of scopolamine and physostigmine on recognition memory in monkeys with ibotenic-acid lesions of the nucleus basalis of Meynert. *Psychopharmacology, 92,* 292–300.

Alzheimer, A. (1907). About a peculiar disease of the cerebral cortex. In H. Greenson & L. Jarvik (Eds.), *Alzheimer Disease and Associated Disorders, 1,* 7–8.

Arai, H., Ichimiya, Y., Kosaka, K, Moroji, T., & Iizuka, R. (1992). Neurotransmitter changes in early- and late-onset Alzheimer-type dementia. *Progress in Neuro-Psychopharmacology and Biological Psychiatry, 16,* 883–890.

Arai, H., Terajima, M., Miura, M., Higuchi, S., Muramatsu, T., Machida, N., Seiki, H., Takase, S., Clark, C. M., Lee, V. M.-Y., Trojanowski, J. Q., & Sasaki, H. (1995). Tau in cerebrospinal fluid: A potential diagnostic marker in Alzheimer's disease. *Annals of Neurology, 38,* 649–652.

Arriagada, P. V., Growdon, J. H., Hedley-Whyte, E. T., & Hyman, B. T. (1992). Neurofibrillary tangles but not senile plaques parallel duration and severity of Alzheimer's disease. *Neurology, 42,* 631–639.

Ashford, J. W., & Fuster, J. M. (1985). Occipital and inferotemporal responses to visual signals in the monkey. *Experimental Neurology, 90,* 444–466.

Ashford, J. W., & Jarvik, L. (1985). Alzheimer's disease: Does neuron plasticity predispose to axonal neurofibrillary degeneration? *New England Journal of Medicine, 313,* 388.

Ashford, J. W., Kolm, P., Colliver, J. A., Bekian, C., & Hsu, L. N. (1989a). Alzheimer patient evaluation and the mini-mental state: Item characteristic curve analysis. *Journal of Gerontology, Psychological Science, 44,* 139–146.

Ashford, J. W., Sherman, K. A., & Kumar, V. (1989b). Advances in Alzheimer therapy: Cholinesterase inhibitors. *Neurobiology of Aging, 10,* 99–105.

Ashford, J. W., Shan, M., Butler, S., Rajasekar, A., & Schmitt, F. A. (1995). Temporal quantification of Alzheimer's disease severity: 'Time Index' model. *Dementia, 6,* 269–280.

Axel, R. (1995, October). The molecular logic of smell. *Scientific American, 273,* 154–159.

Bailey, C. H., & Kandel, E. R. (1995). Molecular and structural mechanisms underlying long-term memory. In M. S. Gazzaniga (Ed.), *The cognitive neurosciences* (pp. 19–36). Cambridge, MA: MIT Press.

Bancher, C., Braak, H., Fischer, P., & Jellinger, K. A. (1993). Neuropathological staging of Alzheimer lesions and intellectual status in Alzheimer's and Parkinson's disease patients. *Neuroscience Letters, 162,* 179–182.

Bartus, R. T., Dean, R. L., Beer, B., & Lippa, A. S. (1982). The cholinergic hypothesis of geriatric memory dysfunction. *Science, 217,* 408–417.

Beal, M. F. (1992). Does impairment of energy metabolism result in excitotoxic neuronal death in neurodegenerative illnesses? *Annals of Neurology, 31,* 119–130.

Beal, M. F. (1995). Aging, energy, and oxidative stress in neurodegenerative diseases. *Annals of Neurology, 38,* 357–366.

Beal, M. F., Mazurek, M. F., Chattha, G. K., Svendsen, C. N., Bird, E. D., & Martin, J. B. (1986a). Neuropeptide Y immunoreactivity is reduced in cerebral cortex in Alzheimer's disease. *Annals of Neurology, 20,* 282–288.

Beal, M. F., Mazurek, M. F., Svendsen, C. N., Bird, E. D., & Martin, J. B. (1986b). Widespread reduction of somatostatin-like immunoreactivity in the cerebral cortex in Alzheimer's disease. *Annals of Neurology, 20,* 489–495.

Benzi, G., & Moretti, A. (1995). Are reactive oxygen species involved in Alzheimer's disease? *Neurobiology of Aging, 16,* 661–674.

Bertholf, R. L. (1987). Aluminum and Alzheimer's disease: Perspectives for a cytoskeletal mechanism. *Critical Reviews in Clinical Laboratory Sciences, 25,* 195–210.

Bigl, V., Arendt, T., & Biesold, D. (1990). The nucleus basalis of Meynert during ageing and in dementing neuropsychiatric disorders. In M. Steriade & D. Biesold (Eds.), *Brain cholinergic systems* (pp. 364–386). New York: Oxford University Press.

Bissette, G., & Myers, B. (1992). Somatostatin in Alzheimer's disease and depression. *Life Sciences, 51,* 1389–1410.

Bobinski, M., Wegiel, J., Wisniewski, H. M., Tarnawski, M., Reisberg, B., Mlodzik, B., de Leon, M. J., & Miller, D. C. (1995). Atrophy of hippocampal formation subdivisions correlates with stage and duration of Alzheimer disease. *Dementia, 6,* 205–210.

Bowen, D. M., Smith, C. B., White, P., & Davison, A. N. (1976). Neurotransmitter related enzymes and indices of hypoxia in senile dementia and other abiotrophics. *Brain, 99,* 459–596.

Braak, H., & Braak, E. (1991). Neuropathological staging of Alzheimer-related changes. *Acta Neuropathologica, 82,* 239–259.

Braak, H., & Braak, E. (1995). Staging of Alzheimer's disease-related neurofibrillary changes. *Neurobiology of Aging, 16,* 271–284.

Breitner, J. C. S., Welsh, K. A., Helms, M. J., Gaskell, P. C., Gau, B. A., Roses, A. D., Pericak-Vance, M. A., & Saunders, A. M. (1995). Delayed onset of Alzheimer's disease with nonsteroidal anti-inflammatory and histamine H2 blocking drugs. *Neurobiology of Aging, 16,* 523–530.

Brewer, G. J., & Ashford, J. W. (1992). Human serum stimulates Alzheimer markers in cultured hippocampal neurons. *Journal of Neuroscience Research, 33,* 355–369.

Brewer, G. J., & Cotman, C. W. (1989). NMDA receptor regulation of neuronal morphology in cultured hippocampal neurons. *Neuroscience Letters, 99,* 268–273.

Brodal, A. (1969). *Neurological anatomy: In relation to clinical medicine.* New York: Oxford University Press.

Brun, A., & Englund, E. (1981). Regional pattern of degeneration in Alzheimer's disease: Neuronal loss and histopathological grading. *Histopathology, 5,* 549–564.

Buchsbaum, M. S., Kessslak, J. P., Lynch, G., Chui, H., Wu, J., Sicotte, N., Hazlett, E., Teng, E., & Cotman, C. W. (1991). Temporal and hippocampal metabolic rate during an olfactory memory task assessed by positron emission tomography in patients with dementia of the Alzheimer type and controls. *Archives of General Psychiatry, 48,* 840–847.

Burdette, J. H., Minoshima, S., Borght, T. V., Tran, D. D., & Kuhl, D. E. (1996). Alzheimer disease: Improved visual interpretation of PET images by using three-dimensional stereotaxic surface projections. *Radiology, 198,* 837–843.

Butcher, L. C., & Wolff, N. J. (1989). Neurotrophic agents may exacerbate the pathological cascade of Alzheimer's disease. *Neurobiology of Aging, 10,* 557–570.

Butterfield, D. A., Hensley, K., Harris, M., Mattson, M., & Carney, J. (1994). beta-Amyloid peptide free radical fragments initiate synaptosomal lipoperoxidation in a sequence-specific fashion: Implications to Alzheimer's disease. *Biochemical and Biophysical Research Communications, 200,* 710–715.

Carlesimo, G. A., & Oscar-Berman, M. (1992). Memory deficits in Alzheimer's patients: A comprehensive review. *Neuropsychology Review, 3,* 119–169.

Coburn, K. L., Ashford, J. W., & Fuster, J. M. (1990). Visual response latencies in temporal lobe structures as a function of stimulus information load. *Behavioral Neuroscience, 104,* 62–73.

Cohen, D., & Eisdorfer, C. (1980). Serum immunoglobulins and cognitive status in the elderly: Pt. I. A population study. *British Journal of Psychiatry, 136,* 33–39.

Cohen, D., Eisdorfer, C., Gorelick, P., Paveza, G., Luchins, D. J., Freels, S., Ashford, J. W., Semla, T., Levy, P., & Hirschman, R. (1993). Psychopathology associated with Alzheimer's disease and related disorders. *Journal of Gerontology: Medical Sciences, 48,* M255–M260.

Coyle, J. T., Price, D. L., & DeLong, M. R. (1983). Alzheimer's disease: A disorder of cortical cholinergic innervation. *Science, 219,* 1184–1190.

Davies, D. C., Brooks, J. W., & Lewis, D. A. (1993). Axonal loss from the olfactory tracts in Alzheimer's disease. *Neurobiology of Aging, 14,* 353–357.

Davies, C. A., Mann, D. M. A., Sumpter, P. W., & Yates, P. O. (1987). A quantitative morphometric analysis of the neuronal and synaptic content of the frontal and temporal cortex in patients with Alzheimer's disease. *Journal of the Neurological Sciences, 78,* 151–164.

Davies, P., & Maloney, A. J. F. (1976). Selective loss of central cholinergic neurons in Alzheimer's disease. *Lancet, ii,* 1403.

DeKosky, S. T., Harbaugh, R. E., Schmitt, F. A., Bakay, R. A. E., Chui, H. C., Knopman, D. S., Reeder, T. M., Shetter, A. G., Senter, H. J., & Markesbery, W. R. (1992). Intraventricular Bethanecol Study Group: Cortical biopsy in Alzheimer's disease: Diagnostic accuracy and neurochemical, neuropathological, and cognitive correlations. *Annals of Neurology, 32,* 625–632.

DeKosky, S. T., & Scheff, S. W. (1990). Synapse loss in frontal cortex biopsies in Alzheimer's disease: Correlation with cognitive severity. *Annals of Neurology, 27,* 457–464.

De Lacoste, M. C., & White, C. L. (1993). The role of cortical connectivity in Alzheimer's disease pathogenesis: A review and model system. *Neurobiology of Aging, 14,* 1–16.

Di Patre, P. L. (1991). Cytoskeletal alterations might account for the phylogenetic vulnerability of the human brain to Alzheimer's disease. *Medical Hypotheses, 34,* 165–170.

Drachman, D. A. (1977). Memory and cognitive function in man: Does the cholinergic system have a specific role? *Neurology, 27,* 783–790.

Ellison, G. (1995). The N-methyl-D-aspartate antagonists phencyclidine, ketamine and dizocilpine as both behavioral and anatomical models of the dementias. *Brain Research Review, 20,* 250–267.

Fillenbaum, G. G., Wilkinson, W. E., Welsh, K. A., & Mohs, R. C. (1994). Discrimination between stages of Alzheimer's disease with subsets of mini-mental state examination items. *Archives of Neurology, 51,* 916–921.

Forbes, W. L., Gentleman, J. F., & Maxwell, C. J. (1995). Concerning the role of aluminum in causing dementia. *Experimental Gerontology, 30,* 23–32.

Francis, P. T., Palmer, A. M., Sims, N. R., Bowen, D. M., Davison, A. N., Esiri, M. M., Neary, D., Snowden, J. S., & Wilcock, G. K. (1985). Neurochemical studies of early-onset Alzheimer's disease. *New England Journal of Medicine, 313,* 7–11.

Francis, P. T., Sims, N. R., Proctor, A. W., & Bowen, D. M. (1993). Cortical pyramidal neuron loss may cause glutamatergic hypoactivity and cognitive impairment in Alzheimer's disease: Investigative and therapeutic perspectives. *Journal of Neurochemistry, 60,* 1589–1604.

Friedlich, A. L., & Butcher, L. L. (1994). Involvement of free oxygen radicals in β-amyloidosis: An hypothesis. *Neurobiology of Aging, 15,* 443–455.

Fuster, J. M. (1995). *Memory in the cerebral cortex: An empirical approach to neural networks in the human and nonhuman primate.* Cambridge, MA: MIT Press.

Geddes, J. W., Anderson, K. J., & Cotman, C. W. (1986). Senile plaques as aberrant sprout-stimulating structures. *Experimental Neurology, 94,* 767–776.

Geddes, J. W., & Cotman, C. W. (1991). Plasticity in Alzheimer's disease: Too much or not enough? *Neurobiology of Aging, 12,* 330–333.

Geddes, J. W., Monaghan, D. T., Cotman, C. W., Lott, I. T., Kim, R. C., & Chui, H. C. (1985). Plasticity of hippocampal circuitry in Alzheimer's disease. *Science, 230,* 1179–1181.

German, D. C., White, C. L., & Sparkman, D. R. (1987). Alzheimer's disease: Neurofibrillary tangles in nuclei that project to the cerebral cortex. *Neuroscience, 21,* 305–312.

Goodman, Y., Bruce, A. J., Cheng, B., & Mattson, M. P. (1996). Estrogens attenuate and corticosterone exacerbates excitotoxicity, oxidative injury, and amyloid β-peptide toxicity in hippocampal neurons. *Journal of Neurochemistry, 66,* 1836–1844.

Goodman, Y., & Mattson, M. P. (1994). Secreted forms of β-amyloid precursor protein protect hippocampal neurons against amyloid β-peptide-induced oxidative injury. *Experimental Neurobiology, 128,* 1–12.

Gottfries, C. G., Adolfsson, R., Aquilonius, S. M., Carlsson, A., Eckernas, S. A., Nordberg, A., Oreland, L., Svennerholm, L., Wiberg, A., & Winblad, B. (1983). Biochemical changes in dementia disorders of Alzheimer type (AD/SDAT). *Neurobiology of Aging, 4,* 261–271.

Grady, C. L., McIntosh, A. R., Horwitz, B., Maisog, J. M., Ungerleider, L. G., Mentis, M. J., Pietrini, P., Schapiro, M. B., & Haxby, J. V. (1995). Age-related reductions in human recognition memory due to impaired encoding. *Science, 269,* 218–221.

Gratton, A., & Wise, R. A. (1988). Comparisons and refractory periods for medial forebrain bundle fibers subserving stimulation-induced feeding and brain stimulation reward: A psychophysical study. *Brain Research, 438,* 256–263.

Haberly, L. B. (1990). Comparative aspects of olfactory cortex. In E. G. Jones & A. Peters (Eds.), *Cerebral cortex* (Vol. 8-B, pp. 137–160). New York: Plenum Press.

Harrington, C. R., Wischik, C. M., McArthur, F. K., Taylor, G. A., Edwardson, J. A., & Candy, J. M. (1994). Alzheimer's disease-like changes in tau protein processing: Association with aluminum accumulation in brains of renal dialysis patients. *Lancet, 343,* 993–997.

Harrison, P. J. (1986). Pathogenesis of Alzheimer's disease—beyond the cholinergic hypothesis [Discussion paper]. *Journal of the Royal Society of Medicine, 79,* 347–352.

Henderson, V. W., Paganini-Hill, A., Emanuel, C. K., Dunn, M. E., & Buckwalter, J. G. (1994). Estrogen replacement therapy in older women. *Archives of Neurology, 51,* 896–900.

Hensley, K., Carney, J. M., Mattson, M. P., Aksenova, M., Harris, M., Wu, J. F., Floyd, R., & Butterfield, D. A. (1994). A model for β-amyloid aggregation and neurotoxicity based on free radical generation by the peptide: Relevance

to Alzheimer's disease. *Proceedings of the National Academy of Sciences, USA, 91,* 3270–3274.
Hirano, A., & Zimmerman, H. M. (1962). Alzheimer's neurofibrillary changes. *Archives of Neurology, 7,* 227–242.
Hock, C., Golombowski, S., Naser, W., & Müller-Spahn, F. (1995). Increased levels of τ protein in cerebrospinal fluid of patients with Alzheimer's disease—correlation with degree of cognitive impairment. *Annals of Neurology, 37,* 414–415.
Horwitz, B. (1988). Neuroplasticity and the progression of Alzheimer's disease. *International Journal of Neuroscience, 41,* 1–14.
Hoyer, S., Oesterreich, K., & Wagner, O. (1988). Glucose metabolism as the site of the primary abnormality in early-onset dementia of Alzheimer type. *Journal of Neurology, 235,* 143–148.
Hyman, B. T. (1994). Studying the Alzheimer's disease brain: Insights, puzzles, and opportunities. *Neurobiology of Aging, 15,* S79–S83.
Hyman, B. T., Van Hoesen, G. W., Damasio, A. R., & Barnes, C. L. (1984). Alzheimer's disease: Cell specific pathology isolates the hippocampal formation in Alzheimer's disease. *Science, 225,* 1168–1170.
Itagaki, S., McGeer, P. L., Akiyama, H., Zhu, S., & Selkoe, D. (1989). Relationship of microglia and astrocytes to amyloid deposits of Alzheimer disease. *Journal of Neuroimmunology, 24,* 173–182.
Jacobs, B. L., & Azmitia, E. C. (1992). Structure and function of the brain serotonin system. *Physiological Review, 721,* 165–229.
Jagust, W. J. (1994). Functional imaging in dementia: An overview. *Journal of Clinical Psychiatry, 55,* 5–11.
Jagust, W. J., Friedland, R. P., Budinger, T. F., Koss, E., & Ober, B. (1988). Longitudinal studies of regional cerebral metabolism in Alzheimer's disease. *Neurology, 38,* 909–912.
Jagust, W. J., Reed, B. R., Seab, J. P., & Budinger, T. F. (1990). Alzheimer's disease: Age at onset and single-photon emission computed tomography patterns of regional cerebral blood flow. *Archives of Neurology, 47,* 628–633.
Jarvik, L., & Greenson, H. (1987). About a peculiar disease of the cerebral cortex, by Alois Alzheimer. *Alzheimer Disease and Associated Disorders, 1,* 7–8.
Jensen, M., Basun, H., & Lannfelt, L. (1995). Increased cerebrospinal fluid tau in patients with Alzheimer's disease. *Neuroscience Letters, 186,* 189–191.
Jette, N., Cole, M. S., & Fahnestock, M. (1994). NGF mRNA is not decreased in frontal cortex from Alzheimer's disease patients. *Molecular Brain Research, 25,* 242–250.
Joachim, C. L., Mori, H., & Selkoe, D. J. (1989). Amyloid β-protein deposition in tissues other than brain in Alzheimer's disease. *Nature, 341,* 226–230.
Jobst, K. A., Smith, A. D., Szatmari, M., Esiri, M. M., Jaskowski, A., Hindley, N., McDonald, B., & Molyneux, A. J. (1994). Rapidly progressing atrophy of medial temporal lobe in Alzheimer's disease. *Lancet, 343,* 829–830.

Kaba, H., Hayashi, Y., Higuchi, T., & Nakanishi, S. (1994). Induction of an olfactory memory by the activation of a metabotropic glutamate receptor. *Science, 265,* 262–264.

Kauer, J. S. (1991). Contributions of topography and parallel processing to odor coding in the vertebrate olfactory pathway. *Trends in Neurosciences, 14,* 79–85.

Kesslak, J. P., Nalcioglu, O., & Cotman, C. W. (1991). Quantification of magnetic resonance scans for hippocampal and parahippocampal atrophy in Alzheimer's disease. *Neurology, 41,* 51–54.

Kuhl, D. E., Metter, E. J., Benson, D. F., Ashford, J. W., Riege, W. H., Fujikawa, D. G., Markham, C. H., Maziotta, J. C., Maltese, A., & Dorsey, D. (1985). Similarities of cerebral glucose metabolism in Alzheimer's and Parkinsonian dementia. *Journal of Cerebral Blood Flow and Metabolism, 5,* S169–S170.

Kuhl, D. E., Small, G. W., Riege, W. H., Fujikawa, D. G., Metter, E. J., Benson, D. F., Ashford, J. W., Mazziotta, J. C., Maltese, A., & Dorsey, D. A. (1987). Cerebral metabolic patterns before the diagnosis of probable Alzheimer's disease [Abstract]. *Journal of Cerebral Blood Flow and Metabolism, 7,* S406.

Kumar, M., Cohen, D., & Eisdorfer, C. (1988). Serum IgG brain reactive antibodies in Alzheimer disease and Down syndrome. *Alzheimer Disease and Associated Disorders, 2,* 50–55.

Landfield, P. W., Applegate, M. D., Schmitzer-Osborne, S. E., & Naylor, C. E. (1991). *Journal of Neurological Science, 106,* 221–229.

Larner, A. J. (1995). The cortical neuritic dystrophy of Alzheimer's disease: Nature, significance, and possible pathogenesis. *Dementia, 6,* 218–224.

Lewandowsky, S., & Murdock, B. B. (1989). Memory for serial order. *Psychological Review, 96,* 25–57.

Lewis, D. A., Campbell, M. J., Terry, R. D., & Morrison, J. H. (1987). Laminar and regional distributions of neurofibrillary tangles and neuritic plaques in Alzheimer's disease: A quantitative study of visual and auditory cortices. *Journal of Neuroscience, 7,* 1799–1808.

Lovell, M. A., Ehmann, W. D., & Markesbery, W. R. (1993). Laser microprobe analysis of brain aluminum in Alzheimer's disease. *Annals of Neurology, 33,* 36–42.

Mark, R. J., Hensley, K., Butterfield, D. A., & Mattson, M. P. (1995). Amyloid β-peptide impairs ion-motive ATPase activities: Evidence for a role in loss of neuronal Ca^{2+} homeostasis and cell death. *Journal of Neuroscience, 15,* 6239–6249.

Masur, D. M., Sliwinski, M., Lipton, R. B., Blau, A. D., & Crystal, H. A. (1994). Neuropsychological prediction of dementia and the absence of dementia in healthy elderly persons. *Neurology, 44,* 1427–1432.

Mattson, M. P. (1990). Antigenic changes similar to those seen in neurofibrillary tangles are elicited by glutamate and calcium influx in cultured hippocampal neurons. *Neuron, 4,* 105–117.

Mattson, M. P. (1992). Calcium as sculptor and destroyer of neural circuitry. *Experimental Gerontology, 27,* 29–49.
Mattson, M. P., Barger, S. W., Cheng, B., Lieberburg, I., Smith-Swintosky, V. L., & Rydel, R. E. (1993a). β-amyloid precursor protein metabolites and loss of neuronal calcium homeostasis in Alzheimer's disease. *Trends in Neurosciences, 16,* 409–415.
Mattson, M. P., Cheng, B., & Smith-Swintosky, V. L. (1993b). Growth factor-mediated protection from excitotoxicity and disturbances in calcium and free radical metabolism. *Seminars in the Neurosciences, 5,* 295–307.
Mattson, M. P., Dou, P., & Kater, S. B. (1988). Outgrowth-regulatory actions of glutamate in isolated hippocampal pyramidal neurons. *Journal of Neuroscience, 8,* 2087–2100.
Mazurek, M. F., Beal, F., Bird, E. D., & Martin, J. B. (1986). Vasopressin in Alzheimer's disease: A study of postmortem brain concentrations. *Annals of Neurology, 20,* 665–670.
McClelland, J. L., Rumelhart, D. E., & the PDP Research Group. (1989). *Parallel distributed processing: Explorations in the microstructure of cognition: Vol. 2. Psychological and biological models.* Cambridge, MA: MIT Press.
McCormick, W. C., Kukull, W. A., van Belle, G., Bowen, J. D., Teri, L., & Larson, E. B. (1994). Symptom patterns and comorbidity in the early stages of Alzheimer's disease. *Journal of the American Geriatric Society, 42,* 517–521.
McRae-Degueurce, A., Booj, S., Haglid, K., Rosengren, L., Karlsson, J. E., Karlsson, I., Wallin, A., Svennerholm, L., Gottfries, C. G., & Dahlstrom, A. (1987). Antibodies in cerebrospinal fluid of some Alzheimer disease patients recognize cholinergic neurons in the rat central nervous system. *Proceedings of the National Academy of Sciences, USA, 84,* 9214–9218.
Mesulam, M. M., Mufson, E. J., Levey, A. I., & Wainer, B. H. (1983). Cholinergic innervation of cortex by the basal forebrain: Cytochemistry and cortical connections of the septal area, diagonal band nuclei, nucleus basalis (substantia innominata), and hypothalamus in the rhesus monkey. *Journal of Comparative Neurology, 214,* 170–197.
Mishkin, M. (1982). A memory system in the monkey. *Philosophical Transactions of the Royal Society of London (Biology), 298,* 85–95.
Mori, H., Hosoda, K., Matsubara, E., Nakamoto, T., Furiya, Y., Endoh, R., Usami, M., Shoji, M., Maruyama, S., & Hirai, S. (1995). Tau in cerebrospinal fluids: Establishment of the sandwich ELISA with antibody specific to the repeat sequence in tau. *Neuroscience Letters, 186,* 181–183.
Motter, R., Vigo-Pelfrey, C., Kholodenko, D., Barbour, R., Johnson-Wood, K., Galasko, D., Chang, L., Miller, B., Clark, C., Green, R., Olson, D., Southwick, P., Wolfert, R., Munroe, B., Lieberburg, I., Seubert, P., & Schenk, D. (1995). Reduction of β-amyloid Peptide$_{42}$ in the cerebrospinal fluid of patients with Alzheimer's disease. *Annals of Neurology, 38,* 643–648.

Mullan, M., & Crawford, F. (1993). Genetic and molecular advances in Alzheimer's disease. *Trends in Neurosciences, 16,* 398–403.
Murdock, B. B., Jr. (1982). A theory for the storage and retrieval of item and associative information. *Psychological Review, 89,* 609–626.
Nagy, Z., Esiri, M. M., Jobst, K. A., Morris, J. H., King, E. M.-F., McDonald, B., Litchfield, S., Smith, A., Barnetson, L., & Smith, A. D. (1995). Relative roles of plaques and tangles in the dementia of Alzheimer's disease: Correlations using three sets of neuropathological criteria. *Dementia, 6,* 21–31.
Nauta, W. J. H., & Karten, H. J. (1970). A general profile of the vertebrate brain with sidelight on the ancestry of the cerebral cortex. In G. C. Quarton et al. (Eds.), *The Neurosciences, Second Study Program* (pp. 7–26). New York: Rockefeller University Press.
Ohm, T. G., Muller, H., Braak, H., & Bohl, J. (1995). Close-meshed prevalence rates of different stages as a tool to uncover the rate of Alzheimer's disease-related neurofibrillary changes. *Neuroscience, 64,* 209–217.
O'Keefe, J., & Nadel, L. (1978). *The Hippocampus as a cognitive map.* Oxford, England: Clarendon Press.
Oppenheim, G. (1994). The earliest signs of Alzheimer's disease. *Journal of Geriatric Psychiatry and Neurology, 7,* 118–122.
Palmer, A. M., Francis, P. T., Benton, J. S., Sims, N. R., Mann, D. M. A., Neary, D., Snowden, J. S., & Bowen, D. M. (1987). Presynaptic serotonergic dysfunction in patients with Alzheimer's disease. *Journal of Neurochemistry, 48,* 8–15.
Palmer, A. M., Procter, A. W., Stratmann, G. C., & Bowen, D. M. (1986). Excitatory amino acid-releasing and cholinergic neurons in Alzheimer's disease. *Neuroscience Letters, 66,* 199–204.
Pearson, R. C. A., Esiri, M. M., Hiorns, R. W., Wilcock, G. K., & Powell, T. P. S. (1985). Anatomical correlates of the distribution of the pathological changes in the neocortex in Alzheimer's disease. *Proceedings of the National Academy of Sciences, USA, 82,* 4531–4534.
Perry, E. K., Perry, R. H., Blessed, G., & Tomlinson, B. G. (1977). Necropsy evidence of central cholinergic defects in senile dementia. *Lancet, 1,* 189.
Represa, A., Duyckaerts, C., Tremblay, E., Hauw J., & Ben-Ari, Y. (1988). Is senile dementia of the Alzheimer type associated with hippocampal plasticity? *Brain Research, 457,* 355–359.
Roberts, E. (1986). Alzheimer's disease may begin in the nose and may be caused by aluminosilicates. *Neurobiology of Aging, 7,* 561–567.
Rosene, D. L., & Van Hoesen, G. W. (1987). The hippocampal formation of the primate brain: A review of some comparative aspects of cytoarchitecture and connections (Vol. 6, pp. 345–456). In E. G. Jones & A. Peters (Eds.), *Cerebral Cortex.* New York: Plenum Press.

Roses, A. D. (1994). The Alzheimer diseases. *Current Neurology, 14,* 111–141.
Rossor, M. N. (1982). Neurotransmitters and CNS Disease: Dementia. *Lancet, ii,* 1200–1204.
Sadowski, M., Morys, J., Barcikowska, M., & Narkiewicz, O. (1995). Astrocyte and microglia reaction in Alzheimer's disease in the hippocampal formation—a quantitative analysis. *Alzheimer's Research, 1,* 71–76.
Saper, C. B., Wainer, B. H., & German, D. C. (1987). Axonal and transneuronal transport in the transmission of neurological disease: Potential role in system degenerations, including Alzheimer's disease. *Neuroscience, 23,* 389–398.
Saunders, A. M., Strittmatter, W. J., Schmechel, D., St. George-Hyslop, P. H., Pericak-Vance, M. A., Joo, S. H., Rosi, B. L., Gusella, J. F., Crapper-MacLachlan, D. R., Alberts, M. J., Hulette, C., Crain, B., Goldgaber, D., & Roses, A. D. (1993). Association of apolipoprotein E allele ∈4 with late-onset familial and sporadic Alzheimer's disease. *Neurology, 43,* 1467–1472.
Scheff, S. W., DeKosky, S. T., & Price, D. A. (1990). Quantitative assessment of cortical synaptic density in Alzheimer's disease. *Neurobiology of Aging, 11,* 29–37.
Scheff, S. W., & Price, D. A. (1993). Synapse loss in the temporal lobe in Alzheimer's disease. *Annals of Neurology, 33,* 190–199.
Scott, S. A., Mufson, E. J., Weingartner, J. A., Skau, K. A., & Crutcher, K. A. (1995). Nerve growth factor in Alzheimer's disease: Increased levels throughout the brain coupled with declines in nucleus basalis. *Journal of Neuroscience, 15,* 6213–6221.
Selkoe, D. J. (1993). Physiological production of the β-amyloid protein and the mechanism of Alzheimer's disease. *Trends in Neurosciences, 16,* 403–409.
Selkoe, D. J. (1994). Alzheimer's disease: A central role for amyloid. *Journal of Neuropathology and Experimental Neurology, 53,* 438–447.
Serby, M., Larson, P., & Kalkstein, D. (1991). The nature and course of olfactory deficits in Alzheimer's disease. *American Journal of Psychiatry, 148,* 357–360.
Shin, R. W., Lee, F. M. Y., & Trojanowski, J. Q. (1994). Aluminum modifies the properties of Alzheimer's disease PHF proteins in vivo and in vitro. *Journal of Neuroscience, 14,* 7221–7233.
Small, G. W., La Rue, A., Komo, S., Kaplan, A., & Mandelkern, M. A. (1995). Predictors of cognitive change in middle-aged and older adults with memory loss. *American Journal of Psychiatry, 152,* 1757–1764.
Smith-Swintosky, V. L., Pettigrew, L. C., Sapolsky, R. M., Phares, C., Craddock, S. D., Brooke, S. M., & Mattson, M. P. (in press). Metyrapone, an inhibitor of glucocorticoid production, reduces brain injury induced by focal and global ischemia and seizures. *Journal of Cerebral Blood Flow and Metabolism.*
Squire, L. R., & Zola-Morgan, S. (1991). The medial temporal lobe memory system. *Science, 253,* 1380–1386.

Stäubli, U., Le, T. T., & Lynch, G. (1995). Variants of olfactory memory and their dependencies on the hippocampal formation. *Journal of Neuroscience, 15*, 1162–1171.

Stein-Behrens, B., Mattson, M. P., Chang, I., Yeh, M., & Sapolsky, R. M. (1994). Stress exacerbates neuron loss and cytoskeletal pathology in the hippocampus. *Journal of Neuroscience, 14*, 5373–5380.

Stern, Y., Gurland, B., Tatemichi, T. K., Tang, M. X., Wilder, D., & Mayeux, R. (1994). Influence of education and occupation on the incidence of Alzheimer's disease. *Journal of the American Medical Association, 271*, 1004–1010.

Steward, O., & Banker, G. A. (1992). Getting the message from the gene to the synapse: Sorting and intracellular transport of RNA in neurons. *Trends in Neurosciences, 15*, 180–186.

Streit, W. J., & Kincaid-Colton, C. A. (1995, November). The brain's immune system. *Scientific American, 273*, 54–61.

Struble, R. G., & Clark, H. B. (1992). Olfactory bulb lesions in Alzheimer's disease. *Neurobiology of Aging, 13*, 469–473.

Su, J. H., Cummings, B. J., & Cotman, C. W. (1994). Early phosphorylation of tau in Alzheimer's disease occurs at Ser-202 and is preferentially located within neurites. *NeuroReport, 5*, 2358–2362.

Sugaya, K., Giacobini, E., & Chiappinelli, V. A. (1990). Nicotinic acetylcholine receptor subtypes in human frontal cortex: Changes in Alzheimer's disease. *Journal of Neuroscience Research, 27*, 349–359.

Talamo, B. R., Rudel, R. A., Kosik, K. S., Lee, V. M.-Y., Neff, S., Adelman, L., & Kauer, J. S. (1989). Pathological changes in olfactory neurons in patients with Alzheimer's disease. *Nature, 337*, 736–739.

Tato, R. E., Frank, A., & Hernanz, A. (1995). Tau protein concentrations in cerebrospinal fluid of patients with dementia of the Alzheimer type. *Journal of Neurology, Neurosurgery, and Psychiatry, 59*, 280–283.

Teri, L. Hughes, J. P., & Larson, E. B. (1990). Cognitive deterioration in Alzheimer's disease: Behavioral and health factors. *Journal of Gerontology: Psychological Sciences, 45*, 58–63.

Terry, R., Masliah, E., Salmon, D. P., Butters, N., DeTeresa, R., Hill, R., Hansen, L. A., & Katzman, R. (1991). Physical basis of cognitive alterations in Alzheimer's disease: Synapse loss is the major correlation of cognitive impairment. *Annals of Neurology, 30*, 572–580.

Trojanowski, J. Q., & Lee, V. M.-Y. (1995). Phosphorylation of paired helical filament tau in Alzheimer's disease neurofibrillary lesions: Focusing on phosphatases. *FASEB, 9*, 1570–1576.

Trombley, P. Q., & Shepherd, G. M. (1993). Synaptic transmission and modulation in the olfactory bulb. *Neurobiology, 3*, 540–547.

Ungerleider, L. G. (1995). Functional brain imaging studies of cortical mechanisms for memory. *Science, 270*, 769–775.

van Gool, W. A., Kuiper, M. A., Walstra, G. J. M., Wolters, E. Ch., & Bolhuis, P. A. (1995). Concentrations of amyloid β protein in cerebrospinal fluid of patients with Alzheimer's disease. *Annals of Neurology, 37,* 277–278.
Van Hoesen, G. W., Pandya, D. N., & Butters, N. (1975). Some connections of the entorhinal (Area 28) and perirhinal (Area 35) cortices of the Rhesus monkey. *Brain Research, 95,* 25–38.
Vigo-Pelfrey, C., Seubert, P., Barbour, R., Blomquist, C., Lee, M., Lee, D., Coria, F., Chang, L., Miller, B., Lieberburg, I., & Schenk, D. (1995). Elevation of microtubule-associated protein tau in the cerebrospinal fluid of patients with Alzheimer's disease. *Neurology, 45,* 788–793.
Welsh, K., Butters, N., Hughes, J., Mohs, R., & Heyman, A. (1991). Detection of abnormal memory decline in mild cases of Alzheimer's disease using CERAD neuropsychological measures. *Archives of Neurology, 48,* 278–281.
Whitehouse, P. J., & Kellar, K. J. (1987). Nicotinic and muscarinic cholinergic receptors in Alzheimer's disease and related disorders. *Journal of Neural Transmission, 24,* 175–182.
Whitehouse, P. J., Price, D. L., Struble, R. G., Clark, A. W., Coyle, J. T., & DeLong, M. R. (1982). Alzheimer's disease and senile dementia: Loss of neurons in the basal forebrain. *Science, 215,* 1237–1239.
Wolf-Klein, G. P., Silverstone, F. A., Broad, M. S., Levy, A., Foley, C. J., Termotto, V., & Breuer, J. (1988). Are Alzheimer patients healthier? *Journal of the American Geriatric Society, 36,* 219–224.
Wolozin, B., Lesch, P., Lebovics, R., & Sunderland, T. (1993). Olfactory neuroblasts from Alzheimer donors: Studies on APP processing and cell regulation. *Biological Psychiatry, 34,* 824–838.
Woody, C. D., & Gruen, E. (1993). Cholinergic and glutamatergic effects on neocortical neurons may support rate as well as development of conditioning. *Progress in Brain Research, 98,* 365–370.
Woolf, N. J., & Butcher, L. L. (1990). Dysdifferentiation of structurally plastic neurons initiates the pathologic cascade of Alzheimer's disease: Toward a unifying hypothesis. In M. Steriade & D. Biesold (Eds.), *Brain cholinergic systems* (pp. 387–438). New York: Oxford University Press.
Yan, S. D., Chen, X., Schmidt, A. M., Brett, J., Godman, G., Zou, Y. S., Scott, C. W., Caputo, C., Frappier, T., Smith, M. A., Perry, G., Yen, S. H., & Stern, D. (1994). Glycated tau protein in Alzheimer disease: A mechanism for induction of oxidant stress. *Proceedings of the National Academy of Sciences, USA, 91,* 7787–7791.
Zattore, R. J. (1990). Memory loss following domoic acid intoxication from ingestion of toxic mussels. *Canada Diseases Weekly Report, 16,* 101–103.

CHAPTER **4**

Genetics of Alzheimer's Disease

Steven S. Matsuyama

Familial clustering of Alzheimer disease (AD) is well known, and there is a consensus that a positive family history of dementia is a risk factor for AD. Classical genetic studies and more recent molecular genetic investigations have provided evidence for the role of genetic factors underlying AD.

In reviewing the genetics of AD, it is important to point out that investigations have been hampered by several factors:

1. Because of its late-age at onset, many family members may have died prior to or during the risk period, thus making it difficult to determine in any given individual if the disease was genetically transmitted or represents a sporadic occurrence;
2. the possibility of genetic heterogeneity; and
3. inaccuracy of the clinical diagnosis.

This work was supported in part by VA Medical Research Funds and the UCLA Alzheimer Disease Center (NIA P30 AG10123). The opinions expressed are those of the author and not necessarily those of the Department of Veterans Affairs.

Even with the most restrictive research diagnostic criteria, 10% to 20% of clinically diagnosed AD patients are classified as false positives on neuropathological examination.

CLASSICAL GENETIC STUDIES

Family Studies

A number of studies on familial risk for AD have been published (see review in Matsuyama, Jarvik, & Kumar, 1985). These early studies often differentiated between presenile and senile onset on the basis of age at onset either before or after age 65, and this distinction has been maintained in this chapter. Among five presenile onset studies (including one study with age at onset ≤ 70), three with autopsy data, the risk for parents ranged from 1.4% to 33.5% and that for siblings from 2.2% to 13.9%. Data from these studies ($N = 144$ families) provided information on secondary cases: 53 secondary cases were reported in 38 families (26.4%), and 26 secondary cases (18.1%) exhibited transmission through two generations. In three senile onset studies, two with autopsy data, the risk for parents ranged from 2.2% to 20.8% and for siblings, from 3.4% to 18.4% (risk figures from a single study based on the combined sample of presenile and senile onset cases is not included). Among the total of 372 families in these studies, 117 secondary cases were reported in 75 families (20.2%), and 33 (8.9%) exhibited transmission through two generations. Overall, the risk of AD to first-degree relatives does not support an autosomal dominant mode of inheritance. However, suggestive genetic transmission is more apparent in presenile than in senile onset families (18.1% vs. 8.9%).

Several family studies published since that review report morbid risk among first-degree relatives approaching 50% by age 90, consistent with an autosomal dominant mode of inheritance (Breitner & Folstein, 1984; Mohs, Breitner, Silverman, & Davis, 1987). However, caution must be used in interpreting a 50% risk, because in calculating such risks, there is a paucity of individuals at later ages resulting in large standard errors.

Segregation analysis is a widely used statistical method to determine the mode of inheritance in which the observed frequency of illness in a family is compared to the pattern expected from hypothesized modes of inheritance. The power of segregation analysis is compromised by etiologic heterogeneity and accuracy of diagnosis. Segregation analyses have confirmed a genetic component in AD (Farrer, Myers, Connor, Cupples, & Growdon, 1991; Rao, et al., 1994). Familial patterns consistent with an autosomal, dominant gene emerged, but data also suggested the possible existence of two or more major genes as well as evidence for a polygenic background.

The limitations of the family study method must be borne in mind when evaluating such studies. They include:

1. difficulties in obtaining accurate information, especially for older individuals whose memory may be impaired and whose parents, siblings, and friends have died—no one is left to provide information about the family;
2. small family sizes, making it difficult to determine the mode of inheritance; and
3. the selection bias—probands are usually brought to the attention of investigators because of dramatic illnesses, often unusually severe, or because of multiple affected family members, and therefore, they are not representative of the group afflicted with a given illness.

To complicate matters even more, familial does not necessarily mean genetic; some familial cases may be due to common environmental factors rather than to an underlying gene defect.

Twin Studies

Twin studies report a 40% to 50% concordance rate among monozygotic (MZ) twins and 8% to 50% for duozygotic (DZ) twins (Small, et al., 1993). Although these concordance rates argue against a simple genetic etiology in AD, there are several limitations in interpreting these data, including:

1. the small number of twin pairs investigated (total of 50 MZ and 10 DZ);
2. questions regarding the accuracy of clinical diagnosis; and
3. the cross-sectional nature of these studies.

Widely disparate ages at onset of the disease in concordant MZ twin pairs (up to 15 years) have been reported, and we must await the results of longitudinal follow-up studies of twins. The absence of 100% concordance in MZ twins suggests that environmental factors also play a role in the etiology of a disease.

Family and twin studies, although providing evidence that AD has a genetic etiology at least in some families, do not provide information as to the location of the genetic defect. Other approaches are needed for that purpose. Application of molecular genetic techniques is appropriate, and as reviewed next, has provided exciting new findings. To understand the principles of this technology, it is important to review some basic fundamentals of genetics.

MOLECULAR GENETICS AND LINKAGE: BASIC BIOLOGY

The genetic material is deoxyribonucleic acid (DNA), a long polymerized structure composed of four kinds of nucleotides. Each nucleotide is made up of the five-carbon sugar deoxyribose, phosphoric acid, and one of four nitrogenous bases—adenine (A), thymine (T), guanine (G), and, cytosine (C). The DNA molecule consists of two polynucleotide chains in a double helix configuration. Base pairing is precise and always complementary: A with T, and G with C. The sequence of the bases provides the code for the genetic information: it is read in non-overlapping groups of three nucleotides (i.e., codons) from a fixed starting point. Each codon specifies an amino acid, the building block of proteins. Substitution of a single base changes only the codon in which the base is located and affects only that amino acid in the protein. Deletion or insertion of a single nucleotide changes the reading frame subsequent to that change, thus altering the amino acid sequence beyond the site of the mutation and is likely to result in loss of protein function.

DNA segments coding for the proteins (exons) are interrupted by intervening segments (introns). In protein synthesis, the first step is transcription of DNA to a messenger RNA (mRNA), which represents a copy of the sequence of the gene. The mRNA is then processed, that is, introns are removed, bringing together the exons, and this processed mRNA is then translated into protein.

Genes are located at identifiable positions (loci) on a particular chromosome. The genetic information of cells is contained within their chromosomes located in the cell nucleus. Two basic laws underlie genetic investigations. The first law states that alleles, that is, different genetic alternatives at the same locus on homologous chromosomes, segregate; and, the second that different pairs of alleles assort independently. This second law applies only to genes residing on separate chromosomes or sufficiently distant from each other on the same chromosome to behave independently. Thus genes do not always segregate independently; some of them remain associated in inheritance, that is, they cosegregate. The propensity of some genes to remain associated in inheritance is called linkage, and the transmission of two loci together is used for linkage analysis and is the basis of the strategy used to localize a disease gene to a region of a specific chromosome. The pattern of transmission of a disease gene can be followed through families if markers (i.e., variants that mark nearby positions on the chromosome) are available in close proximity to the disease gene. The transmission of a trait with a known marker within families suggests that the two genes are located on the same chromosome in close proximity to each other. If a particular marker is consistently inherited with the disease, then the disease gene must be located near the marker. The closer the two loci are, the more frequently they are transmitted together; the farther apart the two loci are, the more likely they are to form new combinations (recombinations), and this recombination frequency provides a measure of the distance between loci.

Evidence for linkage is derived from a statistical analysis of the observed association between two loci, that is, the probability of observing the segregation of the two loci (or combination of traits) over a range of recombination fractions assuming linkage, compared with the probability of observing the two traits together in the absence of linkage (i.e., the loci are segregating independently). The logarithm of this ratio of likelihoods is the lod score. Evidence for linkage is generally accepted if the lod score exceeds 3.0 (linkage is 1,000 times more likely than no linkage). Lod scores are additive across families, but this assumes that it is the same gene segregating in these families. Thus genetic heterogeneity can affect linkage studies seriously.

Early linkage studies utilized highly polymorphic genetic loci (e.g., HLA, blood group antigens, and serum proteins) to determine if a disease cosegregated more frequently than expected by chance with a specific marker. However, known protein polymorphisms cover only approximately 20% of the human genome.

Molecular Genetics

Human genetic linkage analysis was revolutionized in 1978 with the application of molecular genetic techniques and the discovery of new types of markers based on large amounts of DNA base sequence variations, that is, polymorphisms that occur at random in the human genome. Briefly, the technique utilizes restriction enzymes (endonucleases) that recognize specific short sequences of DNA (usually four to six base pairs) and cleave the DNA each time the recognition sequence occurs. Variations in the DNA base sequence (e.g., polymorphisms in the genome or mutation in the DNA recognition site) create or eliminate such recognition sites and lead to DNA fragments of varying lengths. The DNA fragments of distinct lengths are visualized by separating the DNA fragments on the basis of size by gel electrophoresis (small fragments move faster than large ones). Further analysis of the DNA is done by the technique of Southern blotting, wherein the DNA separated in the gel is denatured to single stranded DNA and then transferred onto a membrane filter. This filter is incubated with a labeled DNA probe, that is, a short section of DNA with a known chromosomal location; this probe combines (hybridizes) only with its complementary sequence in a sea of noncomplementary DNA. This labeled complex can then be localized to a particular DNA fragment of a specific molecular weight. A large variety of restriction enzymes with different recognition sequence specificities is known, and by utilizing different restriction enzymes alone or in combinations, one can construct a restriction map of the area recognized by the probe of interest.

Comparing such restriction maps for two different individuals gives restriction fragment length polymorphisms (RFLPs). These RFLPs behave like Mendelian traits and are, therefore, useful genetic markers. When restriction polymorphisms occur in close proximity to the mutated gene, the gene can be used for detection of the disease gene. However, markers that identify RFLPs are capable of detecting only two alleles (based on the presence or absence of an endonuclease recognition site). Recently, highly informative genetic markers have been developed that can detect multiple alleles. This is called short tandem repeat (STR) polymorphism and is based on the variations in numbers of copies of a tandemly repeated DNA sequence of a few nucleotides. The most common STR polymorphism is the CA dinucleotide repeat. The CA repeats have numerous alleles and are randomly distributed in the genome, making them ideal genetic markers for linkage studies.

Molecular genetic approaches utilize the technique of polymerase chain reaction (PCR), which amplifies the DNA by chemical rather than biologic proliferation. In addition, PCR can amplify DNA in frozen or fixed postmortem specimens as well as neuropathologic and cytogenetic slides, and thus may provide a source of DNA from relatives who are no longer alive.

The current molecular genetic approach is to localize, identify, and sequence the gene in question and determine the gene product and its normal function. The advantages of this approach are that neither knowledge of the biochemical nature nor of the altered gene sequence responsible for the trait is necessary to locate the gene.

FAD Genes and Gene Mutations

CHROMOSOME 21. The well-known association between Down syndrome (DS) and AD suggested chromosome 21 as a candidate for AD genes. DS patients who live beyond age 35 invariably develop the hallmark AD neuropathological lesions of senile plaques and neurofibrillary tangles (although not all DS individuals are demented), and there are reports of an increased frequency of DS individuals in AD families (Heston, 1977; Heyman, et al., 1983). In 1987 the initial report of positive linkage with cosegregation of a putative familial AD (FAD) gene with DNA markers on chromosome 21 was published (St. George-Hyslop, et al., 1987). The data were based on four early-onset FAD families. However, examination of the linkage data revealed that none of the families independently gave lod scores > 3, and only one family contributed primarily to the lod score. Since that time, both positive and negative linkage results have been obtained. Two published reports may include most of the families. The first reported on 48 families (30 early-onset [< 65] and 18 late-onset [> 65]), and included nine from earlier studies (St. George-Hyslop et al., 1990). The 30 early-onset cases collectively gave a positive lod score, suggesting linkage to chromosome 21 DNA markers, whereas no evidence for linkage was found for the 18 late-onset families. The second report, also on 48 families (19 early-onset, including 7 Volga Germans and 29 late-onset), found no evidence for a gene on chromosome 21 in early-onset Volga families and late-onset families (Schellenberg, et al., 1991b). However, six early-onset families gave small positive lod scores with chromosome 21 markers. These initial chromosome 21 linkage studies suggested that early-onset AD is genetically heterogeneous with other genetic loci to be determined (see the sections that follow on the amyloid precursor protein gene, chromosome 14, and chromosome 1).

Amyloid Precursor Protein Gene

One of the hallmark neuropathological lesions of AD is the senile plaque with a central core of amyloid, a 39–43 amino acid fragment that is known as the β-amyloid protein, which is the proteolytic product of the larger amyloid precursor protein (APP). APP is a transmembrane protein that resembles a cell surface receptor. One third of the β-amyloid peptide is in the transmembrane domain, and two thirds protrudes into the extracellular space. The APP gene is comprised of 18 exons with three major isoforms produced by alternative splicing; APP 770 and APP 751 contain the Kunitz protease inhibitor, and APP 695 does not. The major pathway of APP processing is the secretory pathway, which cleaves APP extracellularly within the β-amyloid peptide, thus no intact β-amyloid is produced, and this pathway is nonamyloidogenic and not responsible for the AD pathology. Another pathway, the lysosomal/endosomal pathway, however, does produce carboxyl-terminal fragments of APP containing β-amyloid. Several lines of evidence now suggest that this pathway is unlikely to contribute to the production of β-amyloid. A second secretory pathway was recently proposed with cleavage of the APP at the amino-terminal side of β-amyloid. Furthermore, proteolytic breakdown of the β-amyloid containing fragments may lead to AD pathology. The amyloid gene was localized to chromosome 21 at the same time that the putative FAD gene was localized to the same vicinity. An initial report of duplication of the amyloid gene in sporadic AD cases led to the hypothesis that the amyloid gene was the candidate FAD gene. However, recombinations between the FAD locus and the amyloid locus were reported, and duplication of the amyloid gene in sporadic cases was not replicated in additional cases. Nonetheless, the amyloid gene has continued to be the subject of intense research investigation.

There is evidence that the APP gene is the site of mutations predisposing an individual to AD, at least in some early-onset families (see Table 4.1). The first mutation reported was a missense mutation resulting in a valine to isoleucine change at codon 717 (APP 770) in 2 of 17 early-onset FAD families (Goate, et al., 1991). This mutation cosegregated with the disease (all affected family members had the mutation), but was not found in unaffected family members, suggesting that it is an early-onset FAD gene. Other investigators found four additional early-onset families with the same missense mutation, and two families were reported to have different missense mutations at the same site, one leading to a change from valine to glycine and the other from valine to phenylalanine amino acid substitution. These APP 717 mutations are in the transmembrane domain of the APP just outside the carboxyl terminus of the β-amyloid peptide.

Collectively, only 8 of 308 early-onset FAD families examined had a missense mutation in codon 717, but none of 61 late-onset FAD families, 50 FAD families of undetermined onset, 319 sporadic AD patients, 795 normals, and 16 Down syndrome (DS) individuals (Matsuyama, 1995) (see Table 4.1). Thus these mutations are very rare and account for AD in only 2%–3% of early-onset FAD.

A double mutation at codons 670 and 671 resulting in a lysine to asparagine and methionine to leucine substitution, respectively, was reported in two related Swedish families (Mullan, et al., 1992a). This mutation is outside the amino terminus of the β-amyloid peptide. Further, a missense mutation at codon 692, resulting in an alanine to glycine substitution, was reported in one family (Hendriks, et al., 1992). Interestingly, there was variable clinical expression with family members presenting either presenile dementia or recurrent cerebral hemorrhage, suggesting the possibility of a second genetic component. There is precedence for this in the literature, where a mutation in the prion protein gene was found to be identical in two different conditions, fatal familial insomnia and Creutzfeldt-Jakob disease, but clinical expression was determined by a polymorphism at another site in the gene (Goldfarb, et al., 1992). Recently, an APP mutation was reported at codon 665, resulting in a glutamine to aspartate substitution in a patient with late-onset FAD, but the clinical significance remains unknown (Peacock, et al., 1994).

Mutations within the APP gene are not unique to AD. In hereditary cerebral hemorrhage with amyloidosis, Dutch type (HCHWA-D), a rare autosomal dominant condition (described in four families from two coastal villages in The Netherlands) characterized by recurrent intracerebral hemorrhages resulting in severe disability, mental impairment, and eventual death between the ages of 45 and 65, there is extensive cerebral amyloid angiopathy with parenchymal deposits resembling immature plaques. The amyloid is a 39 amino acid fragment derived from APP. The genetic defect in HCHWA-D is a base substitution leading to replacement of glutamate with glutamine at codon 693, which is in the β-amyloid peptide (Levy, et al., 1990), thus leading to speculation that this amino acid substitution interferes with its metabolism.

The expression of these APP mutations leading to AD remains unknown. APP mutations may result in overproduction of β-amyloid, or, alternatively, they may change the configuration of APP and facilitate abnormal cleavage, resulting in increased formation and deposition of β-amyloid.

TABLE 4.1 Amyloid Precursor Protein Gene Mutations

Study	FAD Onset Early-	FAD Onset Late-	Sporadic	Normals	DS
Codon 717 valine ----> isoleucine					
Goate et al., 1991	2/17	0/9	—	0/100	—
Naruse et al., 1991	2/3	—	0/12	0/30	—
Lucotte et al., 1991	1/2	—	—	—	—
Yoshioka et al., 1991	1/7	—	0/3	0/6	—
Codon 717 valine ----> glycine					
Chartier-Harlin et al., 1991b	1/25	—	—	0/52	—
Codon 717 valine ----> phenylalanine					
Murrell et al., 1991	1/1	—	—	0/100	—
No Codon 717 mutations					
Chartier-Harlin et al., 1991a	0/5	—	—	0/100	—
Van Duijn et al., 1991	0/52	—	0/48	—	—
Schellenberg et al., 1991a	0/41[a]	0/35	0/127	0/256	0/16
Crawford et al., 1991	0/14[a]	—	—	—	—
Sorbi et al., 1992	0/7[b]	—	—	—	—
Tanzi et al., 1992	0/39[a]	0/17	0/81	—	—
Jones et al., 1992	0/105	—	—	0/100	—
Kamino et al., 1992	0/50[c]	—	0/153[d]	0/307[d]	—

[a]Includes FAD 1, 2 & 4 reported previously.
[b]Includes FAD 4 reported previously.
[c]Breakdown by onset not provided.
[d]Includes 105 sporadic and 256 controls from Schellenberg et al., 1991a. See "APP_{717}, APP_{693}, and PRIP Gene Mutations are Rare in Alzheimer Disease," by G. D. Schellenberg, et al., 1991, *American Journal of Human Genetics, 49*, pp. 571–517. Copyright 1991 by the *American Journal of Human Genetics*. Reprinted with permission.

CHROMOSOME 14. The absence of linkage of most early-onset AD families to chromosome 21 and the rare frequency of APP gene mutations suggested the existence of at least one additional FAD genetic locus. In 1992, four independent research groups reported linkages of early-onset

AD with genetic markers on chromosome 14 (Schellenberg, et al., 1992; Mullan, et al., 1992b; van Broeckhoven, et al., 1992; St. George-Hyslop, et al., 1992). Among the families included in these studies were the two families previously reported to show weak linkage to chromosome 21. Families with the AD gene on chromosome 14 account for 70%–80% of early-onset familial cases. No linkage was observed between chromosome 14 and late-onset FAD. Further, the absence of linkage in early-onset Volga Germans suggests that a third locus for early-onset AD needs to be determined.

Recently, a multi-institutional international team of investigators reported the successful cloning of the early-onset FAD gene on chromosome 14 (Sherrington, et al., 1995). DNA sequencing of this putative gene, S182 (also known as presenilin 1 or PS-1), found five different missense mutations in seven families, and these mutations were present in AD patients and some at-risk relatives but not in asymptomatic family members more than two standard deviations beyond the mean age at onset and neurological normal controls. The gene appears to code for a transmembrane protein, and its sequence similarity to the membrane protein SPE-4 of C. elegans suggests that it may be involved in protein transport within cells or may be a receptor or channel protein.

CHROMOSOME 1. The gene for AD in early-onset Volga Germans has now been localized to chromosome 1 (Levy-Lahad, et al., 1995a). The candidate gene has been identified as a homolog of S182, the AD gene on chromosome 14 (Levy-Lahad, et al., 1995b). Like S182, it has a transmembrane domain and is referred to as STM2 (second transmembrane gene associated with AD) and recently as presenilin 2 or PS-2. A missense mutation in codon 141 was found in affected individuals in five of seven families. This finding of only a single mutation is consistent with a common ancestor. Like S182, its normal cellular function is unknown.

CHROMOSOME 19. While data about early-onset FAD have been accumulating rapidly, the vast majority of AD patients (more than 75%) develop the disease after the age of 65. Linkage analysis with chromosome 21 markers found no evidence for a late-onset gene on this chromosome. However, evidence for linkage of late-onset FAD to chromosome 19 has been reported (Pericak-Vance, et al., 1991). These investigators used the affected-pedigree-member method, which, unlike lod score analyses, makes no assumption about the mode of transmission and utilizes data on affected individuals only.

A recently identified APP-like protein, APLP1, which maps to chromosome 19 in the area postulated to contain the late-onset FAD gene, is a candidate gene (Wasco, Bupp, & Magendantz, 1990). APLP1 resembles a membrane-associated glycoprotein and has a predicted structure that is similar to APP but does not contain a β-amyloid domain. Nonetheless, the conservation of amino acid sequence and domain structure in APLP and APP suggests that they may share common functions, and APLP processing may have profound effects on APP expression or processing.

Apolipoprotein E Gene

An association of late-onset AD with the apolipoprotein E (Apo E) gene located on chromosome 19 has been reported (Corder, et al., 1993). Specifically, there is an increased frequency of the e4 allele in late-onset sporadic and familial AD. Apo E has three major alleles: e2, e3, and e4, resulting in six genotypes, 2/2, 2/3, 2/4, 3/3, 3/4, and 4/4. The alleles differ by single amino acid substitutions at positions 112 and 158 of the gene: e2 has cysteine at 112 and 158, e3 has cysteine at 112 and arginine at 158, and e4 has arginine at 112 and 158. The e3 allele is the most common, more than 90% of the general population inherits one copy, and about 60%, two copies of the gene. By contrast, only about 30% have at least one e4 allele compared with 64% of sporadic and 80% of familial late-onset AD. Further, individuals with two copies of the e4 allele are much more likely to manifest AD and appear to develop it much earlier than those who have none or one. The risk for AD increased from 20% to 90% and mean age at onset decreased from 84 to 68 years with increasing numbers of e4 alleles. The overall risk was more than eight times greater than that of individuals without e4 and homozygosity for e4 was virtually sufficient to cause AD by age 80. Since that initial report, confirmation has been obtained by other investigators in many different populations. Overall, the APOE-e4 gene variant appears to be the first genetic risk factor to have been identified for late-onset AD. However, normal aged individuals also are e4 positive, and a large proportion of late-onset AD patients do not have an e4 allele.

The risk for AD associated with the e2 and e3 alleles are not as clear. A significant protective effect of the e2 allele for early- and late-onset AD has been reported (Corder, et al., 1994). But a recent study reported that the e2 allele is associated with an increased risk for early-onset AD and reduced survival (van Duijn, et al., 1995). An increased e2 allele frequency was found in African American AD patients but not in Caucasians (Maestre, et al., 1995). Further investigations are warranted to examine the relationship between the e2 allele and AD.

The role of APOE in the pathophysiology of AD remains unknown. The direct involvement of apoE4 in the pathogenesis of AD is supported by its higher avidity for β-amyloid than the apoE3 isoform, and AD patients with two APOE-e4 alleles exhibit greater β-amyloid staining at autopsy than AD patients with two e3 alleles (Strittmatter, et al., 1993). Apo E immunoreactivity is also observed in neurofibrillary tangles, the major component of which is the microtubule-associated protein tau.

It also has been proposed that individuals with the APOE-e4 gene are at an increased risk of AD, not from a deleterious effect of e4, but rather from the absence of e3 (Strittmatter, et al., 1994). These investigators hypothesized that apoE3 stabilizes microtubules (protein filaments needed for normal neuronal functioning) by binding to tau, a protein that promotes the polymerization and stabilization of microtubules, thus preventing the abnormal addition of phosphate groups and protecting the microtubules and the cell integrity. Phosphorylation decreases the efficiency of tau, and hyperphosphorylated tau is the major constituent of the paired helical filaments that make up the neurofibrillary tangles. This hypothesis is provocative because it reduces the role of β-amyloid protein, which many researchers believe causes the neurodegeneration in AD.

The possible association between AD and the human lymphocyte antigen (HLA) histocompatibility complex (located on chromosome 6) has been investigated. Early studies suggested that the A2 allele may be associated with early onset AD (Small & Matsuyama, 1986; Payami, Kaye, Becker, Norman, & Wetzsteon, 1991). Recently, a multi-institutional collaborative study (Payami, et al., 1997) reported a significant shift to earlier age at onset associated with the presence of the A2 allele and independent of APOE-e4.

In summary, classical family and twin studies have provided support for genetic factors underlying AD, and having an afflicted relative increases one's risk for developing AD. Although the proportion of AD cases that are familial is not known with certainty, some families exhibit an autosomal, dominant inheritance pattern, and those with extended pedigrees have been used in molecular genetic studies leading to significant advances in our understanding of the genetics of AD. In the small proportion of early-onset families examined to date, there is a suggested linkage of a FAD gene to chromosomes 14 and 1, as well as reports of mutations within the APP gene on chromosome 21. Further, there is a suggested association between HLA-A2 allele and early-onset AD. In late-onset FAD, there is a suggested linkage to chromosome 19 and strong evidence that the APOE-e4 allele is a major risk factor for late-onset sporadic and familial AD. Collectively, genetic analyses suggest allelic and nonallelic genetic heterogeneity in FAD, with evidence for the involvement of at least five genes.

The recent cloning of the early-onset FAD genes on chromosomes 14 and 1 promises to provide insight into the underlying basis for AD, including clinical and neuropathologic expression. Since all cells in an affected individual contain the same genetic information, the selective vulnerability of neuronal populations in the brain remains to be explained. Although cloning of the genes on chromosomes 14 and 1 offers the potential for predictive presymptomatic testing for some individuals, it raises the ethical issues associated with such testing (i.e., whether to offer testing, and when, whom to test, and how to interpret the findings). Clearly, it is an exciting time in research in the genetics of AD as the application of molecular genetic and other state-of-the-art techniques (e.g., transgenic and knockout mice) offer new hope to concerned relatives, basic scientists, and clinicians for an increased understanding of AD.

REFERENCES

Breitner, J. C. S, & Folstein, M. F. (1984). Familial Alzheimer dementia: A prevalent disorder with prominent clinical features. *Psychology of Medicine, 14,* 63–80.

Chartier-Harlin, M.-C., Crawford, F., Hamandi, K., Mullan, M., Goate, A., Hardy, J., Backhovens, H., Martin, J.-J., & Broeckhoven, C.-V. (1991a). Screening for the β-amyloid precursor protein mutation (APP717:Val- > Ile) in extended pedigrees with early onset Alzheimer's disease. *Neuroscience Letter, 129,* 134–135.

Chartier-Harlin, M.-C., Crawford, F., Houlden, H., Warren, A., Hughes, D., Fidani, L., Goate, A., Rossor, M., Rogues, P., Hardy, J., & Mullan, M. (1991b). Early-onset Alzheimer's disease caused by mutations at codon 717 of the β-amyloid precursor protein gene. *Nature, 353,* 844–846.

Chartier-Harlan, M.-C., Parfitt, M., Legrain, S., Perez-Tur, J., Brousseau, T., Evans, A., Berr, C., Vidal, O., Rogues, P., Gourlet, V., Fruchart, J.-C., Delacourte, A., Rossor, M., & Amouyel, P. (1994). Apolipoprotein E, E4 allele as a major risk factor for sporadic early and late onset form of Alzheimer's disease: Analysis of the 19q13.2 chromosomal region. *Human Molecular Genetics, 3,* 569–574.

Corder, E. H., Saunders, A. M., Risch, N. J., Strittmatter, W. J., Schmechel, D. M., Gaskell, Jr., P. C., Rimmler, J. B., Locke, P. A., Conneally, P. M., Schmader, K. E., Small, G. W., Roses, A. D., Haines, J. L., & Pericak-Vance, M. A. (1994). Protective effect of apolipoprotein E type 2 allele for late onset Alzheimer disease. *Nature Genetics, 7,* 180–184.

Corder, E. H., Saunders, A. M., Strittmatter, W. J., Schmechel, D. E., Gaskell, Jr., P. C., Small, G. W., Roses, A. D., Haines, J. L., & Pericak-Vance, M. A. (1993). Gene dose of apolipoprotein E type 4 allele and the risk of Alzheimer's disease in late onset families. *Science, 261,* 921–923.

Crawford, F., Hardy, J., Mullan, M., Goate, A., Hughes, D., Fidani, L., Rogues, P., Rossor, M., & Chartier-Harlin, M.-C. (1991). Sequencing of exons 16 and 17 of the β-amyloid precursor protein gene in 14 families with early onset Alzheimer's disease fails to reveal mutations in the β-amyloid sequence. *Neuroscience Letter, 133,* 1–2.

Farrer, L., Myers, R. H., Connor, L., Cupples, A., & Growdon, J. H. (1991). Segregation analysis reveals evidence of a major gene for Alzheimer's disease. *American Journal of Human Genetics, 48,* 1026–1033.

Goate, A., Chartier-Harlin, M.-C., Mullan, M., Brown, J., Crawford, F., Fidani, L., Giuffra, L., Haynes, A., Irving, N., James, L., Mant, R., Newton, P., Rooke, K., Rogues, P., Talbot, C., Pericak-Vance, M., Roses, A., Williamson, R., Rossor, M., Owen, M., & Hardy, J. (1991). Segregation of a missense mutation in the amyloid precursor protein gene with familial Alzheimer's disease. *Nature, 349,* 704–706.

Goldfarb, L. G., Petersen, R. B., Tabaton, M., Brown, P., LeBlanc, A. C., Montagna, P., Cortelli, P., Julien, J., Vital, C., Pendelbury, W. W., Haltia, M., Wills, P. R., Hauw, J. J., McKeever, P. E., Monari, L., Schrank, B., Swergold, G. D., Autilio-Gambetti, L., Gajdusek, D. C., Lugaresi, E., & Gambetti, P. (1992). Fatal familial insomnia and familial Creutzfeldt-Jakob disease: Disease phenotype determined by a DNA polymorphism. *Science, 258,* 806–808.

Haines, J. L., St. George-Hyslop, P. H., Rimmler, J. B., Yamaoka, L., Kazantsev, A., Tanzi, R. E., Gusella, J. F., Roses, A. D., & Pericak-Vance, M. A. (1992). Inheritance of multiple loci in familial Alzheimer disease. *Neurobiology of Aging, 13*(Suppl. 1), S67.

Hendriks, L., van Duijn, C. M., Cras, P., Cruts, M., Hal, W. V., vanHarskamp, F., Warren, A., McInnis, M. G., Antonarakis, S. E., Martin, J. J.,, Hofman, A., & Van Broeckhoven, C. (1992). Presenile dementia and cerebral hemorrhage linked to a mutation at codon 692 of the β-amyloid precursor protein gene. *Nature of Genetics, 1,* 218–221.

Heston, L. L. (1977). Alzheimer's disease, trisomy 21, and myeloproliferative disorders: Associations suggesting a genetic diathesis. *Science, 196,* 322–323.

Heyman, A., Wilkinson, W. E., Hurwitz, B. J., Schmechel, D., Sigmon, A. H., Weinberg, T., Helms, M. J., & Swift, M. (1983). Alzheimer's disease: Genetic aspects and associated clinical disorders. *Annals of Neurology, 14,* 507–515.

Jones, C. T., Morris, S., Yates, C. M., Moffoot, A., Sharpe, C., Brock, D. J. H., & St. Clair, D. (1992). Mutation in codon 713 of the β-amyloid precursor protein gene presenting with schizophrenia. *Nature of Genetics, 1,* 306–309.
Kamino, K., Orr, H. T., Payami, H., Wijsman, E. M., Alonso, M. E., Pulst, S. M., Anderson, L., O'dahl, S., Nemens, E., White, J. A., Sadovnick, A. D., Ball, M. J., Kaye, J., Warren, A., McInnis, M., Antonarkis, S. E., Korenberg, J. R., Sharma, V., Kukull, W., Larson, E., Heston, L. L., Martin, G. M., Bird, T. D., & Schellenberg, G. D. (1992). Linkage and mutational analysis of familial Alzheimer disease kindreds for the APP gene region. *American Journal of Human Genetics, 51,* 998–1014.
Levy, E., Carman, M. D., Fernandez-Madrid, I. J., Power, M. D., Lieberburg, I., Van Duinen, S. G., Bots, G. T. A. M., Luyendijk, W., & Frangione, B. (1990). Mutation of the Alzheimer's disease amyloid gene in hereditary cerebral hemorrhage, Dutch type. *Science, 248,* 1124–1126.
Levy-Lahad, E., Wasco, W., Poorkaj, P., Romano, D. M., Oshima, J., Pettingell, W. H., Yu, C., Jondro, P. D., Schmidt, S. D., Wang, K., Crowley, A. C., Fu, Y.-H., Guenette, S. Y., Galas, D., Nemens, E., Wijsman, E. M., Bird, T. D., Schellenberg, G. D., & Tanzi, R. E. (1995b). Candidate gene for the chromosome 1 familial Alzheimer's disease locus. *Science, 269,* 973–977.
Levy-Lahad, E., Wijsman, E., Nemens, E., Anderson, L., Goddard, K. A. B., Weber, J. L., Bird, T. D., & Schellenberg, G. D. (1995a). A familial Alzheimer's disease locus on chromosome 1. *Science, 269,* 970–973.
Lucotte, G., Berriche, S., & David, F. (1991). Alzheimer's mutation. *Nature, 351,* 530.
Maestre, G., Ottman, R., Stern, Y., Gurland, B., Chun, M., Tang, M. X., Shelanski, M., Tycko, B., & Mayeux, R. (1995). Apolipoprotein E and Alzheimer's disease: Ethnic variation in genotypic risks. *Annals of Neurology, 37,* 254–259.
Matsuyama, S. S. (1995). Genetics of dementias. In H. I. Kaplan & B. J. Sadock (Eds.), *Comprehensive textbook of psychiatry* (pp. 2519–2527). New York: Williams and Wilkins.
Matsuyama, S. S., Jarvik, L. F., & Kumar, V. (1985). Dementia: Genetics. In T. Arie (Ed.), *Recent advances in psychogeriatrics* (pp. 45–69). New York: Churchill Livingstone.
Mohs, R. C., Breitner, J. C. S., Silverman, J. M., & Davis, K. L. (1987). Alzheimer's disease. Morbid risk among first degree relatives approximates 50% by 90 years of age. *Archives of General Psychiatry, 44,* 405–408.
Mullan, M., Crawford, F., Axelman, K., Houlden, H., Lilius, L., Winblad, B., & Lannfelt, L. (1992a). A pathogenic mutation for probable Alzheimer's disease in the APP gene at the N-terminus of β-amyloid. *Nature of Genetics, 1,* 345–347.
Mullan, M., Houlden, H., Windelspecht, M., Fidani, L., Lombardi, C., Diaz, P., Rossor, M., Crook, R., Hardy, J., Duff, K., & Crawford, F. (1992b). A locus

for familial early-onset Alzheimer's disease on the long arm of chromosome 14, proximal to the 1-antichymotrypsin gene. *Nature of Genetics, 2,* 340–342.

Murrell, J., Farlow, M., Ghetti, B., & Benson, M. (1991). A mutation in the amyloid precursor protein associated with hereditary Alzheimer's disease. *Science, 254,* 97–99.

Naruse, S., Igarashi, S., Aoki, K., Kaneko, K., Iihara, K., Miyatake, T., Kobayashi, H., Inuzuka, T., Shimizu, T., Kojima, T., & Tsuji, S. (1991). Mis-sense mutation Val- > Ile in exon 17 of amyloid precursor protein gene in Japanese familial Alzheimer's disease. *Lancet, 337,* 978.

Payami, H., Schellenberg, G. D., Zareparsi, S., Kaye, J., Sexton, G. J., Head, M. A., Matsuyama, S. S., Jarvik, L. F., Miller, B., McManus, D. Q., Bird, T. D., Katzman, R., Heston, L., Norman, D., & Small, G. W. (1997). Evidence for association of the major histocompatibility complex allele A2 with onset age of Alzheimer disease. *Neurology, 49,* 512–518.

Payami, H., Kaye, J., Becker, W., Norman, D., & Wetzsteon, P. (1991). HLA-A2, or a closely linked gene, confers susceptibility to early-onset sporadic Alzheimer's disease in men. *Neurology, 41,* 1544–1548.

Peacock, M. L., Murman, D. L., Sima, A. A. F., Warren, J. T., Roses, A. D., & Fink, J. K. (1994). Novel amyloid precursor protein gene mutation (codon 665^{Asp}) in a patient with late-onset Alzheimer disease. *Annals of Neurology, 35,* 432—438.

Pericak-Vance, M. A., Bebout, J. L., Gaskell, Jr., P. C., Yamaoka, L. H., Hung, W. Y., Alberts, M. J., Walker, A. P., Bartlett, R. J., Haynes, C. A., Welsh, K. A., Earl, N. L., Heyman, A., Clark, C. M., & Roses, A. D. (1991). Linkage studies in familial Alzheimer Disease: Evidence for chromosome 19 linkage. *American Journal of Human Genetics, 48,* 1034–1050.

Rao, V. S., van Duijn, C., Connor-Lacke, L., Cupples, L. A., Growdon, J. H., & Farrer, L. A. (1994). Multiple etiologies for Alzheimer disease are revealed by segregation analysis. *American Journal of Human Genetics, 55,* 991–1000.

Saunders, A. M., Strittmatter, W. J., Schmechel, D. E., St. George Hyslop, P. H., Pericak-Vance, M. A., Joo, S. H., Rosi, B. L., Gusella, J. F., Crapper-MacLachlan, D. R., Alberts, M. J., Hulette, C., Crain, B., Goldgaber, D., & Roses, A. D. (1993). Association of apolipoprotein E allele e4 with late-onset familial and sporadic Alzheimer's disease. *Neurology, 43,* 1467–1472.

Schellenberg, G. D., Anderson, L., O'dahl, S., Wijsman, E., Sadovnick, A., Ball, M., Larson, E., Kukull, W., Martin, G., Roses, A., & Bird, T. (1991a). APP$_{717}$, APP$_{693}$, and PRIP gene mutations are rare in Alzheimer disease. *American Journal of Human Genetics, 49,* 511–517.

Schellenberg, G. D., Bird, T. D., Wijsman, E. M., Orr, H. T., Anderson, L., Nemens, E., White, J. A., Bonnycastle, L., Weber, J. L., Alonso, M. E., Potter, H., Heston, L. L., & Martin, G. M. (1992). Genetic linkage evidence for a familial Alzheimer's disease locus on chromosome 14. *Science, 258,* 668–671.

Schellenberg, G. D., Pericak-Vance, M. A., Wijsman, E. M., Moore, D. K., Gaskell, P. C., Yamaoka, L. A., Bebout, J. L., Anderson, L., Welsh, K. A., Clark, C. M., Martin, G. M., Roses, A. D., & Bird, T. D. (1991b). Linkage analysis of familial Alzheimer disease using chromosome 21 markers. *American Journal of Human Genetics, 48,* 563–583.

Sherrington, R., Rogaev, E. I., Liang, Y., Rogaeva, E. A., Levesque, G., Ikeda, M., Chi, H., Lin, C., Li, G., Holman, K., Tsuda, T., Mar, L., Foncin, J.-F., Bruni, A. C., Montesi, M. P., Sorbi, S., Rainero, I., Pinessi, L., Nee, L., Chumanov, I., Pollen, D., Brookes, A., Sanseau, P., Polinsky, R. J., Wasco, W., Da Silva, H. A. R., Haines, J. L., Pericak-Vance, M. A., Tanzi, R. E., Roses, A. D., Fraser, P. E., Rommens, J. M., & St. George-Hyslop, P. H. (1995). Cloning of a gene bearing missense mutations in early-onset familial Alzheimer's disease. *Nature, 375,* 754–761.

Small, G. W., Leuchter, A., Mandelkern, M., LaRue, A., Okonek, A., Lufkin, R. B., Jarvik, L. F., Matsuyama, S. S., & Bondareff, W. (1993). Clinical, neuroimaging, and environmental risk differences in monozygotic female twins appearing discordant for dementia of the Alzheimer type. *Archives of Neurology, 50,* 209–219.

Small, G. W., & Matsuyama, S. S. (1986). HLA-A2 as a possible marker for early-onset Alzheimer's disease in men. *Neurobiology of Aging, 7,* 211–214.

Sorbi, S., Tesco, G., Nacmias, B., Mortilla, M., Forleo, P., Latorraca, S., Piersanti, P., Piacentini, S., & Amaducci, L. (1992). Absence of APP_{717} mutation in Italian FAD families. *International Journal of Geriatric Psychiatry, 7,* 304.

St. George-Hyslop, P. H., Haines, J. L., Farrer, L. A., Polinsky, R., van Broeckhoven, C., Goate, A., Crapper McLachlan, D. R., Orr, H., Bruni, A. C., Sorbi, S., Rainero, I., Foncin, J.-F., Pollen, D., Cantu, J.-M., Tupler, R., Voskresenskaya, N., Mayeux, R., Growdon, J., Fried, V. A., Myers, R. H., Nee, L., Backhovens, H., Martin, J.-J., Rossor, M., Owen, M. J., Mullan, M., Percy, M. E., Karlinsky, H., Rich, S., Heston, L., Montesi, M., Mortila, M., Nacmias, N., Gusella, J. F., Hardy, J. A., & FAD Collaborative Study group. (1990). Genetic linkage studies suggest that Alzheimer's disease is not a single homogeneous disorder. *Nature, 347,* 194–197.

St. George-Hyslop, P. H., Haines, J. L., Rogaev, E., Mortilla, M., Vaula, G., Pericak-Vance, M., Foncin, J. F., Montesi, M., Bruni, A. C., Sorbi, S., Rainero, I., Pinessi, L., Pollen, D., Nee, L., Kennedy, J., Macciardi, F., Rogaeva, E., Liang, Y., Alexandrova, N., Lukiw, W., Schlumpf, K., Tanzi, R., Tsuda, T., Farrer, L. A., Cantu, J. M., Duara, R., Amaducci, L., Bergamini, L., Gusella, J., Roses, A., & Crapper McLachlan, D. R. (1992). Genetic evidence for a novel familial Alzheimer's disease locus on chromosome 14. *Nature of Genetics, 2,* 330–333.

St. George-Hyslop, P. H., Tanzi, R. E., Polinsky, R., Haines, J. L., Nee, L., Watkins, P. C., Myers, R. H., Feldman, R. G., Pollen, D., Drachman, D.,

Growdon, J., Bruni, A., Foncin, J. F., Salmon, D., Frommelt, P., Amaducci, L., Sorbi, S., Piacentini, S., Stewart, G. D., Hobbs, W. J., Conneally, P. M., & Gusella, J. F. (1987). The genetic defect causing familial Alzheimer's disease maps on chromosome 21. *Science, 235,* 885–890.

Strittmatter, W. J., Saunders, A. M., Schmechel, D. E., Pericak-Vance, M. A., Enghild, J., Salvesen, G. S., & Roses, A. D. (1993). Apolipoprotein E: High-avidity binding to β-amyloid and increased frequency of type 4 allele in late-onset familial Alzheimer disease. *Proceedings of the National Academy of Sciences, 90,* 1977–1981.

Strittmatter, W. J., Weisgraber, K. H., Goedert, M., Saunders, A. M., Huang, D., Corder, E. H., Dong, L.-M., Jakes, R., Alberts, M. J., Gilbert, J. R., Han, S.-H., Hulette, C., Einstein, G., Schmechel, D. E., Pericak-Vance, M. A., & Roses, A. D. (1994). Hypothesis: Microtubule instability and paired helical filament formation in Alzheimer disease brain are related to apolipoprotein E genotype. *Experimental Neurology, 125,* 163–171.

Tanzi, R. E. (1991). Invited editorial: Gene mutations in inherited amyloidopathies of the nervous system. *American Journal of Human Genetics, 49,* 507–510.

Tanzi, R., Vaula, G., Romano, D., Mortilla, M., Huang, T., Tupler, R., Wasco, W., Hyman, B., Haines, J., Jenkins, B., Kalaitsidaki, M., Warren, A., McInnis, M., Antonarakis, S., Karlinsky, H., Percy, M., Connor, L., Growdon, J., Crapper-McLachlan, D., Gusella, J., & St. George-Hyslop, P. H. (1992). Assessment of amyloid β-protein precursor gene mutations in a large set of familial and sporadic Alzheimer disease cases. *American Journal of Human Genetics, 51,* 273–282.

van Broeckhoven, C., Backhovens, H., Cruts, M., De Winter, G., Bruyland, M., Cras, P., & Martin, J.-J. (1992). Mapping of a gene predisposing to early-onset Alzheimer's disease to chromosome 14q24.3. *Nature of Genetics, 2,* 335–339.

van Duijn, C. M., de Kniff, P., Wehnert, A., DeVoecht, J., Bronzova, J. B., Havekes, L. M., Hofman, A., & Van Broeckhoven, C. (1995). The apolipoprotein E e2 allele is associated with an increased risk of early-onset Alzheimer's disease and a reduced survival. *Annals of Neurology, 37,* 605–610.

van Duijn, C., Hendriks, L., Cruts, M., Hardy, J., Hofman, A., & Van Broeckhoven, C. (1991). Amyloid precursor protein gene mutation in early-onset Alzheimer's disease. *Lancet, 337,* 978.

Wasco, W., Bupp, K., Magendantz, M., Gusella, J., Tanzi, R. E., & Solomon, F. (1990). Identification of a mouse brain's cDNA that encodes a protein related to the Alzheimer-associated amyloid β precursor protein. *Proceedings of the National Academy of Sciences, 87,* 2405–2408.

Yoshioka, K., Miki, T., Katsuya, T., Ogihara, T., & Sakaki, Y. (1991). The ^{717}Val-> Ile substitution in amyloid precursor protein is associated with familial Alzheimer's disease regardless of ethnic groups. *Biochemistry and Biophysics Research Commission, 178,* 1141—1146.

PART TWO

Diagnosis: Update

APHASIA - difficulty speaking or writing, naming errors, unable to repeat sentences correctly.

AGNOSIA

APRAXIA - able to move muscles involved in speech & understands what is to be done but has difficulty speaking.

CHAPTER 5

Diagnosis of Alzheimer's Disease

J. Wesson Ashford
Frederick Schmitt
Vinod Kumar

Impairment of mental function with aging has been alluded to throughout history; however, Alois Alzheimer was the first to describe the clinical course of dementia and associate it with specific pathological changes in the brain (Alzheimer, 1907; see also Jarvik & Greenson, 1987; Katzman, 1996). His case concerned a 55-year-old female whose symptoms began as a paranoid delusion regarding her husband. This initial symptom was followed by memory deterioration and the development of other psychiatric symptoms, including general paranoia and social dysfunction. There was a marked loss of the ability to encode information, with additional neuropsychiatric signs of aphasia, agnosia, and apraxia. Yet her neurologic reflexes were unremarkable. As the disease became more severe, Alzheimer noted bewilderment, psychosis, screaming, and fluctuation of symptoms. After 4.5 years of illness, the patient was bedfast, contracted, and incontinent, and soon died. At autopsy, her brain showed atrophy, arteriosclerotic changes, neurofibrillary changes, senile plaques, and gliosis. With regard to the clinical presentation with its progressive course and the neuropathology, the description of this patient is typical of the clinical features that are manifested by patients with Alzheimer's disease. Recently, several review articles have discussed the approach to diagnosing this disease, now commonly referred to as dementia of the Alzheimer type (DAT) (Ashford, Schmitt, & Kumar, 1996; Corey-Bloom et al., 1995; Eisdorfer, Sevush, Barry, Kumar, & Loewenstein, 1994; Fleming, Adams, & Petersen, 1995; Geldmacher & Whitehouse, 1996; Katzman & Jackson, 1991; Khachaturian & Radebaugh, 1996; Raskind & Brower, 1996; Siu, 1991).

DAT has features that are common across all patients including an early and insidious development of memory difficulty, which evolves into impairments of language, visual spatial, psychomotor, and executive function (American Psychiatric Association, 1994; McKhann et al., 1984). Diagnostic confirmation requires certain pathological criteria at autopsy, which are consistent with Alzheimer's description of the histopathological changes (Khachaturian, 1985; Mirra & Markesbery, 1996). However, it is now recognized that Alzheimer's disease is a heterogeneous group of disorders (for reviews, see Ashford, Shan, Butler, Rajasekar, & Schmitt, 1995; Boller, Forett, Khachaturian, Poncet, & Christen, 1992; Fisher et al., 1996; Heyman, 1996; Mirra & Markesbery, 1996; Morris, 1996; Roses, 1996). There are variations in this disease's clinical presentation. The initial cognitive impairments are sometimes dominated by language or visual spatial dysfunction (Fisher et al., 1996), or by psychiatric symptoms, including depression and psychosis (Cohen et al., 1993b). Further, the presence of aphasia seems to be associated with an earlier onset and a more rapid disease course (Heyman, 1996; Lawlor, Ryan, Schmeidler, Mohs, & Davis, 1994; Yesavage, Brooks, Taylor, & Tinklenberg, 1993). Also, Parkinsonian or extrapyramidal symptoms are associated with a more rapid progression of the dementia (Chui, Lyness, Sobel, & Schneider, 1994; Mayeux, 1996; Morris, 1996; Stern et al., 1996a), and these symptoms may be associated neuropathologically with the presence of Lewy bodies in the cortex. The concentration of the Alzheimer neuropathological changes in various regions of the brain also can vary in a given patient (Arnold et al., 1991; Arriagada, Growdon, Hedley-White, & Hyman, 1992; Braak & Braak, 1991; Mirra & Markesbery; Ulrich & Stahelin, 1984; Van Hoesen & Solodkin, 1994). For example, the degree to which occipital cortical areas are affected by senile plaques and neurofibrillary tangles varies considerably from case to case (Lewis, Campbell, Terry, & Morrison, 1987), and visual cortical involvement may be associated with visual spatial deficits (Pietrini et al., 1996) as well as vivid visual hallucinations (Pliskin et al., 1996).

The genetic heterogeneity of DAT is also a well-known disease factor (Roses, 1996). There are at least four chromosomal loci (presenilin-II on chromosome 1; presenilin-I on chromosome 14; apolipoprotein-E on chromosome 19; and the amyloid preprotein on chromosome 21) that contain genetic mutations associated with familial Alzheimer's disease (see chap. 4 of this volume for a discussion of genetic issues in DAT). Specific environmental factors that increase the risk for DAT, such as head injury (Mayeux et al., 1993, 1995; Rasmusson, Brandt, Martin, & Folstein, 1995) and possibly aluminum content in the water supply (Forbes, Gentleman, & Maxwell, 1995), also have been identified, as well as other factors, such as thyroid dysfunction and a history of depressive disorder. Other factors may protect against DAT, such as arthritis or use of anti-inflammatory drugs (Mayeux, 1996). These various factors may result in differences in presentation or onset of DAT symptoms. Nevertheless, there are considerable limitations in the current knowledge base about the precise causes of DAT.

The heterogeneity of DAT leaves diagnosticians with several dilemmas, including early recognition, differential diagnosis, assessment of severity, and distinction of comorbid conditions. As knowledge about DAT grows, clinicians will be able to define particular variants of DAT and how specific factors, including genetic mechanisms, contribute to this syndrome's development and symptom progression. They also will be able to use established clinical criteria to make accurate prognostic statements and therapeutic recommendations.

THE PRECLINICAL AND EARLY PHASE OF DAT

Family members frequently report specific instances that they recollect as marking the beginning of a patient's dementing illness. The initial symptoms frequently relate to an episode of memory dysfunction (Ashford, Kolm, Colliver, Bekian, & Hsu, 1989; Masur, Sliwinski, Lipton, Blau, & Crystal, 1994; McCormick et al., 1994; Oppenheim, 1994; Persson & Skoog, 1992; Welsh, Butters, Hughes, Mohs, & Heyman, 1991). However, it is possible that the neural degeneration associated with DAT begins years, perhaps even decades, before the first symptoms are observed (Katzman, 1993; Ohm, Muller, Braak, & Bohl, 1995; Snowdon et al., 1996). For example, one pathological study examining the deposition of amyloid in the brain suggested that the pathological process may begin early in life (Rumble et al., 1989). Alternatively, high levels of education and initial ability many protect against intellectual decline (Blum & Jarvik, 1974; Stern et al., 1994); however, there are other interpretations, including the possibility that education may mask the early detection of symptoms or lead to a lifestyle associated with less stress or lower likelihood of head trauma or other risk factors (Katzman, 1993, 1996; Mortimer & Graves, 1993). A reasonable speculation is that the hippocampus, which supports new learning and is severely affected in DAT, undergoes a progressive deterioration with age (de Leon et al., 1996; Gallagher et al., 1996), but memory impairments do not occur until fewer than a critical minimal number of neurons remain in the hippocampus (Seab et al., 1988). Further, this threshold of hippocampal neuron loss for emergence of the symptoms of DAT is related to age (Jobst, Hindley, King, & Smith, 1994). However, there is no clear indication of when or how DAT begins or how it progresses to clinical diagnosis.

After the initial cognitive symptom of DAT appears, other cognitive and social dysfunctions develop gradually over a prolonged period of time. During this time period, the emergence of cognitive dysfunction slowly begins to affect the family or those closest to the patient. In most cases, during this early phase of DAT, the persons closest to the patient gradually become concerned, eventually discuss the problem with each other, and finally seek professional advice.

The patient may present the clinician with one or more of many neuropsychiatric symptoms, though the most common difficulty is recent memory dysfunction. Occasionally, DAT patients may present with depression or psychosis, or other predominantly behavioral symptoms. Other neurological symptoms, particularly aphasia, agnosia, apraxia, and disturbance of executive function, frequently occur in DAT patients. In some cases, these symptoms are the presenting features of the disease; however, many of these problems can occur in nondemented elderly individuals with other neurological diseases.

EARLY RECOGNITION OF DAT

An important challenge for clinical medicine is to recognize patients' problems before the crisis that brings them to physicians. Clinicians can recognize with considerable accuracy in the office cognitive changes associated with dementia using short mental status tests (Meiran, Stuss, Guzman, Lafleche, & Willmer, 1996; Mulligan, Mackinnon, Jorm, Giannakopoulos, & Michel, 1996; Reid et al., 1996; Stuss, Meiran, Guzman, Lafleche, & Willmer, 1996). The most widely used test for screening for early dementia is the Mini-Mental State Exam (MMSE) (Crum, Anthony, Bassett, & Folstein, 1993; Folstein, Folstein, & McHugh, 1975; Tombaugh & McIntyre, 1992). Many studies have examined the performance of elderly individuals on the MMSE and have generally supported the use of a score of 23 or below as a threshold for impaired cognition. However, this test is limited in its ability to distinguish normal individuals from those suffering from mild dementia (Ashford et al., 1989; Fillenbaum, Wilkinson, Welsh, & Mohs, 1994; see chap. 6 of this volume for an additional discussion).

Further, cross-sectional studies have found MMSE scores to decrease with advanced age, and scores also are affected by education (Butler, Ashford, & Snowdon, 1996; Crum et al., 1993; Katzman, 1993, 1996; Teresi et al., 1995). Accordingly, age and education should be used in interpreting a patient's MMSE score (see Table 5.1; Tangalos et al., 1996). However, DAT increases in incidence with age (Katzman, 1996), and DAT may be more prevalent in populations with less education or less occupational attainment (Mortimer & Graves, 1993; Stern et al., 1994).

TABLE 5.1 Mini-Mental State Exam Cutoff Scores for Impaired Cognition and Diagnostic Consideration of Dementia (scores equal to or less than those shown indicate further evaluation)

	Education		
Age	6–11	12–16	16 +
60–69	26	27	29
70–79	24	26	27
80–89	23	24	26
90+	23	23	25

Source: Adapted from "The Mini-Mental State Examination in General Medicine Practice: Clinical Utility and Acceptance," by Tangalos et al., 1996; *Mayo Clinic Proceedings, 71,* pp. 829–837. Copyright 1996 by the *Mayo Clinic Proceedings.* Reprinted with permission; and "Age, Education, and Changes in the Mini-Mental State Exam Scores of Older Women," by Butler et al., 1996, *Journal of the American Geriatrics Society, 44,* pp. 675–681. Copyright 1996 by the *Journal of the American Geriatrics Society.* Reprinted with permission.

Thus an early diagnosis of DAT should take into account the patient's age and education as well as other potentially contributing or confounding conditions (Katzman & Jackson, 1991). Accordingly, DAT diagnosis is generally approached as a dichotomous decision that can be aided by the epidemiologically determined sensitivity and specificity of the cognitive tests using "receiver operating characteristics" (Kukull et al., 1994; Mulligan et al., 1996). However, in early DAT cognitive function diverges from the normal range, not as a dichotomous event, and a patient's status should be calculated on a temporal progression (Ashford et al., 1995), with probability of disease estimated according to the variables that are available (see Table 5.2).

The MMSE is an examination composed of a cross section of items, each with measurable characteristics relevant to the assessment of the DAT patient (Ashford et al., 1989; Fillenbaum, Wilkinson, Welsh, & Mohs, 1994; Teresi et al., 1995), even though these items were not specifically selected for assessing this group of patients. The MMSE can be modified for better utility in the DAT population (Molloy, Alemayehu, & Roberts, 1991), but the original version is so widely used that a change from the present pattern of usage will require the development of a paradigm of major significance. Simple screening questions also may be adapted from the MMSE for telephone screening (Gatz et al., 1995; Lanska, Schmitt, Stewart, & Howe, 1993). However, for initial detection of DAT in the clinician's office, the MMSE may be supplemented with items to strengthen its diagnostic value (Ashford et al., 1992; Cummings & Benson, 1983; Geldmacher & Whitehouse, 1996). For example, the number of animals named in 1 minute is a valuable index for discriminating between DAT patients and normal individuals (Monsch et al., 1994), with most normal individuals able to name at least 15. Also, most normal individuals will know the name of the U.S. president and the immediate past U.S. president, though many mildly demented patients will claim that they do not keep track of such political issues. Abstractions, for example, similarities (oranges and bananas, cats and dogs, tables and chairs), are often difficult for even very mildly impaired patients, but usually present no problem for even very elderly normal people. Modifications of the Boston Naming Test (Knesevich, LaBarge, & Edwards, 1986) can be used to identify the dysnomia associated with DAT. To test visual spatial functions more completely, clock drawing (Watson, Arfken, & Birge, 1993) and drawing a range of objects, such as a circle, a diamond, intersecting rectangles, and a cube, are also useful (Mohs, 1996), though

TABLE 5.2 Dementia Stage Descriptions

Dementia Stage (Type of impairment with clinical findings)	Time-Index (yrs. of disease)	MMSE (range 0–30)	CDRm (range 0–5)	GDS/FAST (range 0–7)
Early Dementia	−2 to 0*	24 to 28	0.5	Stages 2–3

Memory—new learning impaired, slight forgetfulness
Language—occasional word loss, paraphasia
Visuospatial—problems with complex designs, unusual objects
Orientation—difficulty with exact date and time
ADLs—slight impairment at job, shopping, finances, hobbies
Psychiatric—depressive symptoms in up to 1/3 of cases
CT/MRI—minimal cortical atrophy (may not be noted)
PET/SPECT—mild temporoparietal hypometabolism/hypoperfusion (unilateral or bilateral)

Mild Dementia	0 to 2.0	19 to 23	1.0	Stage 4

Memory—moderate learning difficulty; defects in remote recall
Language—reticent, simple conversation, mild anomia
Visuospatial—mild difficulty identifying, using complex objects
Orientation—misses date, may become lost in unfamiliar place
ADLs—less independent function, some prompting in personal care
Psychiatric—sadness, may have delusions and/or hallucinations
CT/MRI—mild cortical atrophy, hippocampal thinning apparent
PET/SPECT—decrease of temporoparietal metabolism/perfusion

Moderate Dementia	2 to 3.5	11 to 18	2.0	Stage 5

Memory—new information rapidly lost, personal history deficits
Language—vocabular limitations in conversation, naming deficit
Visuospatial—difficulty copying simple drawings, using objects
Orientation—disoriented to time, often to place, becomes lost in less familiar places
ADLs—no function outside of home, requires assistance with personal care
Psychiatric—occasional delusions, hallucinations (in 50% of cases with AD)
CT/MRI—atrophy with ventricular dilatation, large temporal horn
PET/SPECT—metabolism/perfusion defect begins to affect frontal regions

Severe Dementia	3.5 to 5	5 to 10	3.0	Stages 6a–6e

Memory—complete loss of recent information, most of remote
Language—uses simple words, sentences, may name simple objects

(continued)

TABLE 5.2 *(continued)*

Dementia Stage (Type of impairment with clinical findings)	Time-Index (yrs. of disease)	MMSE (range 0–30)	CDRm (range 0–5)	GDS/FAST (range 0–7)

Visuospatial—severe difficulty using common objects (conceptual & ideational apraxia)
Orientation—orientation only to person, may not know birth date
ADLs—no activities, inadequate self-grooming, often incontinent
Psychiatric—uncooperativity, may get agitated, restless, pace
CT/MRI—moderate sulcal atrophy, ventricular dilation
PET/SPECT—patchy loss of temporoparietal & frontal activity

Profound Dementia   5 to 6.5   0 to 4   4.0   Stages 7a–c

Attention—wandering, patient can be engaged only briefly
Memory—essentially no memory function, cannot remember family members
Language—may use single words only, poor comprehension
Visuospatial—responds meaningfully only to very simple objects
Orientation—no orientation to self, family members, space, time
ADLs—full assistance dressing/eating, bowel/bladder incontinent
Psychiatric—frequent agitation, obliviousness, pacing, or pronounced sleep disturbance
CT/MRI—severe sulcal atrophy, temporal lobe shriveling
PET/SPECT—severe loss of temporoparietal & frontal activity

Complete Dementia   6.5 to 8   0   5.0   Stage 7d–f

Attention—patient is bed/wheelchair bound, no communication
Language—unintelligible sounds, screaming
ADLs—unable to ambulate, difficulties with feeding, swallowing
Psychiatric—screaming, hitting/pinching/biting during ADL care
  Death occurs because of aspiration pneumonia, urinary tract infection, occult severe medical condition: cardiac, ulcer, etc.

Note. DAT is a progressive disorder not manifesting discrete stages. However, epochs of this illness can be described conveniently using divisions delineated according to severity. The scheme presented in this table was adapted from Reisberg et al., 1994, and Ashford et al., 1995. Time-Index (calculated from data of Ashford et al., 1995); MMSE (Mini-Mental State Exam, Folstein et al., 1975); CDRm (Clinical Dementia Rating Scale, Hughes et al., 1982), modified according to Ashford et al., 1992; GDS/FAST (Global Deterioration Scale/Functional Assessment Staging Measure, Reisberg et al., 1994). Note that the Time-Index is estimated to begin 2 years before diagnosis. Although illness duration is frequently estimated to last 7 to 8 years (see Jost & Grossberg, 1996), the Time-Index carries the assessment to severe levels of dementia that are associated with a high mortality. Reprinted with permission.

the critical issue for mild DAT patients is whether they can draw these shapes from memory.

In an analysis of the items from the "Functional Activities Questionnaire," the question "Do you require assistance remembering appointments, family occasions, or holidays and in taking medications?" was the most accurate screening test (Shankle, Dillencourt, & Pazzani, 1996). With such additions, a clinician can make a fairly comfortable determination that a patient has a clinically significant impairment. Other brief items can be used to enhance further the initial detection of dementia (Mohs, Marin, Green, & Davis, 1996; Welsh et al., 1991). However, all of these tests must be used judiciously and are more meaningful when they are used with respect to values from confirmed normal individuals of similar backgrounds (Sliwinski, Lipton, Buschke, & Stewart, 1996) to determine the point of dysfunction in the time course of the patient's decline (Table 5.2; see also Ashford et al., 1995).

Neuropsychological assessment can often detect early DAT even before family members have recognized symptoms of early DAT or the disease process has significantly impaired day-to-day functions (Schmitt & Sano, 1994). Short cognitive test batteries that focus on associative learning appear to distinguish very mild Alzheimer cases from the normal aging process (Petersen, Smith, Ivnik, Kokmen, & Tangalos, 1994; Welsh et al., 1991) and diagnose DAT with up to 85% accuracy 4 years before it is possible to make a standard clinical diagnosis (Masur et al., 1994; Petersen, et al., 1995). Also, PET brain scanning techniques can identify patients with early DAT with considerable reliability (Kuhl et al., 1987; Small et al., 1989), and further specificity is achieved when apolipoprotein E genotype is considered in relation to the PET scan changes (Reiman et al., 1996; Small et al., 1995; see chap. 7 in this volume for further details). However, at this time, clinicians and health care agencies have not established a practical reason (e.g., preventive interventions or pharmacotherapy) for urging widespread implementation of these early recognition tools.

CLINICAL EXAMINATION OF THE PATIENT WITH DEMENTIA

In the clinical setting, when the patient presents a cognitive problem and a diagnosis of dementia is under consideration, there is a well-accepted diagnostic regimen (see Table 5.3).

TABLE 5.3 Standard Laboratory Tests for Dementia Evaluation

Medical history
Family history
Physical exam
Neurological exam
Mental status exam/neuropsychological assessment
Complete blood count
Estimated sedimentation rate (check for inflammatory processes)
Blood chemistry panel (including liver and kidney function tests)
Serum electrolytes (including magnesium and zinc)
Thyroid function tests
Vitamin B-12/folic acid levels
Serological test for syphilis, HIV
Routine urinalysis
Chest X ray
Electrocardiogram
Brain scan (CT at minimum; MRI and SPECT if available)

Medical History

The first step in the diagnostic regimen is to obtain a complete medical history. Because of the unreliability of the patient's memory, information from a third party is essential. The first issue is to determine the nature of the chief complaint. If memory dysfunction is present, it is critical to determine if this was the first symptom. Memory impairment is a presenting symptom about 50% of the time, but another psychiatric problem such as depression or suspiciousness is present about 30% of the time, while a different cognitive dysfunction or an impairment of day-to-day functions occurs as the symptom that precipitates the initial visit 10% of the time (Oppenheim, 1994).

The next step is to determine whether any specific events or stresses were associated with the occurrence of the first symptom (Guterman et al., 1993). Careful attention must be given to the course of the decline, including an estimation of the accuracy of the retrospective information, to determine if the disease course is progressive or characterized by abrupt changes, such as might be caused by vascular events, metabolic changes, or affective disorders.

A review of the patient's medical history should focus on illnesses that could have caused or contributed to the cognitive impairment. Of particular concern is the use of centrally active medications or toxins. Any medication with anticholinergic side effects could contribute to cognitive dysfunction, including anti-Parkinsonian agents (benztropine, trihexyphenidyl), tricyclic antidepressants (amitriptyline), older antipsychotics (thioridazine), antispasmodics (atropine, scopolamine, l-hyoscyamine, oxybutynin), or antihistamines (diphenhydramine, chlorpheniramine). Several medical conditions, such as head injury and arthritis, and possibly hay fever or asthma and metal work, seem to influence the risk and age at the onset of DAT (Breitner, 1994).

It also is important to obtain a family history of cognitive problems. There has been less interest in recent years in the family history of lymphoma and Down's syndrome although links with DAT have been reported (Heston, Mastri, Anderson, & White, 1981). Although the determination of genetic factors does not have a clear role in the routine diagnostic evaluation, about 40% of patients with Alzheimer's disease have a family history of dementia. The cumulative risk in first-degree relatives of DAT patients is about 50% by 80 years of age, whereas it is about 20% for controls (Breitner, Murphy, Silverman, Mohs, & Davis, 1988). Often, the familial association seems to be related more to longevity than to dementia, but a parent or sibling who had an onset of dementia before 75 years of age strengthens the suspicion of DAT.

Physical Examination

A complete examination is a recommended component of the dementia evaluation. Not only can a variety of systemic conditions, including heart, lung, liver, and kidney disorders contribute to cognitive impairment, but a demented patient may not report medical difficulties adequately. After listening to the heart for murmurs and arrhythmias, the carotids and cranium should be auscultated carefully for bruits. Examination of the retinal fundi can give an estimation of arterial, hypertensive, or diabetic disease, which may suggest a vascular component of the dementia. Retinal photographs can make this exam much easier and more reliable, and contribute more to the diagnosis.

Neurological Examination

While the neurological examination of the DAT patient is usually unremarkable and devoid of focal signs, there are several signs that are typical of DAT patients, and other tests must be performed to rule out important differential issues (Corey-Bloom et al., 1995; Fleming et al., 1995; Gilman, 1996). A cranial nerve exam should include testing for olfactory function (coffee, cinnamon, etc.). DAT patients are noted for early loss of the ability to identify odors, later losing the capacity to detect smell sensation (Doty, Reyes, & Gregor, 1987; Murphy, Gilmore, Seery, Salmon, & Lasker, 1990; Serby, Larson, & Kalkstein, 1991; Nordin, Monsch, & Murphy, 1995), though many normal adults have difficulty identifying scents as well. The patient's vision (corrected Jaeger reading level) and hearing (tuning fork and rubbing fingers) should be determined because impairment of either visual or auditory function can hamper cognitive performance.

A motor examination usually reveals normal strength and coordination in mild DAT patients, but later there is difficulty following simple commands for testing motor performance along with incoordination. Extrapyramidal motor system signs such as rigidity and tremor can be indications of Parkinson's disease or suggestive of diffuse Lewy body disease, and are associated with a more rapid course of dementia (Chui et al., 1994; Heyman, 1996; Mayeux, 1996; Morris; Stern et al., 1996a). Although DAT patients may not have increased tone, they do have a tendency to not relax, and try to help with passive manipulation, a condition called Gegenhalten. Adventitious movements suggest consideration of Huntington's disease. Gait dysfunction may indicate a variety of problems, but should lead to consideration of normal pressure hydrocephalus, especially with the additional history of bladder control difficulties. Gait problems due to Alzheimer pathology usually develop late in the disease course.

Reflexes in the DAT patient tend to be mildly brisk (Franssen et al., 1991), an indication of cortical dysfunction. Though the snout reflex is frequently present in the normal elderly individual, it is invariably found in the DAT patient and becomes more severe as the disease progresses. Other pathological reflexes are not typically seen in the mild DAT patient and may be more indicative of frontal (palmo-mental, grasp) or Parkinsonian (glabellar) pathology (Galasko, Kwo-on-Yuen, Klauber, & Thal, 1990).

A sensory exam should include testing for vibration. Impairment may indicate a peripheral neuropathy due to vitamin B-12 deficiency or diabetes. The sensory exam is usually intact in the DAT patient, and specific abnormalities should trigger an investigation of the cause.

Focal neurological signs and symptoms should be noted carefully because of their potential relation to stroke and tumor. They are not usually caused by Alzheimer pathology. Particular phenomena that indicate focality are visual field defects, hemiparesis, asymmetric deep tendon reflexes, and an extensor plantar response. Myoclonus and rapid dementia progression suggest Creutzfeldt-Jakob disease.

Neuropsychological Testing

Neuropsychological assessment is an important component of the dementia evaluation. This component of the clinical examination gives the most explicit and objective description of the patient's difficulties and contributes considerably to the differential diagnosis. Neuropsychological measures most directly reflect the loss of brain function caused by Alzheimer pathology. Neuropsychological deficits in DAT reflect the effect of the Alzheimer pathological processes on memory structures and mechanisms. Since DAT primarily involves a loss of memory processing capabilities, other cognitive losses seem to occur in relation to the destruction of memory substrates (see chap. 3 of this volume for a further discussion of this issue). For any measure of DAT to be demonstrated to have reliability, it must correlate with the neuropsychological measures. (For a more extensive discussion of neuropsychological testing, see chap. 6 of this volume.)

Laboratory Tests

A specific list of tests is commonly employed as part of the DAT evaluation (see Table 5.3). However, this regimen should be adjusted for the individual patient (Eisdorfer et al., 1994; Fleming et al., 1995; Siu, 1991).

A cerebrospinal fluid (CSF) examination is usually done only in those cases where cancer or a cerebral infection is considered, particularly syphilis (Corey-Bloom et al., 1995). Several recent studies of CSF have shown that DAT patients have significantly increased levels of the microtubule-associated tau (e.g., Arai et al., 1995) and diminished concentrations of β-amyloid (e.g., Motter et al., 1995). Although these two changes may not constitute a positive diagnosis of DAT, they can give support to consideration of this disease in the differential diagnosis.

Brain Imaging in DAT Diagnosis

Indirect examination of the brain, from pneumoencephalograms and arteriograms of the past to CT/MRI and PET/SPECT scans of the present, has long been advocated as part of the dementia evaluation. Brain imaging techniques have been improving rapidly for diagnosing Alzheimer's disease. There is general agreement among experts in this field that a brain scan is a justifiable procedure to rule out a tumor, stroke, normal pressure hydrocephalus, or subdural hematoma, in a patient with mild or moderate cognitive dysfunction (Corey-Bloom et al., 1995).

This clinical objective can be accomplished with cerebral tomography (CT) without contrast. However, shrinkage in the medial temporal lobe also can be assessed with this technique to give an accurate estimation of the atrophy associated with Alzheimer's disease (Jobst et al., 1994). The justification for a more extensive or expensive examination such as magnetic resonance imaging (MRI), single photon emission computed tomography (SPECT), or positron emission tomography (PET) is a contested issue. However, techniques for brain imaging and computer analysis are rapidly improving interpretation (Smith, 1996). MRI, particularly of the coronal sections in DAT, shows atrophy of the hippocampus and temporal lobe, which can support the diagnosis of Alzheimer's disease and give an estimation of the severity of the disease process (Jagust, 1994; Jobst et al., 1994), but quantification using this technique is not standardized. PET, measuring metabolic activity, and SPECT, measuring cerebral blood flow, both show characteristic decreases of activity in the temporal and parietal regions of the brain (Herholz, 1995; Schmitt, Shih, & DeKosky, 1992; Small et al., 1989; Stollberger, Fazekas, Payer, & Flooh, 1995; Waldemar et al., 1994).

The combination of morphologic imaging and SPECT can further improve diagnostic power (Jobst et al., 1994; Stollberger et al., 1995), and three-dimensional rendering of PET images also improves DAT diagnosis substantially (Burdette, Minoshima, Borght, Tran, & Kuhl, 1996). PET in conjunction with genotyping also provides better assessment of DAT (Reiman et al., 1996; Small et al., 1995) and may reveal persons who are at risk for DAT. In the future, there will be increased use of the more advanced imaging techniques, especially if radioactive agents to selectively tag neurotransmitter systems or neuropathology are developed, and this approach may lead to definite diagnosis in the living patient. However, the practical utilization of the range of imaging tools available in current clinical practice requires judicious consideration of the diagnostic requirement. (See chap. 7 of this volume for a discussion of the advances in neuroimaging.)

Other approaches to assessing brain function are the electroencephalogram (EEG) and the event-related potential (ERP). The EEG is characteristically slowed in DAT, and this is a reliable, but nonspecific, indicator of cerebral dysfunction, including lateralization. The ERP at a latency of about 300 msec in response to a surprising stimulus (P300) is diminished in amplitude with aging and even more so with dementia, but this change also is considered nonspecific. Topographic mapping can enhance electrophysiological techniques. For example, DAT seems to be associated with a selective loss of P300 energy posteriorly (Ashford et al., 1993), consistent with the posterior temporoparietal dysfunction seen on functional brain scans and the distribution of the pathology at autopsy. With further refinements, these measures may be of more diagnostic utility in the future.

CLINICAL DIAGNOSIS OF DAT

The DSM-IV (American Psychiatric Association, 1994) provides a useful set of criteria to aid in the diagnosis of DAT (see Table 5.4). The central criterion in the clinical diagnosis of DAT is deterioration of memory. However, memory impairment must be accompanied by a disturbance in another higher cognitive function. This disturbance of cognition must represent a decline from a previous higher level of function and interfere

TABLE 5.4 DSM-IV Criteria for Dementia of Alzheimer Type

A. Development of multiple cognitive deficits including both:
    1. memory impairment
    2. one or more additional cognitive disturbances:
        (a) aphasia; (b) apraxia; (c) agnosia; (d) disturbance in executive functioning.
B. These cognitive deficits each cause significant functional impairment and represent a significant decline from a previous level of functioning.
C. Course characterized by gradual onset and continuing decline.
D. The cognitive deficits are not due to:
    1. other central nervous system conditions
    2. systemic conditions
    3. substance-induced conditions.
E. The deficits are not exclusively related to delirium.
F. Another Axis I (psychiatric) disorder does not better account for the disturbance.

Source: Adapted from the American Psychiatric Association, 1994. Copyright 1994 by the American Psychiatric Association. Reprinted with permission.

with social and occupational function. Additionally, the dementia cannot be diagnosed as part of a delirium or another psychiatric disturbance. While these criteria are clinically obvious in moderately to severely demented patients, they may be unclear in patients with very mild DAT or other medical or psychiatric problems (where the diagnosis of DAT is of greatest concern).

Assessment of cognitive dysfunction by the clinician should be based on historical report, direct observation, and objective testing. The memory loss in DAT is specifically a disorder of the ability to encode or learn new information (Ashford et al., 1989; Welsh et al., 1991). As the disease advances, there is a progressive destruction of the fundamental neural substrate of memory, which results in the eventual loss of previously formed memories. As mentioned previously, a structured neuropsychological examination also can give an organized formulation of the cognitive strengths and deficits of the patient, track symptom progression, and aid in early differential diagnosis (Schmitt & Sano, 1994; see also chap. 6 of this volume).

The associated social dysfunction can be estimated effectively through a caregiver report, using the Instrumental and Basic Activities of Daily Living (ADL) scales (Ashford, Kumar, et al., 1992; Galasko, Bennett, & the Alzheimer's Disease Cooperative Study, 1996), the Blessed Dementia Scale (Blessed, Tomlinson, & Roth, 1968), the Alzheimer's Disease Assessment Scale—Noncognitive Battery (Mohs, 1996; Mohs et al., 1996), or other structured interviews. The Blessed Dementia Scale also has been correlated with pathological changes. Some ADL tests are performance based and require the direct observation of patient performance (see chap. 6 of this volume for further discussion of functional assessment). Such tools determine specific skills related to higher level functions such as shopping and management of finances or basic functions such as grooming and toileting. In patients with DAT, scores on cognitive rating scales and ADL scales correspond highly with each other, suggesting that the underlying brain deficit is reflected accurately by both types of measurement (Ashford, Kumar, et al., 1992).

DIFFERENTIAL DIAGNOSIS OF DEMENTIA

Although DAT accounts for at least half of the cases of dementia, the diagnostic criteria for dementia are generic and apply to a syndrome that can be caused by a multitude of conditions. The routine battery of examinations (Table 5.3) is a practical approach to investigating the possible causes of dementia other than Alzheimer's disease. However, this battery frequently does not clarify the diagnosis because several dementing conditions may coexist (Ashford, Rosenblatt, Bekian, & Hayes, 1987; Chui, Zhang, Victoroff, & Zaias, 1996; Risse et al., 1990; Victoroff, Mack, Lyness, & Chui, 1995). The principal justification for this battery of tests is the search for a reversible or treatable form of dementia (Table 5.5). For example, a frequently discovered problem is the use of centrally active medications whose elimination improves the patient's cognitive function. In the clinical setting, there is a major urgency to discover potentially reversible causes of dementia, because such conditions will become progressively more difficult to arrest or reverse (Eisdorfer et al., 1994). Of most concern are the diagnoses of subdural hematoma, normal pressure hydrocephalus, hypothyroidism, and B-12 deficiency.

An important clinical feature of DAT is the slow and insidious development of the symptoms, while head trauma, surgery, stroke, or a specific hypoxic or hypoglycemic episode can result in a rapid onset of symptoms. Creutzfeldt-Jakob disease, brain tumor, and depression have gradual onset, but usually progress at faster rates than DAT. However, the naturally slow development of other insidious diseases (e.g., thyroid disorder, normal pressure hydrocephalus) may mimic the onset and course of DAT. Further, a series of small strokes without focal neurological findings might induce a progressive loss of cognitive function that is difficult to distinguish from the DAT symptom constellation even with neuropsychological testing and

TABLE 5.5 Reversible and Treatable Dementias

Types
Depression
B-12/folate deficiency
Tumor (especially meningioma)
Subdural hematoma
Normal pressure hydrocephalus
Infections
Toxins
Endocrinopathy

neuroimaging. Consequently, there are no definite clinical features of DAT that can confirm the diagnosis of Alzheimer's disease. For the benefit of the family, a clear diagnosis of dementia should be emphasized, while maintaining the consistent position that a definite diagnosis at this time requires autopsy confirmation; but the possibility or probability of Alzheimer's disease can be estimated clinically based on the typicality of the presentation and the lack of other possible causes of dementia (McKhann et al., 1984). Using this clinical standard, diagnostic accuracy established at autopsy ranges from 60% for "possible" cases to 90% for "probable" cases (Galasko et al., 1994).

As mentioned previously, an important diagnostic and management consideration is the co-occurrence of different types of medical problems in the elderly individual that could account for symptoms of dementia (Ashford et al., 1987; Eisdorfer et al., 1994; Katzman & Jackson, 1991; Risse et al., 1990). Although DAT accounts for more than half of the cases of dementia at autopsy, there are a host of other common conditions that occur in dementia patients, including pulmonary disease, a history of falls and of surgery, any of which also could account for all or even part of the patient's cognitive dysfunction. A history of head injury occurs five times more frequently in DAT patients than the general population, leading to the speculation that certain injuries or stresses may initiate the Alzheimer process, especially when they occur in elderly individuals. Multi-infarct disease, alcoholism, diffuse Lewy-body disease (Weiner et al., 1996), and Parkinson's disease (Aarsland, Tandberg, Larsen, & Cummings, 1996b) also are commonly associated with dementia (Mirra & Markesbery, 1996; Morris, 1996; Victoroff et al., 1995), and the prevalence of these conditions seems to vary according to location (or at least to the institutions conducting the studies).

Argyrophilic grain disease, Pick's disease, and other frontotemporal dementias can be distinguished from DAT due to the initial personality changes and disinhibitions (Mendez, Selwood, Mastri, & Frey, 1993), but these distinctions are not reliable. Other important conditions to consider are Huntington's disease, HIV infection, and Creutzfeldt-Jakob disease. However, existence of these other conditions does not rule out the independent co-occurrence of Alzheimer's disease in a particular patient.

There are other factors that commonly complicate the diagnosis of Alzheimer's disease, such as the history of alcohol abuse. As discussed previously, dementia in the presence of the triad of incontinence, gait disturbance, and memory impairment, accompanied by a characteristic enlargement of the ventricles seen on brain scans, suggests normal pressure hydrocephalus, which should be excluded by cisternography. Improvement after shunting can be demonstrated by SPECT scanning (Shih & Tasdemiroglu, 1995; Wong, Luciano, MacIntyre, Brunken, Hahn, & Go, 1997).

IMPORTANCE OF VASCULAR CHANGES

The distinction of dementia due to vascular disease is the issue that most complicates the diagnosis of DAT (Katzman & Jackson, 1991). This differentiation has represented a broad focus of study and has served as the primary issue in the study of the diagnostic accuracy of DAT. This issue is critical because there are about 500,000 cases of stroke each year, 150,000 of these being fatal (Bronner, Kanter, & Manson, 1995), whereas there are about 500,000 new cases of DAT each year, with about 500,000 patients dying with DAT. Recently, specific criteria have been proposed for identifying vascular dementias (American Psychiatric Association, 1994; Chui et al., 1992; Roman et al., 1993). However, these diagnostic approaches provide no specific criteria to determine relative combinations of these two common entities. Arteriosclerotic pathology was even described in the first case reported by Alzheimer. Punctate white matter changes on MRI scans, suggestive of pathology in small penetrating arteries, are seen frequently in demented patients, even when the onset and progression have been reported as slow and progressive (Skoog, Palmertz, & Andreasson, 1994). White matter changes are associated with increasing age, hypertension, heart disease, and diabetes (Kent, Haynor, Longstreth, & Larson, 1994), but not with an Alzheimer diagnosis (Erkinjuntti et al., 1994). At the present time, the clinical significance of these white matter changes remains unclear.

An important consideration about vascular dementia is that there are many mechanisms through which vascular abnormalities can impair brain function (Chui et al., 1992; Roman et al., 1993). Blood flow to the brain is exquisitely regulated according to cortical activation (Parks et al., 1989), independently of blood pressure. "Hardening of the arteries" of the brain, alone, though common, is not likely to impair cognition as dramatically as DAT. The most direct concern is embolism, which may originate in the heart or in an atheromata or other lesion of the aorta, the carotid arteries, the circle of Willis, the cerebral arteries, or the small penetrating arteries directly supplying the cortex or white matter. Large emboli can cause massive strokes, whereas small emboli may cause small lesions, though the extent of cell death in tissue that has suffered ischemia also may vary. Of concern in the differential diagnosis of DAT is that small vessels branch off the middle cerebral artery close to its exit from the circle of Willis and travel long distances to supply the hippocampus, the basal ganglia, and deep white matter. Small lesions associated with emboli or atheromata in these vessels may damage the same region of the brain most affected by DAT, the hippocampus, as well as causing primary loss of long cortico-cortical white matter tracts. Also, strokes affecting specific cortical regions may produce a constellation of impairments that are difficult to distinguish from DAT, such as "angular gyrus syndrome" (Benson, Cummings, & Tsai, 1982). Further, many small strokes could produce a clinical picture indistinguishable from DAT. However, it is no longer considered likely that cognitive impairment requires a nonspecific loss of a definite quantity of brain tissue, such as 100 ml. Also, any nonspecific assortment of large and small strokes is unlikely to present a clinical picture highly similar to DAT. Differences between DAT and vascular dementia are even reported for MMSE performances (Magni et al., 1996).

The Hachinsky Scale was developed to determine the presence of embolic dementia (Hachinski et al., 1975). This scale was modified according to pathological outcome criteria (Rosen, Terry, Fuld, Katzman, & Peck, 1980). Although this scale can help to clarify the diagnosis, a high score does not mean the patient does not have Alzheimer's disease, and a low score may be found in some stroke patients.

Other vascular diatheses must be considered such as hypoperfusion, especially after cardiac or pulmonary arrest or severe hypotension, particularly in "watershed regions" of the cortex that may have naturally poor perfusion. Also, hemorrhagic lesions may cause a variety of symptoms, though they are usually severe and fatal. Hypoperfusion also may be caused by gradual thickening of cerebral artery walls. Any of these processes that leads to brain tissue damage can cause some cognitive impairment. Thus it is often a challenge to separate the clinical presentation of a vascular dementia from the slow, selective decline of memory and other cognitive functions seen in DAT.

There is uncertainty about whether Alzheimer's disease may produce amyloid, which can infiltrate blood vessels and cause vascular insults, or if vascular insults may stress the brain and initiate the Alzheimer pathological process. Microangiopathy is a vascular condition caused by β-amyloid associated with DAT, and can lead to local ischemia, stressing cells and potentially aggravating the DAT process. Also, coronary artery disease seems to be associated with senile plaque formation in the brain (Sparks et al., 1990), and individuals with hypertension have an increased density of neurofibrillary tangles in the brain (Sparks et al., 1995). Consequently, the distinction of vascular dementia and DAT is complicated by primary and mutual causality issues.

In any case, if vascular dementia is suspected, an evaluation, including complete cardiac, aortic, and carotid studies, should be initiated, and all possible efforts should be made to prevent further vascular injury to the brain. Factors associated with stroke should be addressed, including reduction of blood pressure below 135/85, elimination of tobacco exposure and alcohol use, rigorous control of diabetes, obesity, and serum cholesterol, management of diet, supplementation of antioxidants, and appropriate anticoagulation (Bronner et al., 1995). Atrial fibrillation should be treated with warfarin as soon as possible. Notably, cognition may improve after vascular risk factors are controlled (Meyer, Judd, Tawaklna, Rogers, & Mortel, 1986). The appropriate message for the patient and family is that following the recommendations for "stroke-risk reduction" reduces the risk of stroke (Bronner et al., 1995), and there may be some benefit for slowing the Alzheimer process as well.

ASSESSMENT OF DAT SEVERITY AND CLINICAL COURSE

An important component of dementia diagnosis is the assessment of severity. Clinicians have developed a wide range of tools to quantitate dementia severity. The Blessed Dementia Scale (Blessed et al., 1968) was long considered the most reliable because it had been associated with neuropathological changes. Other measures of dementia severity have been developed and studied extensively, such as the Global Deterioration Scale (Reisberg, Sclan, Franssen, Kluger, & Ferris, 1994), the Clinical Dementia Rating Scale (Hughes, Berg, Danziger, Coben, & Martin, 1982), and systematic composites of other scales, which improve precision and reliability of the severity estimate (Ashford, Kumar, et al., 1992).

During the late course of DAT, patients lose so much memory and other cognitive functions that they are no longer able to complete such tests as the MMSE (Ashford et al., 1989; Auer, Sclan, Yaffee, & Reisberg, 1994). Consequently, approaches have been developed to test patients using observations of basic functions (Haycox, 1984; Reisberg et al., 1994; Teresi, Lawton, Ory, & Holmes, 1994; Volicer, Hurley, Lathi, & Kowall, 1994). At the extreme, the Glasgow Coma Scale assesses rudimentary neurologic functions (Benesch, McDaniel, Cox, & Hamill, 1993) and has been applied to assess end-stage DAT. There also have been analyses of patients based on a regression of function through Piagetian developmental stages (Auer et al., 1994; Cole & Dastoor, 1987; Ronnberg & Ericsson, 1994). Other objective tests relying, in part, on nonverbal responses, such as the Severe Impairment Battery (SIB) (Saxton, McGoingle-Gibson, Swihart, Miller, & Boller, 1990) appear to be reliable and useful for assessing moderate and severe patients with greater dynamic range than the MMSE (Schmitt et al., 1996).

Major problems have resulted from the diversity of assessment tools. Use of different tools leads to poor comparability between studies. Consequently, there is also lack of consensus regarding progression rates and patterns. This lack of coordination has led to failure to develop a system for progressively improving assessment techniques. It has been proposed that all dementia measurement scales can be translated into a "Time-Index," and then be compared directly and meaningfully (Ashford et al., 1995).

An important debate in the assessment of DAT is the issue of heterogeneity, whether subgroups may be identified with significantly separate characteristics or different patterns of symptom development (Eisdorfer et al., 1994; Fisher et al., 1996). Clearly, there is variability in the initial onset and course of DAT which is related to many factors such as age, education, genetic typology, medical and neurologic problems, and other stresses (Guterman et al., 1993). However, the reason for analyzing these factors is to account for a continually greater proportion of the extraneous variables so that the core disease process can be observed more closely. Accounting for more variables allows the clinician and researcher to approach the essential issue of DAT, which is the underlying cause of the dementia (Mayeux, 1996). One model proposes that several factors may contribute to the initiation of the Alzheimer process (e.g., age, head trauma, hypoxia, or a multivalent cation toxicity or imbalance); then normal genetic variations, as well as mutations that interfere with the processing of certain proteins, induce progression down a vulnerable final common pathway, which is thought to involve neuroplastic mechanisms in the brain (see chap. 3 of this volume). The attack on neuroplastic mechanisms in DAT, presumably involving the processing of the microtubule-associated protein tau and the amyloid precursor protein, may vary topographically from patient to patient. In some instances, one hemisphere or brain region may be affected more severely or rapidly than the other (Fisher et al., 1996; Haxby et al., 1988). This loss of correspondence between the rates of deterioration in the hemispheres could be related to loss of communication through the corpus callosum, which shrinks during DAT progression (Biegon et al., 1994; Janowsky, Kaye, & Carper, 1996). Also, certain pathological processes, such as Lewy bodies, may only affect some patients, contributing further to heterogeneity of the clinical picture (Mirra & Markesbery, 1996; Victoroff et al., 1995; Weiner et al., 1996). However, this complexity of the DAT picture indicates the need to analyze individual clinical characteristics for their relationship to the long-term disease course (Ashford et al., 1989, 1995; Stern et al., 1996b), as well as their capacity to discriminate among diverse clinical entities and biological factors contributing to the progress of the disease.

The principal reason for the failure to develop a uniform tool for quantification of dementia severity is the lack of a fundamental physical standard against which to calibrate assessment scales. However, severity measurement can be translated into an absolute physical quantity, time course (Ashford et al., 1995; Reisberg et al., 1994; Stern et al., 1996b). The average time course across many DAT patients can be used to estimate the duration of the illness and predict the future pattern of the patient's deterioration. Patients with DAT usually follow a typical downhill course that lasts about 10 years, on average, from the first symptoms until the most profound level of impairment, clearly a devastating decline relative to normal aging (Jost & Grossberg, 1996). The two-standard deviation limits of the rate of deterioration suggest that 95% of patients will deteriorate between 0.5 and 1.5 times this rate, or follow a course lasting between 5 and 15 years. This time-course estimation provides the caregivers with a time line of expected changes and, thus, can help the family to prepare for the future (Table 5.2). Further, this approach could be useful in the evaluation of compounds targeted as treatments for DAT.

PSYCHIATRIC MENTAL STATUS EXAMINATION

The evaluation of the psychiatric mental status is an important part of the dementia evaluation, though its importance and implications are overlooked frequently. Not only may the psychiatric symptoms be associated with the initiation of DAT or a more rapid progression (Chui et al., 1994), but these symptoms are frequently the most distressing to the family and caregivers and are the most amenable to treatment. The psychiatric symptoms that occur most frequently in the DAT patient are agitation, depression, apathy, disorders of behavior, sleep disorders, and psychosis, including paranoia, hallucinations, and delusions (see Table 5.6; Cohen et al., 1993b; Cohen-Mansfield, 1996; Eisdorfer et al., 1994). These symptoms occur as the initial observation in one third of the patients (Oppenheim, 1994), including both depression (Jost & Grossberg, 1996) and psychosis (Pliskin et al., 1996; Rubin & Kinscherf, 1989). In Alzheimer's case, the initial symptom was a paranoid delusion. During the course of the disease, many different psychiatric symptoms can occur, with the frequency of occurrence of different symptoms varying according to the severity of the dementia (Cohen-Mansfield, 1996; Kurita, Blass, Nolan, Black, & Thaler, 1993; Reisberg, Frannssen, Sclan, Kluger, & Ferris, 1989).

Significant depression is commonly reported in DAT, occurring in 25%–30% of the patients (Cohen et al., 1993b; Reifler et al., 1989; Wragg & Jeste, 1989), though major affective disorder is much less common (Bungener, Jouvent, & Derouesne, 1996; Weiner, Edland, & Luszczynska, 1994) and depressive symptomatology is much more common (Cohen et al., 1993b; Teri, 1996). As the dementia becomes more severe, the mood is characterized more by apathy (Devanand et al., 1991), which is associated with frontal and anterior temporal lobe dysfunction (Craig et al., 1996). When evaluating depression, it is important to obtain information from interviews of the patient and a caregiver (Logsdon & Teri, 1995). The Geriatric Depression Scale (Montorio & Izal, 1996), the Hamilton Depression Scale (Hamilton, 1967), or the Cornell Scale for Depression in Dementia (Alexopoulos, Abrams, & Young, 1988) are useful guides for querying the patient and the caregiver about depressive symptoms. Depression is important because depression might be a causative or risk factor in dementia (this is a high stress cerebral state), and the treatment of depression will produce modest improvement of cognitive function in the demented patient (Reifler et al., 1989).

In DAT, agitation is a common problem that defines a wide range of inappropriate behaviors, including aggression, purposeless activity, and verbal disruptiveness (Cohen-Mansfield, 1996; Table 5.6). Agitation is associated with paranoia in men, but with other psychiatric problems in

TABLE 5.6 Domains of Aberrant Behavior in DAT

Mood Disorder
  Inactivity, apathy, indifference, lack of initiative
  Depressed mood
  Excess bodily concern, complaining
  Moaning, crying, tearfulness
  Manic, elevated mood
  Irritable, anxious, nervous

Psychotic Disorder
  Distrustful, avoidant
  Paranoid delusions, suspicious
  Responding to hallucinations

Inappropriate Behavior
  Stealing, destroying property
  Spitting, inappropriate voiding
  Inappropriate robing, disrobing
  Verbal sexual advances, physical sexual advances

Aggression, Nonphysical, Verbal
  Uncooperative, argumentative
  Cursing, angry statements
  Demanding, verbal threats

Aggression, Physical
  Grabbing, pushing, shoving, hitting, slapping, kicking, scratching, pinching, biting
  Throwing things, using weapons, combative, assaultive

Purposeless Motor Activity
  Hand-wringing, picking, fidgeting, overactive, rocking
  Restless, pacing, aimless wandering

Purposeless Verbal Activity
  Repetitive questions
  Repetitive speech, sounds
  Yelling, screeching, screaming
  Moaning, crying, tearfulness

Sleep Disorder
  Excess daytime napping
  Excess nighttime wandering

(continued)

TABLE 5.6 *(continued)*

Shortened circadian rhythm
Prolonged circadian rhythm

Mealtime Behaviors
  Refuses to eat
  Throws food, steals food
  Hordes, hides food, overeats, binges

Source: Partly adapted from Cohen et al., 1993; Cohen-Mansfield, 1996.

women and is more common in women (Cohen et al., 1993a). Aggressive behaviors are more common in male patients (Cohen-Mansfield) and are associated with psychosis (Aarsland et al., 1996a) and underlying medical illness (Malone, Thompson, & Goodwin, 1993), as well as caregiver depression and having an adult child caregiver without a spouse present (Paveza et al., 1992).

Numerous psychotic symptoms occur in DAT patients, but frequent presentations are paranoid delusions and complex visual hallucinations (Pliskin et al., 1996). Psychotic symptoms are associated with more rapid deterioration (Drevets & Rubin, 1989; Chui et al., 1994), but are frequently responsive to therapeutic interventions (Teri, 1996). Preliminary indications suggest that the new antipsychotic medications, such as risperidone and olanzapine, may be more effective in DAT patients while causing fewer extrapyramidal side effects, when they are used for carefully defined psychotic symptoms. The recognition and treatment of agitation and psychosis is important because these symptoms are upsetting and disruptive to the caregivers and a major precipitant of placement in a long-term care setting. In long-term care settings, agitation places heavy demands on staff time, and aggressive behaviors frequently lead to injuries of staff and other patients.

A particularly common and troublesome problem in DAT patients is disruption of the circadian rhythm (Crosby, Wyles, Verran, & Tynan, 1993), which results in excessive daytime sleeping, nocturnal wandering, and cycles that exceed 24 hours, some as long as 72 hours. Nocturnal disruptiveness is particularly difficult for caregivers, and such behavior may be tolerated poorly in a nursing home if the patient is noisy or enters other patients' rooms. However, this symptom is among the most amenable to pharmacotherapy (Ashford & Zec, 1993). The use of melatonin may even be able to keep the patient's cycle in synchrony with the environment (Brezinski, 1997).

In the DAT patient, especially those that are severely impaired or noncommunicative, assessment of mood, psychotic symptoms, and other bodily discomforts is a very difficult task. However, great strides have been made in the field as numerous behavior assessment tools have been developed (Aarsland et al., 1996a; Cummings et al., 1994; Drachman, Swearer, O'Donnell, Mitchell, & Maloon, 1992; Mack & Patterson, 1994; Mungas, Weiler, Franzi, & Henry, 1989; Patterson & Bolger, 1994; Reisberg et al., 1987; Seltzer & Buswell, 1994; Sinha et al., 1992; Sultzer et al., 1994; Tariot et al., 1995; Teri et al., 1992). These instruments establish several different approaches for assessing the array of aberrant behaviors in DAT patients, using frequency of occurrence, severity, and hierarchical scaling (Table 5.2). These instruments need further refinement and testing to establish their utility in assessing pharmacologic and nonpharmacologic treatment responses.

FUTURE CONSIDERATIONS FOR DAT DIAGNOSIS

The most careful application of clinical diagnostic criteria still results in uncertainty. The issues of diagnostic uncertainty lead to the question of how to determine the actual diagnosis. Autopsy is the only means available for establishing the type of dementia. Diagnostic clarification by autopsy is important for the patient's family members, as well as for the advancement of research into the cause and treatment of Alzheimer's disease and the other dementias. Currently, there is no clinical justification for a biopsy in AD for diagnostic purposes. However, future successful treatments may change our views. For research purposes, diagnostic certainty is important to support epidemiological, etiological, and prevention studies. At the present time, the clinical diagnosis of DAT has an accuracy of about 90% in uncomplicated cases, and this rate compares favorably with many other medical diagnoses where definitive tests are not available. For example, for appendicitis, a lower error rate than 10% at surgical pathology indicates that some cases may have been missed and is considered poor practice. Cerebrospinal fluid analyses and computer analyses on anatomical and functional brain images may soon give us more accurate diagnoses.

In the future, research must focus on prevention and early intervention. Accordingly, the clinical diagnosis of DAT must be made during the preclinical phase of this disease. Several recent studies have suggested that Alzheimer's disease can be predicted up to 4 years before a clinical diagnosis can be made (Masur et al., 1994; Petersen et al., 1995). Efficient recognition of preclinical Alzheimer's disease might be achieved by computer tests of cognition or more focused psychological tests until specific biological markers are developed.

REFERENCES

Aarsland, D., Cummings, J. L., Yenner, G., & Miller, B. (1996a). Relationship of aggressive behavior to other neuropsychiatric symptoms in patients with Alzheimer's disease. *American Journal of Psychiatry, 153,* 243–247.

Aarsland, D., Tandberg, E., Larsen, J. P., & Cummings, J. L. (1996b). Frequency of dementia in Parkinson disease. *Archives of Neurology, 53,* 538–542.

Alexopoulos, G. S., Abrams, R. C., & Young, R. C. (1988). Cornell Scale for Depression in Dementia. *Biological Psychiatry, 23,* 271–284.

Alzheimer, A. (1907). About a peculiar disease of the cerebral cortex. (Translated by L. Jarvik and H. Greenson.) *Alzheimer Disease and Associated Disorders, 1*(1), 7–8, 1987.

American Psychiatric Association. (1994). *Diagnostic and Statistical Manual of Mental Disorders* (4th ed.). Washington, DC: American Psychiatric Association.

Arai, H., Terajima, M., Miura, M., Higuchi, S., Muramatsu, T., Machida, N., Seiki, H., Takase, S., Clark, C. M., Lee, V. M.-Y., Trojanowski, J. Q., & Sasaki, H. (1995). Tau in cerebrospinal fluid: A potential diagnostic marker in Alzheimer's disease. *Annals of Neurology, 38,* 649–652.

Arnold, S. E., Hyman, B. T., Flory, J., Damasio, A. R., & Van Hoesen, G. W. (1991). The topographical and neuroanatomical distribution of neurofibrillary tangles and neuritic plaques in the cerebral cortex of patients with Alzheimer's disease. *Cerebral Cortex, 1,* 103–116.

Arriagada, P. V., Growdon, J. H., Hedley-Whyte, E. T., & Hyman, B. T. (1992). Neurofibrillary tangles but not senile plaques parallel duration and severity of Alzheimer's disease. *Neurology, 42,* 631–639.

Ashford, J. W., Coburn, K. L., & Yamashita, K. (1992). P300 power loss in aging and Alzheimer's disease. *Society for Neuroscience, Abstracts, 18,* 306–320.

Ashford, J. W., Kolm, P., Colliver, J. A., Bekian, C., & Hsu, L-N. (1989). Alzheimer patient evaluation and the Mini-Mental State: Item characteristic curve analysis. *Journal of Gerontology, 5,* 139–146.

Ashford, J. W., Kumar, V., Barringer, M., Becker, M., Bice, J., Ryan, N., & Vicari, S. (1992). Assessing Alzheimer severity with a global clinical scale. *International Psychogeriatrics, 4,* 55–74.
Ashford, J. W., Rosenblatt, M. J., Bekian, C., & Hayes, T. (1987). The complete dementia evaluation: Complications and complexities. *American Journal of Alzheimer's Care and Research, 2,* 9–15.
Ashford, J. W., Schmitt, F. A., & Kumar, V. (1996). Diagnosis of Alzheimer's disease. *Psychiatric Annals, 26,* 262–268.
Ashford, J. W., Shan, M., Butler, S., Rajasekar, A., & Schmitt, F. A. (1995). Temporal quantification of Alzheimer's disease severity: 'Time-Index' model. *Dementia, 6,* 269–280.
Ashford, J. W., & Zec, R. F. (1993). Pharmacologic treatment in Alzheimer's disease. In R. Parks, R. Zec, & R. Wilson (Eds.), *Neuropsychology of Alzheimer's disease and other dementias.* New York: Oxford University Press.
Auer, S., Sclan, S., Yaffee, R., & Reisberg, B. (1994). The neglected half of Alzheimer disease: Cognitive and functional concomitants of severe dementia. *Journal of the American Geriatric Society, 42,* 1266–1272.
Benesch, C. G., McDaniel, K. D., Cox, C., & Hamill R. W. (1993). End-stage Alzheimer's disease. *Archives of Neurology, 50,* 1309–1315.
Benson, D. F., Cummings, J. L., & Tsai, S. (1982). Angular gyrus syndrome simulating Alzheimer's disease. *Archives of Neurology, 39,* 616–620.
Brezinski, A. (1997). Melatonin in humans. *New England Journal of Medicine, 336,* 186–195.
Biegon, A., Eberling, J. L., Richardson, B. C., Roos, M. S., Wong, S. T. S., Reed, B. R., & Jagust, W. J. (1994). Human corpus callosum in aging and Alzheimer's disease: A magnetic resonance imaging study. *Neurobiology of Aging, 15,* 393–397.
Blessed, G., Tomlinson, B. E., & Roth, M. (1968). The association between quantitative measures of dementia and of senile change in the cerebral grey matter in elderly subjects. *British Journal of Psychiatry, 114,* 797–811.
Blum, J., & Jarvik, L. (1974). Intellectual performance of octogenarians as a function of education and initial ability. *Human Development, 17,* 364–375.
Boller, F., Forett, F., Khachaturian, Z., Poncet, M., & Christen, Y. (Eds.). (1992). *Heterogeneity of Alzheimer's disease.* New York: Springer-Verlag.
Braak, H., & Braak, E. (1991). Neuropathological staging of Alzheimer-related changes. *Acta Neuropathologica, 82,* 239–259.
Breitner, J. C. S. (1994). New epidemiologic strategies in Alzheimer's disease may provide clues to prevention and cause. *Neurobiology of Aging, 15,* S175–S177.
Breitner, J. C. S., Murphy, E. A., Silverman, J. M., Mohs, R. C., & Davis, K. L. (1988). Age-dependent expression of familial risk in Alzheimer's disease. *American Journal of Epidemiology, 128,* 536–548.

Bronner, L. L., Kanter, D. S., & Manson, J. E. (1995). Primary prevention of stroke. *New England Journal of Medicine, 333,* 1392–1400.

Bungener, C., Jouvent, R., & Derouesne, C. (1996). Affective disturbance in Alzheimer's disease. *Journal of the American Geriatrics Society, 44,* 1066–1071.

Burdette, J. H., Minoshima, S., Borght, T. V., Tran, D. D., & Kuhl, D. E. (1996). Alzheimer disease: Improved visual interpretation of PET images by using three-dimensional stereotaxic surface projections. *Radiology, 198,* 837–843.

Butler, S. M., Ashford, J. W., & Snowdon, D. A. (1996). Age, education, and changes in the Mini-Mental State Exam scores of older women: Findings from the Nun study. *Journal of the American Geriatrics Society, 44,* 675–681.

Chui, H. C., Lyness, S. A., Sobel, E., & Schneider, L. S. (1994). Extrapyramidal signs and psychiatric symptoms predict faster cognitive decline in Alzheimer's disease. *Archives of Neurology, 51,* 676–681.

Chui, H. C., Victoroff, J. I., Margolin, D., Jagust, W., Shankle, R., & Katzman, R. (1992). Criteria for the diagnosis of ischemic vascular dementia proposed by the State of California Alzheimer's Disease Diagnostic and Treatment Centers. *Neurology, 42,* 473–480.

Chui, H., Zhang, Q., Victoroff, J., & Zaias, B. (1996). Differentiating Alzheimer disease and vascular dementia: Reframing the question. In R. Becker & E. Giacobini (Eds.), *Alzheimer disease: From molecular biology to therapy* (pp. 13–17). Cambridge, MA: Birkhauser.

Cohen, D., Eisdorfer, C., Gorelick, P., Luchins, D., Freels, S., Semla, T., Paveza, G., Shaw, H., & Ashford, J. W. (1993a). Sex differences in the psychiatric manifestations of Alzheimer's disease. *Journal of the American Geriatrics Society, 41,* 229–232.

Cohen, D., Eisdorfer, C., Gorelick, P., Paveza, G., Luchins, D., Freels, S., Ashford, J. W., Semla, T., Levy, P., & Hirschman, R. (1993b). Psychopathology associated with Alzheimer's disease and related disorders. *Journal of Gerontology, 48,* M225–M260.

Cohen-Mansfield, J. (1996). Inappropriate behavior. In Z. S. Khachaturian & T. S. Radebaugh (Eds.), *Alzheimer's disease: Cause(s), diagnosis, treatment, and care.* New York: CRC Press.

Cole, M. G., & Dastoor, D. P. (1987). A new hierarchic approach to the measurement of dementia. *Psychosomatics, 28,* 298–304.

Corey-Bloom, J., Thal, L. J., Galasko, D., Folstein, M., Drachman, D., Raskind, M., & Lanska, D. (1995). Diagnosis and evaluation of dementia. *Neurology, 45,* 211–218.

Craig, A., Cummings, J. L., Fairbanks, L., Itti, L., Miller, B., Li, J., & Mena, I. (1996). Cerebral blood flow correlates of apathy in Alzheimer disease. *Archives of Neurology, 53,* 1116–1120.

Crosby, L. J., Wyles, C. L., Verran, J. A., & Tynan, C. M. (1993). Taxonomy of evening and nighttime behavior patterns of persons with Alzheimer's disease. *American Journal of Alzheimer's Care and Related Disorders & Research, 10,* 7–15.

Crum, R. M., Anthony, J. C., Bassett, S. S., & Folstein, M. F. (1993). Population-based norms for the Mini-Mental State Examination by age and education level. *Journal of the American Medical Association, 269,* 2386–2391.

Cummings, J. L., & Benson, D. F. (1983). *Dementia: A clinical approach.* Boston, MA: Butterworths.

Cummings, J. L., Mega, M., Gray, K., Rosenberg-Thompson, S., Carusi, D. A., & Gornbein, J. (1994). The neuropsychiatric inventory: Comprehensive assessment of psychopathology in dementia. *Neurology, 44,* 2308–2314.

De Leon, M. J., Convit, A., George, A. E., Golomb, J., De Santi, S., Tarshish, C., Rusinek, H., Bobinski, M., Ince, C., Miller, D., & Wisniewski, H. (1996). In vivo structural studies of the hippocampus in normal aging and in incipient Alzheimer's disease. *Annals of the New York Academy of Sciences, 777,* 1–13.

Devanand, D. P., Brockinton, C. D., Moody, B. J., Brown, R. P., Mayeux, R., Endicott, J., & Sackeim, H. A. (1992). Behavioral syndromes in Alzheimer's disease. *International Psychogeriatrics, 4,* 161–184.

Doty, R. L., Reyes, P. F., & Gregor, T. (1987). Presence of both odor identification and detection deficits in Alzheimer's disease. *Brain Research Bulletin, 18,* 597–600.

Drachman, D. A., Swearer, J. M., O'Donnell, B. F., Mitchell, A. L., & Maloon, A. (1992). The Caretaker Obstreperous-Behavior Rating Assessment (COBRA) Scale. *Journal of the American Geriatric Society, 40,* 463–470.

Drevets, W. C., & Rubin, E. H. (1989). Psychotic symptoms and the longitudinal course of senile dementia of the Alzheimer type. *Society of Biological Psychiatry, 25,* 39–48.

Eisdorfer, C., Sevush, S., Barry, P. B., Kumar, V., & Loewenstein, D. A. (1994). Evaluation of the demented patient. *Medical Clinics of North America, 78,* 773–793.

Erkinjuntti, T., Gao, F., Lee, D. H., Eliasziw, M., Merskey, H., & Hachinski, V. C. (1994). Lack of difference in brain hyperintensities between patients with early Alzheimer's disease and control subjects. *Archives of Neurology, 51,* 260–268.

Fillenbaum, G. G., Wilkinson, W. E., Welsh, K. A., & Mohs, R. C. (1994). Discrimination between stages of Alzheimer's disease with subsets of Mini-Mental State Examination items. *Archives of Neurology, 51,* 916–921.

Fisher, N. J., Rourke, B. P., Bieliauskas, L., Giordani B., Berent, S., & Foster, N. (1996). Neuropsychological subgroups of patients with Alzheimer's disease. *Journal of Clinical and Experimental Neuropsychology, 18,* 49–370.

Fleming, K. C., Adams, A. A., & Petersen, R. C. (1995). Dementia: Diagnosis and evaluation. *Mayo Clinic Proceedings, 70,* 1093–1107.

Folstein, M. F., Folstein, S. E., & McHugh, P. R. (1975). ''Mini-Mental State'': A practical method for grading the cognitive state of patients for the clinician. *Journal of Psychiatric Research, 12,* 189–198.

Forbes, W. F., Gentleman, J. F., & Maxwell, C. J. (1995). Concerning the role of aluminum in causing dementia. *Experimental Gerontology, 30,* 23–32.

Franssen, E. H., Reisberg, B., Kluger, A., Sinaiko, E., & Boja, C. (1991). Cognition-independent neurologic symptoms in normal aging and probable Alzheimer's disease. *Archives of Neurology, 48,* 148–154.

Galasko, D. R., Bennett, D., & the Alzheimer's Disease Cooperative Study. (1996). An item pool to assess activities of daily living in Alzheimer's disease. In R. Becker & E. Giacobini (Eds.), *Alzheimer disease: From molecular biology to therapy* (pp. 413–417). Boston, MA: Birkhauser.

Galasko, D., Hansen, L. A., Katzman, R., Wiederholt, W., Masliah, E., Terry, R., Hill, L. R., Lessin, P., & Thal, L. J. (1994). Clinical-neuropathological correlations in Alzheimer's disease and related disorders. *Archives of Neurology, 51,* 888–895.

Galasko, D., Kwo-on-Yuen, P., Klauber, M. R., & Thal, L. J. (1990). Neurological findings in Alzheimer's disease and normal aging. *Archives of Neurology, 47,* 625–627.

Gallagher, M., Landfield, P. W., McEwen, B., Meaney, M. M., Rapp, P. R., Sapolsky, R., & West, M. J. (1996). Hippocampal neurodegeneration in aging. *Science, 274,* 484–485.

Gatz, M., Reynolds, C., Nikolic, J., Lowe, B., Karel, M., & Pedersen, N. (1995). An empirical test of telephone screening to identify potential dementia case. *International Psychogeriatrics, 7,* 429–438.

Geldmacher, D. S., & Whitehouse, P. J. (1996). Evaluation of dementia. *New England Journal of Medicine, 335,* 331–336.

Gilman, S. (1996). Clinical assessment of patients with dementia. In Z. S. Khachaturian & T. S. Radebaugh (Eds.), *Alzheimer's disease: Cause(s), diagnosis, treatment, and care* (pp. 85–95). New York: CRC Press.

Guterman, A., Loewenstein, D., Gamez, E., Lermo, M., Weinberg, G., & Cotler, K. (1993). Stressful life experiences and the early detection of Alzheimer's disease: Potential limitations associated with the estimation of illness duration. *Behavior, Health, and Aging, 3,* 43–49.

Hachinski, V. C., Iliff, L. D., Zilhka, E., Du Boulay, G. H., McAllister, V. L., Marshall, J., Russell, R. W. R., & Symon, L. (1975). Cerebral blood flow in dementia. *Archives of Neurology, 32,* 632–637.

Hamilton, M. (1967). Development of a rating scale for primary depressive illness. *British Journal of Social and Clinical Psychology, 6,* 278–296.

Haxby, J. V., Grady, C. L., Koss, E., Horwitz, B., Schapiro, M., Friedland, R. P., & Rapoport, S. I. (1988). Heterogeneous anterior-posterior metabolic patterns in dementia of the Alzheimer type. *Neurology, 38,* 1853–1863.

Haycox, J. A. (1984). A simple, reliable clinical behavioral scale for assessing demented patients. *Journal of Clinical Psychiatry, 45,* 23–24.

Herholz, K. (1995). FDG PET and differential diagnosis of dementia. *Alzheimer's Disease and Associated Disorders, 9,* 6–16.

Heston, L. L., Mastri, A. R., Anderson, E., & White, J. (1981). Dementia of the Alzheimer type. *Archives of General Psychiatry, 38,* 1085–1090.
Heyman, A. (1996). Heterogeneity of Alzheimer's disease. In K. S. Khachaturian & T. S. Radebaugh (Eds.), *Alzheimer's disease: Cause(s), diagnosis, treatment and care* (pp. 105–107). New York: CRC Press.
Hughes, C. P., Berg, L., Danziger, W. L., Coben, L. A., & Martin, R. L. (1982). A new clinical scale for the staging of dementia. *British Journal of Psychiatry, 140,* 566–572.
Jagust, W. J. (1994). Functional imaging in dementia: An overview. *Journal of Clinical Psychiatry, 55*(Suppl. 11), 5–11.
Janowsky, J. S., Kaye, J. A., & Carper, R. A. (1996). Atrophy of the corpus callosum in Alzheimer's disease versus healthy aging. *Journal of the American Geriatrics Society, 44,* 798–803.
Jarvik, L., & Greenson, H. (1987). About a peculiar disease of the cerebral cortex, by Alois Alzheimer. *Alzheimer's Disease and Associated Disorders, 1,* 7–8.
Jobst, K. A., Hindley, N. J., King, E., & Smith, A. D. (1994). The diagnosis of Alzheimer's disease: A question of image? *Journal of Clinical Psychiatry, 55*(Suppl. 11), 22–31.
Jost, B. C., & Grossberg, G. T. (1996). The evolution of psychiatric symptoms in Alzheimer's disease: A natural history study. *Journal of the American Geriatrics Society, 44,* 1078–1081.
Katzman, R. (1996). Current research on Alzheimer's disease in a historical perspective. In Z. S. Khachaturian & T. S. Radebaugh (Eds.), *Alzheimer's disease: Cause(s), diagnosis, treatment, and care* (pp. 15–29). New York: CRC Press.
Katzman, R. (1993). Education and the prevalence of dementia and Alzheimer's disease. *Neurology, 43,* 13–20.
Katzman, R., & Jackson, J. E. (1991). Alzheimer disease: Basic and clinical advances. *Journal of the American Geriatrics Society, 39,* 516–525.
Kent, D. L., Haynor, D. R., Longstreth, W. T., & Larson, E. B. (1994). The clinical efficacy of magnetic resonance imaging in neuroimaging. *Annals of Internal Medicine, 120,* 856–871.
Khachaturian, Z. S. (1985). Diagnosis of Alzheimer's disease. *Archives of Neurology, 42,* 1097–1105.
Khachaturian, Z. S., & Radebaugh, T. S. (Eds.). (1996). *Alzheimer's disease: Cause(s), diagnosis, treatment, and care.* New York: CRC Press.
Knesevich, J. W., LaBarge, E., & Edwards, D. (1986). Predictive value of the Boston naming test in mild senile dementia of the Alzheimer type. *Psychiatry Research, 19,* 155–161.
Kuhl, D. E., Small, G. W., Riege, W. H., Fujikawa, D. G., Metter, E. J., Benson, D. F., Ashford, J. W., Mazziotta, J. C., Maltese, A., & Dorsey, D. A. (1987). Abnormal PET-FDG scans in early Alzheimer's disease. *Journal of Nuclear Medicine, 28,* 645.

Kukull, W. A., Larson, E. B., Teri, L., Bowen, J., McCormick, W., & Pfanschmidt, M. L. (1994). The Mini-Mental State Examination score and the clinical diagnosis of dementia. *Journal of Clinical Epidemiology, 47,* 1061–1067.

Kurita, A., Blass, J. P., Nolan, K., Black, R., & Thaler, H. (1993). Relationship between cognitive status and behavioral symptoms in Alzheimer's disease and mixed dementia. *Journal of the American Geriatrics Society, 41,* 732–736.

Lanska, D. J., Schmitt, F. A., Stewart, J. M., & Howe, J. N. (1993). Telephone-assessed mental state. *Dementia, 4,* 117–119.

Lawlor, B. A., Ryan, T. M., Schmeidler, J., Mohs, R. C., & Davis, K. L. (1994). Clinical symptoms associated with age at onset in Alzheimer's disease. *American Journal of Psychiatry, 151,* 1646–1649.

Lewis, D. A., Campbell, M. J., Terry, R. D., & Morrison, J. H. (1987). Laminar and regional distributions of neurofibrillary tangles and neuritic plaques in Alzheimer's disease: A quantitative study of visual and auditory cortices. *Journal of Neuroscience, 7,* 1799–1808.

Logsdon, R. G., & Teri, L. (1995). Depression in Alzheimer's disease patients: Caregivers as surrogate reporters. *Journal of the American Geriatrics Society, 43,* 150–155.

Mack, J. L., & Patterson, M. B. (1994). The evaluation of behavioral disturbances in Alzheimer's disease: The utility of three rating scales. *Journal of Geriatric Psychiatry and Neurology, 7,* 101–117.

Magni, E., Binetti, G., Padovani, A., Cappa, S. F., Bianchetti, A., & Trabucchi, M. (1996). The Mini-Mental State Examination in Alzheimer's disease and multi-infarct dementia. *International Psychogeriatrics, 8,* 127–134.

Malone, M. L., Thompson, L., & Goodwin, J. S. (1993). Aggressive behaviors among the institutionalized elderly. *Journal of the American Geriatrics Society, 41,* 853–856.

Masur, D. M., Sliwinski, M., Lipton, R. B., Blau, A. D., & Crystal, H. A. (1994). Neuropsychological prediction of dementia and the absence of dementia in healthy elderly persons. *Neurology, 44,* 1427–1432.

Mayeux, R. (1996). Putative risk factors for Alzheimer's disease. In Z. S. Khachaturian and T. S. Radebaugh (Eds.), *Alzheimer's disease: Cause(s), diagnosis, treatment, and care* (pp. 39–49). New York: CRC Press.

Mayeux, R., Ottman, R., Maestre, G., Nagai, C., Tang, M.-X., Ginsberg, H., Chun, M., Tycko, B., & Shelanski, M. S. (1995). Synergistic effects of traumatic head injury and apolipoprotein-epsilon 4 in patients with Alzheimer's disease. *Neurology, 45,* 555–557.

Mayeux, R., Ottman, R., Tang, M., Noboa-Bauza, L., Marder, K., Gurland, B., & Stern, Y. (1993). Genetic susceptibility and head injury as risk factors for Alzheimer's disease among community-dwelling elderly persons. *Annals of Neurology, 33,* 494–501.

McCormick, W. C., Kukull, W. A., van Belle, G., Bowen, J. D., Teri, L., & Larson, E. (1994). Symptom patterns and comorbidity in the early stages of Alzheimer's disease. *Journal of the American Geriatrics Society, 42,* 517–521.

McKhann, C., Drachman, D., Folstein, M., Katzman, R., Price, D., & Stadlan, E. M. (1984). Clinical diagnosis of Alzheimer's disease: Report of the NINCDS-ADRDA Work Group under the auspices of Department of Health and Human Services Task Force on Alzheimer's Disease. *Neurology, 34,* 939–944.

Meiran, N., Stuss, D. T., Guzman, A., Lafleche, G., & Willmer, J. (1996). Diagnosis of dementia: Methods for interpretation of scores of 5 neuropsychological tests. *Archives of Neurology, 53,* 1043–1054.

Mendez, M. F., Selwood, A., Mastri, A. R., & Frey, W. H. (1993). Pick's disease versus Alzheimer's disease: A comparison of clinical characteristics. *Neurology, 43,* 289–292.

Meyer, J. S., Judd, B. W., Tawaklna, T., Rogers, R. L., & Mortel, K. F. (1986). Improved cognition after control of risk factors for multi-infarct dementia. *Journal of the American Medical Association, 256,* 2203–2209.

Mirra, S. S., & Markesbery, W. R. (1996). The neuropathology of Alzheimer's Disease: Diagnostic feature and standardization. In Z. S. Khachaturian & T. S. Radebaugh (Eds.), *Alzheimer's disease: Cause(s), diagnosis, treatment, and care* (pp. 111–123). New York: CRC Press.

Mohs, R. (1996). The use of tests and instruments in the evaluation of patients with dementia. In Z. S. Khachaturian & T. S. Radebaugh (Eds.), *Alzheimer's disease: Cause(s), diagnosis, treatment, and care* (pp. 97–104). New York: CRC Press.

Mohs, R. C., Marin, D., Green, C. R., & Davis, K. L. (1996). The Alzheimer's Disease Assessment Scale: Modifications that can enhance its use in future clinical trials. In R. Becker & E. Giacobini (Eds.), *Alzheimer disease: From molecular biology to therapy* (pp. 407–411). Boston, MA: Birkhauser.

Molloy, D. W., Alemayehu, E., & Roberts R. (1991). Reliability of a standardized Mini-Mental State Examination compared with the traditional Mini-Mental State Examination. *American Journal of Psychiatry, 148,* 102–105.

Monsch, A. U., Bondi, M. W., Butters, N., Paulsen, J. S., Salmon, D. P., Brugger, P., & Swenson, M. R. (1994). A comparison of category and letter fluency in Alzheimer's disease and Huntington's disease. *Neuropsychology, 8,* 25–30.

Montorio, I., & Izal, M. (1996). The Geriatric Depression Scale: A review of its development and utility. *International Psychogeriatrics, 8,* 103–112.

Morris, J. C. (1996). Diagnosis of Alzheimer's disease. In Z. S. Khachaturian & T. S. Radebaugh (Eds.), *Alzheimer's disease: Cause(s), diagnosis, treatment, and care* (pp. 75–84). New York: CRC Press.

Mortimer, J. A., & Graves, A. B. (1993). Education and other socioeconomic determinants of dementia and Alzheimer's disease. *Neurology, 43,* S39–S44.

Motter, R., Vigo-Pelfrey, C., Kholodenko, D., Barbour, R., Johnson-Wood, K., Galasko, D., Chang, L., Miller, B., Clark, C., Green, R., Olson, D., Southwick, P., Wolfert, R., Munroe, B., Lieberburg, I., Seubert, P., & Schenk, D. (1995). Reduction of β-Amyloid Peptide$_{42}$ in the cerebrospinal fluid of patients with Alzheimer's disease. *Annals of Neurology, 38,* 643–648.

Mulligan, R., Mackinnon, A., Jorm, A., Giannakopoulos, P., & Michel, J. (1996). A comparison of alternative methods of screening for dementia in clinical settings. *Archives of Neurology, 53,* 532–536.

Mungas, D., Weiler, P., Franzi, C., & Henry, R. (1989). Assessment of disruptive behavior associated with dementia: The disruptive behavior rating scales. *Journal of Geriatric Psychiatry and Neurology, 2,* 192–202.

Murphy, C., Gilmore, M. M., Seery, C. S., Salmon, D. P., & Lasker, B. R. (1990). Olfactory thresholds are associated with degree of dementia in Alzheimer's disease. *Neurobiology of Aging, 11,* 465–469.

Nordin, S., Monsch, A. U., & Murphy, C. (1995). Unawareness of smell loss in normal aging and Alzheimer's disease: Discrepancy between self-reported and diagnosed smell sensitivity. *Journals of Gerontology, 50B,* 187–192.

Ohm, T. G., Muller, H., Braak, H., & Bohl, J. (1995). Close-meshed prevalence rates of different stage as a tool to uncover the rate of Alzheimer's disease-related neurofibrillary changes. *Neuroscience, 64,* 209–217.

Oppenheim, G. (1994). The earliest signs of Alzheimer's disease. *Journal of Geriatric Psychiatry and Neurology, 7,* 118–122.

Parks, R. W., Crockett, D. J., Tuokko, H., Beattie, B. L., Ashford, J. W., Coburn, K. L., Zec, R. F., Becker, R. E., McGeer, P. L., & McGeer, E. G. (1989). Neuropsychological "systems efficiency" and Positron Emission Tomography. *Journal of Neuropsychiatry, 1,* 269–282.

Patterson, M. B., & Bolger, J. P. (1994). Assessment of behavioral symptoms in Alzheimer disease. *Alzheimer Disease and Associated Disorders, 8,* 4–20.

Paveza, G. J., Cohen, D., Eisdorfer, C., Freels, S., Semla, T., Ashford, J. W., Gorelick, P., Hirschman, R., Luchins, D., & Levy, P. (1992). Severe family violence and Alzheimer's disease: Prevalence and risk factors. *Gerontologist, 32,* 493–497.

Persson, G., & Skoog, I. (1992). Subclinical dementia: Relevance of cognitive symptoms and signs. *Journal of Geriatric Psychiatry and Neurology, 5,* 172–178.

Petersen, R. C., Smith, G. E., Ivnik, R. J., Tangalos, E. G., Schaid, D. J., Thibodeau, S. N., Kokmen, E., Waring, S. C., & Kurland, L. T. (1995). Apolipoprotein E status as a predictor of the development of Alzheimer's disease in memory-impaired individuals. *Journal of the American Medical Association, 273,* 1274–1278.

Petersen, R. C., Smith, G. E., Ivnik, R. J., Kokmen, E., & Tangalos, E. G. (1994). Memory function in very early Alzheimer's disease. *Neurology, 44,* 867–872.

Pietrini, P., Furey, M. L., Graff-Radford, N., Freo, U., Alexander, G. E., Grady, C. L., Dani, A., Mentis, M. J., & Schapiro, M. (1996). Preferential metabolic involvement of visual cortical areas in a subtype of Alzheimer's disease: Clinical implications. *American Journal of Psychiatry, 153,* 1261–1268.
Pliskin, N. H., Kiolbasa, T. A., Towle, V. L., Pankow, L., Ernest, J. T., Noronha, A., & Luchins, D. J. (1996). Charles Bonnet Syndrome: An early marker for dementia? *Journal of the American Geriatric Society, 44,* 1055–1061.
Raskind, M., & Brower, P. (1996, July). Alzheimer's disease: A diagnosis and management update. *Federal Practitioner, 13,* 24–36.
Rasmusson, D., Brandt, J., Martin, D., & Folstein, M. (1995). Head injury as a risk factor in Alzheimer's disease. *Brain Injury, 9,* 213–219.
Reid, W., Broe, G., Creasey, H., Grayson, D., McCusker, E., Bennett, H., Longley, W., & Sulway, M. R. (1996). Age at onset and pattern of neuropsychological impairment in mild early-stage Alzheimer disease. *Archives of Neurology, 53,* 1056–1061.
Reifler, B. V., Teri, L., Raskind, M., Veith, R., Barnes, R., White, E., & McLean, P. (1989). Double-blind trial of imipramine in Alzheimer's disease patients with and without depression. *American Journal of Psychiatry, 146,* 45–49.
Reiman, E. M., Caselli, R. J., Yun, L. S., Chen, K., Bandy, D., Minoshima, S., Thibodeau, S. N., & Osborne, D. (1996). Preclinical evidence of Alzheimer's disease in persons homozygous for the e4 allele for apolipoprotein E. *New England Journal of Medicine, 334,* 752–758.
Reisberg, B., Borenstein, J., Salob, S., Ferris, S., Franssen, E., & Georgotas, A. (1987). Behavioral symptoms in Alzheimer's disease: Phenomenology and treatment. *Journal of Clinical Psychiatry, 48,* 9–13.
Reisberg, B., Frannssen, E., Sclan, S., Kluger, A., & Ferris, S. (1989). Stage specific incidence of potentially remediable behavioral symptoms in aging and Alzheimer disease: A study of 120 patients using the BEHAVE-AD. *Bulletin of Clinical Neurosciences, 54,* 95–112.
Reisberg, B., Sclan, S. G., Franssen, E., Kluger, A., & Ferris, S. (1994). Dementia staging in chronic care populations. *Alzheimer Disease and Associated Disorders, 8*(Suppl. 1), S188–S205.
Risse, S. C., Raskind, M. A., Nochlin, D., Sumi, S. M., Lampe, T. H., Bird, T. D., Cubberley, L., & Peskind, E. (1990). Neuropathological findings in patients with clinical diagnoses of probable Alzheimer's disease. *American Journal of Psychiatry, 147,* 168–172.
Roman, G. C., Tatemichi, T. K., Erkinjuntti, T., Cummings, J. L., Masdeu, J. C., Garcia, J. H., Amaducci, L., Orgogozo, J.-M., Brun, A., Hofman, A., Moody, D. M., O'Brien, M. D., Yamaguchi, T., Grafman, J., Drayer, B. P., Bennett, D. A., Fisher, M., Ogata, J., Kokmen, E., Bermejo, F., Wolf, P. A., Gorelick, P. B., Bick, K. L., Pajeau, A. K., Bell, M. A., DeCarli, C., Culebras, A., Korczyn, A. D., Bogousslavsky, J., Hartmann, A., & Schein-

berg, P. (1993). Vascular dementia: Diagnostic criteria for research studies. *Neurology, 43,* 250–260.

Ronnberg, L., & Ericsson, K. (1994). Reliability and validity of the hierarchic dementia scale. *International Psychogeriatrics, 6,* 87–94.

Rosen, W. G., Terry, R. D., Fuld, P. A., Katzman, R., & Peck, A. (1980). Pathological verification of [the] ischemic score in differentiation of dementias. *Annals of Neurology, 7,* 486–488.

Roses, A. D. (1996). The metabolism of apolipoprotein E and the Alzheimer's diseases. In Z. S. Khachaturian & T. S. Radebaugh (Eds.), *Alzheimer's disease: Cause(s), diagnosis, treatment, and care* (pp. 207–216). New York: CRC Press.

Rubin, E. H., & Kinscherf, D. A. (1989). Psychopathology of very mild dementia of the Alzheimer type. *American Journal of Psychiatry, 146,* 1017–1021.

Rumble, B., Retallack, R., Hilbich, C., Simms, G., Multhaup, G., Martins, R., Hockey, A., Montgomery, P., Beyreuther, K., & Masters, C. L. (1989). Amyloid A4 protein and its precursor in Down's syndrome and Alzheimer's disease. *New England Journal of Medicine, 320,* 1446–1452.

Saxton, J., McGoingle-Gibson, K., Swihart, A., Miller, M., & Boller, F. (1990). Assessment of the severely impaired patient: Description and validation of a new neuropsychological test battery. *Psychological Assessment, 2,* 298–303.

Schmitt, F. A., Ashford, J. W., Ferris, S., Mackell, J., Saxton, J., Schneider, L., Clark, C., Ernesto, C., Schafer, K., & Thal, L. (1996). Severe Impairment Battery: A potential measure for AD clinical trials. In R. Becker & E. Giacobini (Eds.), *Alzheimer disease: From molecular biology to therapy* (pp. 419–423). Boston, MA: Birkhauser.

Schmitt, F. A., & Sano, M. C. (1994). Neuropsychological approaches to the study of dementia. In J. C. Morris (Ed.), *Handbook of dementing illnesses* (pp. 89–123). New York: Marcel Dekker.

Schmitt, F. A., Shih, W.-J., & DeKosky, S. T. (1992). Neuropsychological correlates of single photon emission computed tomography (SPECT) in Alzheimer's disease. *Neuropsychology, 6,* 159–171.

Seab, J. P., Jagust, W. J., Wong, S. T. S., Roos, M. S., Reed, B. R., & Budinger, T. F. (1988). Quantitative NMR measurements of hippocampal atrophy in Alzheimer's disease. *Magnetic Resonance in Medicine, 8,* 200–208.

Seltzer, B., & Buswell, A. (1994). Psychiatric symptoms in Alzheimer's disease: Mental status examination versus caregiver report. *Gerontologist, 34,* 103–109.

Serby, M., Larson, P., & Kalkstein, D. (1991). The nature and course of olfactory deficits in Alzheimer's disease. *American Journal of Psychiatry, 148,* 357–360.

Shankle, W. R., Dillencourt, M., & Pazzani, M. (1996). Improving dementia screening with machine learning methods. *Society for Neuroscience, Abstracts, 4,* 829.

Shih, W.-J., & Tasdemiroglu, E. (1995). Reversible hypoperfusion of the cerebral cortex in normal-pressure hydrocephalus on technetium-99m-HMPAO brain SPECT images after shunt operation. *Journal of Nuclear Medicine, 36,* 470–473.

Sinha, D., Zemlan, F. P., Nelson, S., Bienenfeld, D., Thienhaus, O., Ramaswamy, G., & Hamilton, S. (1992). A new scale for assessing behavioral agitation in dementia. *Psychiatry Research, 41,* 73–88.

Siu, A. L. (1991). Screening for dementia and investigating its causes. *Annals of Internal Medicine, 115,* 122–132.

Skoog, I., Palmertz, B., & Andreasson, L.-A. (1994). The prevalence of white-matter lesions on computed tomography of the brain in demented and nondemented 85-year-olds. *Journal of Geriatric Psychiatry and Neurology, 7,* 169–175.

Sliwinski, M., Lipton, R. B., Buschke, H., & Stewart, W. (1996). The effects of preclinical dementia on estimates of normal cognitive functioning in aging. *Journal of Gerontology, 52B,* 217–225.

Small, G. W., Kuhl, D. E., Riege, W. H., Fujikawa, D. G., Ashford, J. W., Metter, E. J., & Mazziotta, J. C. (1989). Cerebral glucose metabolic patterns in Alzheimer's disease: Effect of gender and age at dementia onset. *Archives of General Psychiatry, 46,* 527–532.

Small, G. W., Mazziotta, J. C., Collins, M., Baxter, L., Phelps, M., Mandelkern, M., Kaplan, A., La Rue, A., Adamson, C., & Chang, L. (1995). Apolipoprotein E type 4 allele and cerebral glucose metabolism in relatives at risk for familial Alzheimer disease. *Journal of the American Medical Association, 273,* 942–947.

Smith, C. (1996). Quantitative computed tomography and magnetic resonance imaging in aging and Alzheimer's disease. *Journal of Neuroimaging, 6,* 44–53.

Snowdon, D. A., Kemper, S. J., Mortimer, J. A., Greiner, L. H., Wekstein, D. R., & Markesbery, W. R. (1996). Linguistic ability in early life and cognitive function and Alzheimer's disease in late life. *Journal of the American Medical Association, 275,* 528–532.

Sparks, D. L., Hunsaker, J. C., Scheff, S. W., Kryscio, R. J., Henson, J. L., & Markesbery, W. R. (1990). Cortical senile plaques in coronary artery disease, aging and Alzheimer's disease. *Neurobiology of Aging, 11,* 601–607.

Sparks, D. L., Scheff, S. W., Liu, H., Landers, T. M., Coyne, C. M., & Hunsaker, J. C. (1995). Increased incidence of neurofibrillary tangles (NFT) in nondemented individuals with hypertension. *Journal of the Neurological Sciences, 131,* 162–169.

Stern, Y., Gurland, B., Tatemichi, T. K., Tang, M. X., Wilder, D., & Mayeux, R. (1994). Influence of education and occupation on the incidence of Alzheimer's disease. *Journal of the American Medical Association, 271,* 1004–1010.

Stern, Y., Liu, X., Albert, M., Brandt, J., Jacobs, D. M., Castillo-Castañeda, C. D., Marder, K., Bell, K., Sano, M., & Bylsma, F. (1996a). Modeling the influence of extrapyramidal signs on the progression of Alzheimer disease. *Archives of Neurology, 53,* 1121–1126.

Stern, Y., Liu, X., Albert, M., Brandt, J., Jacobs, D. M., Castillo-Castañeda, C. D., Marder, K., Bell, K., Sano, M., Bylsma, F., Lafleche, G., & Tsai, W.-Y. (1996b). Application of a growth curve approach to modeling the progression of Alzheimer's disease. *Journal of Gerontology, 51A,* M179–M184.

Stollberger, R., Fazekas, F., Payer, F., & Flooh, E. (1995). Morphology-oriented analysis of cerebral SPET using matched magnetic resonance images. *Nuclear Medicine Communications, 16,* 265–272.

Stuss, D. T., Meiran, N., Guzman, A., Lafleche, G., & Willmer, J. (1996). Do long tests yield a more accurate diagnosis of dementia than short tests? *Archives of Neurology, 53,* 1033–1039.

Sultzer, D. L., Levin, H. S., Mahler, M. E., High, W. M., & Cummings, J. L. (1992). Assessment of cognitive, psychiatric, and behavioral disturbances in patients with dementia: The Neurobehavioral Rating Scale. *Journal of the American Geriatrics Society, 40,* 549–555.

Tangalos, E. G., Smith, G. E., Ivnik, R. J., Petersen, R. C., Kokmen, E., Kurland, L. T., Offord, K. P., & Parisi, J. E. (1996). The Mini-Mental State Examination in general medicine practice: Clinical utility and acceptance. *Mayo Clinic Proceedings, 71,* 829–837.

Tariot, P. N., Mack, J. L., Patterson, M. B., Edland, S. D., Weiner, M. F., Fillenbaum, G., Blazina, L., Teri, L., Rubin, E., Mortimer, J. A., Stern, Y., & the Behavioral Pathology Committee of the Consortium to Establish a Registry for Alzheimer's Disease. (1995). The Behavior Rating Scale of the Consortium to Establish a Registry for Alzheimer's Disease. *American Journal of Psychiatry, 152,* 1349–1357.

Teresi, J. A., Golden, R. R., Cross, P., Gurland, B., Kleinman, M., & Wilder, D. (1995). Item bias in cognitive screening measures: Comparisons of elderly white, Afro-American, Hispanic and high and low education subgroups. *Journal of Clinical Epidemiology, 48,* 473–483.

Teresi, J., Lawton, M. P., Ory, M., & Holmes, D. (1994). Measurement issues in chronic care populations: Dementia special care. *Alzheimer Disease and Associated Disorders, 8*(Suppl. 1), S144–S183.

Teri, L. (1996). Managing problems in dementia patients: Depression and agitation. In Z. S. Khachaturian & T. S. Radebaugh (Eds.), *Alzheimer's disease: Cause(s), diagnosis, treatment, and care* (pp. 297–304). New York: CRC Press.

Teri, L., Truax, P., Logsdon, R., Uomoto, J., Zarit, S., & Vitaliano, P. P. (1992). Assessment of behavioral problems in dementia: The revised memory and behavior problems checklist. *Psychology and Aging, 7,* 622–631.

Tombaugh, T. N., & McIntyre, N. J. (1992). The Mini-Mental State Examination: A comprehensive review. *Journal of the American Geriatrics Society, 40,* 922–935.

Ulrich, J., & Stahelin, H. B. (1984). The variable topography of Alzheimer type changes in senile dementia and normal old age. *Gerontology, 30,* 21–214.

Van Hoesen, G. W., & Solodkin, A. (1994). Cellular and systems neuroanatomical changes in Alzheimer's disease. *Annals of the New York Academy of Sciences, 747,* 12–35.

Victoroff, J., Mack, W. J., Lyness, S. A., & Chui, H. C. (1995). Multicenter clinicopathological correlation in dementia. *American Journal of Psychiatry, 152,* 1476–1484.

Volicer, L., Hurley, A. C., Lathi, D. C., & Kowall, N. W. (1994). Measurement of severity in advanced Alzheimer's disease. *Journal of Gerontology, 49,* M223–M226.

Waldemar, G., Walovitch, R. C., Andersen, A. R., Hasselbalch, S. G., Bigelow, R., Joseph, J. L., Paulson, O. B., & Lassen, N. A. (1994). ^{99m}Tc-Bicisate (Neurolite) SPECT brain imaging and cognitive impairment in dementia of the Alzheimer type: A blinded read of image sets from a multicenter SPECT trial. *Journal of Cerebral Blood Flow and Metabolism, 14,* S99–S105.

Watson, Y. I., Arfken, C. L., & Birge, S. J. (1993). Clock completion: An objective screening test for dementia. *Journal of the American Geriatrics Society, 41,* 1235–1240.

Weiner, M. F., Edland, S. D., & Luszczynska, H. (1994). Prevalence and incidence of major depression in Alzheimer's disease. *American Journal of Psychiatry, 151,* 1006–1009.

Weiner, M. F., Risser, R. C., Cullum, C. M., Honig, L., White, C., Speciale, S., & Rosenberg, R. N. (1996). Alzheimer's disease and its Lewy body variant: A clinical analysis of postmortem verified cases. *American Journal of Psychiatry, 153,* 1269–1273.

Welsh, K., Butters, N., Hughes, J., Mohs, R., & Heyman, A. (1991). Detection of abnormal memory decline in mild cases of Alzheimer's disease using CERAD neuropsychological measures. *Archives of Neurology, 48,* 278–281.

Wong, C.-y. O., Luciano, M. G., MacIntyre, W. J., Brunken, R. C., Hahn, J. F., & Go, R. T. (in press). Viable neurons with luxury perfusion in hydrocephalus. *Journal of Nuclear Medicine.*

Wragg, R. E., & Jeste, D. V. (1989). Overview of depression and psychosis in Alzheimer's disease. *American Journal of Psychiatry, 146,* 577–587.

Yesavage, J. A., Brooks, J. O., Taylor, J., & Tinklenberg, J. (1993). Development of aphasia, apraxia and agnosia and decline in Alzheimer's disease. *American Journal of Psychiatry, 150,* 742–747.

CHAPTER 6

Neuropsychological Assessment of Alzheimer's Disease: An Examination of Important Issues Underlying Current Practice

David A. Loewenstein
Michele Quiroga

Neuropsychology, the study of brain-behavior relationships, is essential for a diagnosis of Alzheimer's Disease (AD). The National Institute of Neurologic and Communicative Disorders and Stroke-Alzheimer's Disease and Related Disorders Association (NINCDS-ADRDA) criteria (McKhann et al., 1984) are among the most widely accepted set of guidelines for the clinical diagnosis of AD. The criteria for a clinical diagnosis of probable AD are:

1. progressive memory impairment and decline of other cognitive abilities;
2. dementia established by clinical evaluation through the use of such instruments as the Folstein Mini-Mental State Evaluation (MMSE) (Folstein, Folstein, & McHugh, 1975), Blessed Dementia Rating

Scale (Blessed, Tomlinson, & Roth, 1968), or a similar instrument and confirmation by neuropsychological evaluation;
3. no disturbance of consciousness;
4. onset between 40 and 90 years of age (most often after the age of 65); and
5. the absence of other disorders that could account for observed cognitive deficits.

A diagnosis of possible AD is made when a patient presents only a single progressive cognitive deficit, or there is an identifiable brain or systemic disorder that could account for the deficit, but is not thought to be the cause of the dementia. An atypical clinical presentation also may result in a diagnosis of possible AD (McKhann et al.).

One of the requirements of the NINCDS-ADRDA criteria is confirmation of neuropsychological deficits for the determination of a dementia syndrome. The domains specified by the NINCDS-ADRDA work group include neuropsychological confirmation of deficits in memory, language, perceptual skills, praxis, attention, orientation, higher order problem-solving abilities, and functional status. To meet criteria for a dementia syndrome, the NINCDS-ADRDA guidelines specify that an individual must score at or below the lowest 5th percentile in two neuropsychological domains (one should be memory) relative to an age, education, gender, and culturally appropriate normative reference group.

Because a clinical diagnosis of AD is one of exclusion, it is essential that cutoffs for each neuropsychological domain be stringent, hence the requirement that cognitive impairment is sufficient in a particular domain and that only 5% of normal controls would have scores equal to or lower than the score obtained by the patient. Unfortunately, this requires an implicit assumption that adequate normative data are available for comparative purposes. La Rue (1987, 1992) points out that many commonly utilized neuropsychological tests do not have established reliability and validity with older adults and that appropriate normative data are frequently unavailable that adjust for gender, age, or level of educational attainment. Further, there is a paucity of normative data for individuals over the age of 80 (Morris & Fulling, 1988). Loewenstein, Arguelles, Arguelles, and Linn-Fuentes (1994) also express concerns that normative data are not available for older, diverse, cultural or language groups that may in turn render these individuals more susceptible to misdiagnosis. Finally, there is a lack of consensus as to the types and number of test instruments that should be used to assess a particular neuropsychological domain, appropriate weightings for each domain, and their relationships to an overall diagnosis of AD (Loewenstein & Rubert, 1992). For example, impairment at the 10th percentile in seven neuropsychological domains (including memory) might constitute the absence of a dementia syndrome, whereas a label of dementia would apply to an individual who scored below the 5th percentile in two domains such as memory and perceptual skills. Empirically driven models would be very helpful in allowing the scientist or clinician to maximize the information obtained from individuals presenting for evaluation of their cognitive functions (Loewenstein & Rubert, 1992).

Other important goals associated with neuropsychological assessment of the older adult include:

1. determining the presence or absence of cognitive impairment;
2. identification of strengths and weaknesses for remediation and behavioral management purposes;
3. suggestion of particular types of disease processes;
4. evaluation of the effects of specific lesions identified in neuroimaging studies;
5. development of cognitive profile analyses for genetic and epidemiological studies; and
6. provision of a baseline by which to evaluate the efficacy of different pharmacologic and treatment strategies.

These important areas must be evaluated with tests that have demonstrated reliability and validity with older adults. In addition, they must be flexible enough to accommodate those individuals who present sensory deficits in such areas as vision and hearing.

In this chapter, it is our intention to address several conceptual issues that are believed to be important in current neuropsychological batteries for evaluation of the older adult.

THE EXTENT OF NEUROPSYCHOLOGICAL EVALUATION REQUIRED TO OBTAIN THE OPTIMAL YIELD OF INFORMATION FOR DIAGNOSIS AND PATIENT MANAGEMENT

In the clinical setting, neuropsychological evaluation must be sufficiently comprehensive to address the eight domains set forth by the NINCDS-

ADRDA work group for confirmation of a dementia syndrome. A question raised by many neuropsychologists is whether one or a specific combination of measures in each neuropsychological domain is sufficient to render an assessment of the patient. Zec (1993) proposes that a successful neuropsychological battery with AD and other dementias must provide early detection of dementia, differential diagnosis, as well as identify the progressive stages of the illness.

Although differences of professional opinion exist, many neuropsychologists would agree that the most comprehensive information regarding brain-behavior relationships is required for an adequate understanding of the older patient presenting for evaluation. For example, memory dysfunction is a principal feature of AD, and an assessment of encoding, storage, retrieval, and recognition memory on selective reminding tests are often beneficial in diagnostic determination. The distinction between memory for recent and more remote events, semantic versus figural memory, declarative versus procedural knowledge, supraspan and even speed of mental processing using computerized tasks can be helpful in characterizing a particular memory disorder or dementia. Similarly, tests of aphasia generally include, at a minimum, tests of confrontation naming, verbal fluency, comprehension skills, repetition of phrases, calculation ability, as well as the ability to read and write. Different tests of praxis, including ideomotor, ideational, and constructional praxis, also are components of the neuropsychology battery. Measures of attention, concentration, higher-order problem-solving abilities, motor skills, orientation, and functional skills also should be assessed.

The issue of how much neuropsychological testing is required is an important question because of emotional stress and economic burden that can occur when a patient is "overtested." There have been instances where the severely demented patient is literally put through hours of unnecessary cognitive or neuropsychological testing that proves frustrating for both the patient and family members. In working with cognitively impaired individuals, it is essential that the point of diminishing returns for testing is clearly formulated as to avoid undue patient burden. Using MMSE scores is one manner in which to determine the appropriate amount of testing required to examine the global level of cognitive impairment represented by the patient. Murden, McRae, Kaner, and Buckman (1991) found that for both African American and white non-Hispanic groups a MMSE of 17 or less is almost always indicative of cognitive impairment or dementia. Sensitivities and specificities were 93% and 100% for those individuals with above an eighth grade education and a MMSE of 23 or greater. Utilizing a cutoff MMSE score of 17 or greater provides sensitivities and specificities of 81% and 100% for those patients who have less than 8 years of education. More recently, Mungas, Marshall, Weldon, Haan, and Reed (1996) developed an age and education correction formula for English- and Spanish-speaking older adults.

Loewenstein and Rubert (1992) also have suggested that the use of different batteries with core overlapping measures for those with different levels of cognitive impairment provides the highest yield of information while minimizing patient burden. Those who score 17 or below on the MMSE in our laboratories (unless aphasic) are typically administered the Fuld Object Memory Evaluation (OME) (Fuld, 1981), the Direct Assessment of Functional Status Scale (DAFS) (Loewenstein et al., 1989), and other select measures as required. These tests may be augmented by a few other measures to provide an analysis of the specific degree of impairment in such areas as language, praxis, and reasoning. Other tests may be considered by the neuropsychologist and the interdisciplinary team in cases where they are warranted. In cases where the MMSE is exceptionally low, provided that this is not a result of sensory impairment, information derived from a brief battery of tests can augment the psychosocial assessment and provide a basis for planning, management, and remediation of a particular patient.

Patients who obtain MMSE scores of 18 or above are generally administered a battery of neuropsychological tests that are sensitive to cognitive impairment. The battery covers all neuropsychological domains specified by the NINCDS-ADRDA work group and includes tests that are culturally appropriate for the Cuban American elderly population. It is important to note that the MMSE score is not sensitive to early dementia in the high ranges, with the tendency to produce false negatives (Loewenstein & Rubert, 1992; Murden et al., 1991). By using batteries appropriate to a patient's level of cognitive status, which are sufficiently flexible to be modified in the presence of extreme dysphasia or sensory impairment, it is possible to employ a core of tests common to each battery. This helps avoid overtaxing the patient while still permitting testing of limits and the addition of specific tests that might be useful in a particular diagnostic case. It also should be stressed that screening measures other than the MMSE also can provide guidance in the selection of appropriate tests.

Different patients pose different questions that can be addressed successfully by neuropsychological assessment. The importance of capturing essential information, while avoiding unnecessary testing (which fails to address the specific aims of the evaluation), is the key to an effective cognitive evaluation of the older adult.

THE SELECTION OF NEUROPSYCHOLOGICAL TESTS AND TEST BATTERIES

There are a number of neuropsychological tests available for the assessment of dementia. Each measure has its particular strengths and weaknesses and may have advantages among certain populations. The reader is referred to Lezak (1995) and La Rue (1992) for an in-depth discussion of specific cognitive measures that have established reliability and validity for the assessment of dementia.

Because of the tremendous variability in the use of neuropsychological tests for the evaluation of dementia, there also have been attempts to develop more specialized batteries so that there is greater uniformity in the testing process. The Consortium to Establish a Registry in Alzheimer's Disease (CERAD) (Morris et al., 1989) has successfully utilized a well-validated brief battery of neuropsychological tests in large numbers of AD patients. The neuropsychological battery was designed to provide clinicians with the minimum information necessary to make a confident diagnosis of probable AD. Results of the 1-year follow-up indicated that tests were sensitive to the progression of illness. The cognitive measures of the CERAD include tests of orientation, word list memory, recognition, word list delayed recall, confrontational naming, animal fluency, tests of constructional praxis, and the Folstein MMSE. Further work is in process to test the usefulness of the CERAD battery with minority groups and in persons with low educational levels. There was limited information on patients with very mild dementia and with severe dementia in this cohort.

Welsh, Butters, Hughes, Mohs, and Heyman (1992) found that the delayed recall of the list-learning task distinguished 90% of mildly demented patients from 92% of control subjects. Further, the battery of tests has shown sensitivity to the severity of dementia. A recent study by Welsh et al., 1995, revealed that African Americans score significantly poorer on visual naming, constructional praxis, and the MMSE after accounting for age and educational attainment. It is commendable that the ethnic and cultural appropriateness of this battery is being examined so that the CERAD can be applicable to diverse groups of older adults presenting for evaluation.

Examples of other batteries that also have been used in the diagnosis and staging of Alzheimer's disease are the Alzheimer's Disease Assessment Scale (ADAS) (Rosen, Mohs, & Davis, 1984), the Washington University Battery (Storandt, Botwinick, Danzinger, Berg, & Hughes, 1984), and a 4-hour assessment battery used at the University of California, San Diego, Alzheimer's Research Center (UCSD-ADRC) (Salmon & Butters, 1992). A limitation of these and similar batteries is that they do not cover all of the domains specified by the NINCDS-ADRDA work group. For example, the CERAD battery in and of itself may not effectively tap perceptual skills, problem-solving abilities, and functional status.

There have been recent attempts to develop specific neuropsychological measures that may better predict the presence or absence of dementia among patients who have sought evaluation for possible cognitive impairment. Moncsh, Bondi, Butters, Salmon, Katzman, and Thal (1992) compared four verbal fluency measures and found that a category fluency test could provide a sensitivity of 100% and a specificity of 92.5% in discriminating mildly demented persons from normal, healthy controls. Knopman and Ryberg (1989) developed a new memory test, a delayed word recall test, and found that a verbal memory test possessed high accuracy for predicting AD. More recently, Loewenstein, Rubert, Arguelles, and Duara (1995) demonstrated that the OME (Fuld, 1981) was found to be a very sensitive test for early AD in both white non-Hispanic and Cuban American Spanish-speaking groups with sensitivities of 95.5% and 95.9%. Specificity was 96.7% and 100% for both groups, respectively.

La Rue (1992) and Zec (1995) propose examples of tests that provide a comprehensive neuropsychological assessment in AD and related disorders. Normative data for tests administered to older adults also can be found in Spreen and Strauss (1991) and La Rue (1992). Comprehensive norms for older adults on subtests of the Halstead Reitan Battery are available in Heaton, Grant, and Matthews (1991), and the original Wechsler Memory Scale (Wechsler & Stone, 1945) has been reviewed extensively by D'Elia, Satz, and Schretlen (1989).

THE EFFECT OF ETHNICITY, CULTURE, AND LANGUAGE

Cultural and language biases have increasingly been recognized as problematic in the assessment of the older adult. This is particularly disturbing in that culturally unfair or inappropriate tests can result in serious diagnostic errors (Loewenstein et al., 1994; Loewenstein, Arguelles, Barker, & Duara, 1993). Lopez and Taussig (1991) demonstrated that non-Hispanic elderly individuals score considerably higher on Digit-Span and Block Design subtests of the WAIS-R (Wechsler, 1981) relative to Spanish-speaking subjects who were administered these tests in their native language. Moreover, non-Hispanic elderly patients perform much better on WAIS-R subtests such as Similarities and Vocabulary relative to Spanish-speaking elderly patients who were administered the Escala de Inteligencia Wechsler Para Adultos (EIWA) (Wechsler, 1968). Loewenstein, Ardilla, et al. (1992) found that normal, elderly Spanish speakers scored lower on a 10-minute delayed recognition memory for grocery items relative to a white non-Hispanic elderly comparison group. In another study, Fillenbaum, Heyman, Williams, Prosnitz, and Burchett (1990) demonstrated that the sensitivity/specificity of the MMSE for detecting dementia in Anglo-Americans was 100% and 94%. For African Americans, the sensitivity and specificity was 100% and 58.5% respectively. Moreover, Escobar et al. (1986) concluded that both cultural and linguistic artifacts affected test performance when evaluating a community population of mixed ethnicity.

In this and a number of other studies, level of educational attainment has played a major role in differences between diverse ethnic and cultural groups. Murden et al. (1991) evaluated 100 white non-Hispanic and 258 black individuals and found that there were no significant differences between these groups with regard to MMSE scores. A cutoff score of 24 or above was recommended if a patient had 8 or more years of education, and a cutoff score of 17 or more was most effective for persons with 8 years or less of education. In another study, Unverzagt et al. (1994) collected normative data for 83 healthy, normal, elderly individuals and revealed that there were very strong educational influences on test performance, with less powerful effects for age that were primarily related to memory. Mungas et al. (1996) developed a formula that was effective for the correction of age and education on the MMSE for English- and Spanish-speaking normal, elderly controls.

Loewenstein et al. (1993) found that the FAS Controlled Word Association Test, Digit-Span, and the Comprehension Test were substantially lower in Cuban American, Spanish-speaking subjects when compared with a white non-Hispanic group matched for dementia severity. These differences were still apparent after adjusting for level of educational attainment. The results concerning the FAS verbal fluency task can be best explained by the fact that these letters occur at different frequencies in Spanish and in English. Furthermore, this test may pose an orthographic as well as a verbal fluency test in that the subject must make a judgment as to whether a phonologically correct word actually meets the criteria for beginning with a certain letter. For example, in non-Castillian Spanish, the s sound also can be produced by the letters z and even c. Because subjects are required to produce words that begin with a particular letter and, at the same time, suppress letters with a similar sound, Spanish-speaking individuals might be placed at a disadvantage because this represents a more difficult task for them than for their English-speaking counterparts. Not only would this result in more time required to make a correct response but also in inappropriate responses that could result in a lower verbal fluency score. In this case, one could collect culturally appropriate normative data for this task or switch to a test of animal or category fluency that likely would possess minimal cultural and language biases.

Digit-Span of the WAIS-R has been shown to be different for a wide array of cultural groups (Loewenstein et al., 1993; Lopez & Taussig, 1991). It is possible that the 1-second presentation of digits engenders different chunking strategies among elderly white non-Hispanic and Cuban American groups. This possibility is bolstered by the fact that factoring syllable length (which is typically longer for digits in Spanish) did not affect outcomes. Recent pilot work in our laboratories suggests that Cuban American elderly perform more closely to white non-Hispanic groups when digits are chunked into 2s. In this as well as similar research, one must question whether tests derived from a European-American perspective have validity with other ethnic and cultural groups. That is, does the test measure what it is supposed to measure when used by different ethnic and cultural groups?

The Comprehension subtest of the Wechsler Adult Intelligence Scale-Revised (WAIS-R) also can be a difficult test for Cuban American elderly patients because it includes proverbs and customs associated with the white non-Hispanic culture, which likely has low saliency and validity for Cuban American groups. A more detailed analysis of cross-cultural bias in dementia can be found in Loewenstein et al. (1994).

It is apparent that the indiscriminate use of neuropsychological tests that have been normed on white non-Hispanic populations (which are heterogeneous in and of themselves) can place individuals from different ethnic and cultural groups at a distinct disadvantage. The implicit assumption that the results of clinical research on Mexican Americans, Cuban Americans, Puerto Rican-Americans, and individuals from different Latin American countries can be generalized to *all Spanish speakers* can be just as deleterious in the evaluation of a particular individual. Neuropsychological tests should not be merely translated by an examiner as he or she goes along or uses translated versions. Rather, all measures should be properly translated, back translated, and committee translated, as well as pilot tested, as described in Loewenstein et al. (1994).

Loewenstein et al. (1994) also conclude, based on their work and research with culturally diverse groups, that it is imperative to:

1. modify or discontinue tests that are not relevant or salient for different cultural and language groups.
2. construct tests that are more culturally fair, appropriate, and salient for diverse cultural groups.
3. develop age and education normative data that are fair as well as local norms that are appropriate for specific cultural groups.

A promising development is normative data that are being collected for the CERAD battery. Prineas et al. (1995) are currently conducting a large epidemiological prevalence study among white non-Hispanics, African Americans and Cuban American elderly that also should provide meaningful comparative cognitive/neuropsychological data for diagnostic purposes.

One instrument that appears to be especially promising is the OME (Fuld, 1981), which was described previously. This is a measure of memory function that requires the individual to recall 10 common household objects identified by touch, sight, and name prior to recall. Interspersing recall and distractor trials, the subject is selectively reminded of those targets not recalled, then administered a distractor test, and then again is asked to recall the 10 target items. The score is the total number of targets summed across the five recall trials. Five minute delayed recall and recognition memory for the targets are also assessed. The summed total of targets recalled across the five trials of the test has been shown to be culturally fair and has equivalently high sensitivities and specificities (.95 to 1.0) for elderly Cuban American and white non-Hispanic groups (Loewenstein et al., 1995). The OME is likely more culturally fair than other measures because it uses 10 common household objects that are salient for individuals from diverse cultural backgrounds and is not susceptible to educational confounds. Pilot data collected as part of the Prineas et al. (1995) epidemiological study suggest that this measure may be culturally fair for elderly African Americans residing in the community. This instrument has already been shown to be culturally appropriate for the Japanese elderly (Fuld, Osamu, Blau, Westbrook, & Katzman, 1988). The generalizability of these findings to other diverse ethnic and cultural groups is presently unknown.

THE ROLE OF FUNCTIONAL ASSESSMENT

There has been some debate as to whether there is a need for formal functional assessment in the neuropsychological evaluation of the older adult. Many proponents of neuropsychological testing believe that neuropsychological test scores alone can provide the necessary information extending beyond brain-behavior relationships. This includes, but is not limited to, predicting levels of functional capacities, providing remediation strategies, and making judgments about an individual's abilities to drive an automobile, manage his or her finances, and to live independently. Such functional judgments may have a significant effect on important issues related to long-term care, placement, and health services utilization. Studies demonstrating high levels of association between neuropsychological and functional tasks as well as principal components analyses demonstrating a strong relationship between specific arrays of neuropsychological and functional variables often fail to address the modest degree of shared variance between neuropsychological and functional measures. This renders generalization to a particular case most difficult. The available data are simply too limited to provide guidance for the clinician as how to make use of specific neuropsychological instruments to make meaningful functional judgments regarding a cognitively impaired patient. In their review of the literature, Butler, Anderson, Furst, Namerow, and Satz (1989) described how poorly formal neuropsychological assessment related to actual functional task performance. Similar results were obtained by Haut, Frazen, Keefover, and Rankin (1991). Loewenstein, Rubert, et al., 1992 found that optimal combinations of neuropsychological tests could not adequately predict or explain the AD patient's performance on a broad array of functional measures that were part of the DAFS Scale. These results were later replicated by Loewenstein et al. (1995), who showed that although there were statistically significant associations between optimal combinations of neuropsychological/functional variables, the degree of shared variance was minimal and that the majority of patient variability in functional measures could not be predicted by knowledge of important demographic information or by neuropsychological performance.

In an attempt to address these concerns, the DAFS (Loewenstein et al., 1989) was developed to provide an objective, comprehensive evaluation of a broad array of functional capacities such as telling time, using the telephone, preparing a letter for mailing, identifying common traffic signs, identifying and counting currency, writing a check, balancing a checkbook, making change for a purchase, and shopping with a written list. Basic eating, dressing, and grooming skills also are assessed. The reader is referred to Loewenstein et al. (1989) regarding the reliabilities, validities, and full description of each functional subtest.

The advantage of using direct performance-based measures is that performance is based on behavioral tasks that the patient is routinely required to perform in his or her everyday environment. This may be preferable to ratings based on patient or caregiver judgments, which may be susceptible to reporter error or caregiver bias (Magaziner, Basset, & Hebel, 1987; Magaziner, Simonsick, Kashner, & Hebel, 1988; Rubinstein, Schaier, Weiland, & Kane, 1984; Weinberger, Samsa, Schmader, Greenberg, Carr, & Wilderman, 1992; Zimmerman & Magaziner, 1994). On the other hand, there are problems with sole reliance on a performance-based approach. For example, components of functional behaviors required within the environment may not necessarily translate into higher order levels of functional activities that occur in the course of everyday living. If an individual forgets to pay an electric bill when it is due or, conversely, pays the same bill several times during the month, this disability may relate to an ostensible memory deficit rather than to the lack of requisite skills that one needs in comprehending that he or she has to pay a bill, write an appropriate check, prepare a letter for mailing, and place it in the mail.

It is proposed that many sequences of activities such as meal preparation, managing one's finances, cleaning one's house, and issues as basic as personal hygiene involve a variety of overlearned functional and cognitive behaviors. Depressed patients who may be functionally intact may simply lack the motivation to perform such activities of daily living because of their motivational state.

It is clear that an understanding and prediction of specific functional capacities is a difficult, yet integral, part of the neuropsychological evaluation for dementia. As a result, neuropsychological assessment is not in and of itself sufficient to render specific judgments about an individual's ability to manage finances, to live independently, or other important judgments regarding a person's life. At the very least, until better technologies are developed, extensive collateral reports of reliable informants, behaviorally based functional assessments of specific functional capacities within the clinical setting and, when necessary, home visitation can provide optimal data upon which to base clinical decision making.

SUMMARY AND CONCLUSIONS

The neuropsychological assessment of AD and other dementias are of extreme importance in the diagnosis and management of these disorders. Confirmation of a dementia syndrome by NINCDS-ADRDA criteria remains essential because a diagnosis of AD will be rendered in cases where all other causes or etiologies of the condition have been systematically ruled out. If neuropsychologists are to ensure that normal individuals or those with age-associated memory impairment are not mistakingly given a devastating diagnosis such as AD, the NINCDS-ADRDA criteria for impairment must remain stringent and conservative. However, one must prepare to consider important issues such as individuals who may score in the lower 10th percentile in seven neuropsychological domains and be labeled as normal, whereas an individual who obtains a memory and attentional score at the lower 5th percentile would be labeled as demented. This leads us to question the extent to which each neuropsychological area or domain should be assessed (Loewenstein & Rubert, 1992). For example, if 10 or more memory-specific measures are administered, what are the chances that one might show impairment and the person would be classified as impaired in that domain? Further, why are neuropsychological domains in Alzheimer's disease equally weighted? It would appear that specific domains in Alzheimer's disease might carry more weight than other domains. This issue has yet to be addressed.

It is probably not appropriate to administer indiscriminately a large neuropsychological test battery to all patients presenting for evaluation. For those individuals who are significantly demented, this only provides an unnecessary burden to the patient who is already likely stressed and anxious about his or her deficits. If such an individual is in a state of denial, repeatedly administering tests that point out his or her deficits is yet another frustrating experience for the patient.

Despite some of the limitations described previously, the NINCDS-ADRDA guidelines continue to be the most widely accepted criteria for establishing a dementia syndrome. The required confirmation of neuropsychological deficits protects against an erroneous diagnosis of cognitive impairment or dementia syndrome, which could lead to a devastating diagnosis of AD. Therefore, with many patients, all eight neuropsychological domains should be assessed. This does not limit the neuropsychologist in ordering additional testing when there are sensory deficits, dysphasia, or when a more in-depth analysis of praxis is required. What is required is prudence in the ability to make distinctions about that which will provide optimal information regarding:

1. the establishment of cognitive impairment and a dementia syndrome;
2. the definition of specific patterns of deficits to assist in diagnosis;
3. the extent to which specific types of cognitive and functional deficits can provide the basis for useful management or remediation strategies; and
4. the provision of an objective baseline to monitor decline longitudinally.

Another major issue concerns the use of neuropsychological tests for diverse cultural and ethnic groups. As with many assessment instruments before them, neuropsychological testing can be biased against those who speak different languages and belong to diverse ethnic and cultural groups. It also is particularly difficult in evaluating the older adult in which there is often a paucity of normative data. If normative data are lacking, it is incumbent upon us as neuropsychological specialists to develop adequate local norms for different cultural and language populations. Because the effects of education make it even more difficult to interpret neuropsychological test deficits, multicenter trials and the use of epidemiological ascertainment methods should be considered as a means of better serving different minority groups. Loewenstein et al. (1995) have even suggested that neuropsychological and geriatric advocacy groups work hand in hand with major test publishers to develop more standardized tests for older, diverse, ethnic and cultural groups in the United States and abroad. This could provide quality assurance in the standard administration and scoring of neuropsychological measures while opening up new markets.

Finally, there is a need for behaviorally based functional assessment within the clinical setting. While some neuropsychologists may believe that neuropsychology, the study of brain-behavior relationships, should be limited to ostensible neuropsychological tests, the reality of current practice is that neuropsychologists are increasingly asked to render important decisions about an individual's ability to manage his or her finances, drive an automobile, or live independently. Objective assessments of functional abilities within the clinical setting as well as good collateral reports by caregivers or other qualified informants can only serve to better the excellent standard of patient care.

REFERENCES

Blessed, G., Tomlinson, B. E., & Roth, M. (1968). The association between quantitative measures of dementia and of senile changes in the cerebral gray matter of elderly subjects. *British Journal of Psychology, 225,* 797–811.

Butler, R., Anderson, L., Furst, C. J., Namerow, N. S., & Satz, P. (1989). Behavioral assessment in neuropsychological rehabilitation: A method for measuring vocational-related skills. *Clinical Neuropsychologist, 3,* 235–243.

D'Elia, L., Satz, P., & Schretlen, D. (1989). Wechsler Memory Scale: A critical appraisal of the normative studies. *Journal of Clinical and Experimental Neuropsychology, 11,* 551–568.

Escobar, J. I., Burnam, A., Karno, M., Forsythe, A., Landsverk, J., & Golding, J. (1986). Use of the Mini-Mental State Examination (MMSE) in a community population of mixed ethnicity. *Journal of Nervous and Mental Disorders, 174,* 607–614.

Fillenbaum, A., Heyman, A., Williams, K., Prosnitz, B., & Burchett, B. (1990). Sensitivity and specificity of standardized screen of cognitive impairment and dementia among elderly black and white community residents. *Journal of Clinical Epidemiology, 43,* 651–660.

Folstein, M. F., Folstein, S. A., & McHugh, P. R. (1975). Mini-Mental State: A practical method for grading the cognitive state of patients for the clinician. *Journal of Psychiatric Research, 12,* 196–198.

Fuld, P. A. (1981). *The Fuld Object Memory Evaluation.* Chicago: Stoeling Instrument.

Fuld, P. A., Osamu, M., Blau, A., Westbrook, L., & Katzman, R. (1988). Cross-cultural and multi-ethnic dementia evaluation by mental status and memory testing. *Cortex, 24,* 511–519.

Haut, M. W., Franzen, M. D., Keefover, R., & Rankin, E. (1991, July). *Functional status and cognitive functions in dementia.* Paper presented at the 19th Annual Meeting of the International Neuropsychological Society, San Antonio, TX.

Heaton, R. K., Grant, I., & Matthews, C. G. (1991). Differences in neuropsychological test performance associated with age, education, and sex. In I. Grant & K. M. Adams (Eds.), *Neuropsychological assessment of neuropsychiatric disorders* (pp. 100–120). New York: Oxford University Press.
Knopman, D. S., & Ryberg, S. (1989). A verbal memory test with high predictive accuracy for dementia of the Alzheimer type. *Archives of Neurology, 46,* 141–145.
La Rue, A. (1987). Methodological concerns: Longitudinal studies of dementia. *Alzheimer's Disease and Associated Disorders, 1,* 180–192.
La Rue, A. (1992). *Aging and neuropsychological assessment.* New York: Plenum Press.
Lezak, M. D. (1995). *Neuropsychological assessment* (3rd ed.). New York: Oxford University Press.
Loewenstein, D. A., Amigo, E., Duara, R., Guterman, A., Hurwitz, D., Berkowitz, N., Wilkie, F., Weinberg, G., Black, B., Gittleman, B., & Eisdorfer, C. (1989). A new scale for the assessment of functional status in Alzheimer's disease and related disorders. *Journal of Gerontology, 4,* 114–121.
Loewenstein, D. A., Ardilla, A., Roselli, M., Hayden, S., Duara, R., Berkowitz, N., Linn-Fuentes, P., Mintzer, J., Norville, M., & Eisdorfer, C. (1992). A comparative analysis of functional status among Spanish- and English-speaking patients with dementia. *Journal of Gerontology: Psychological Sciences, 47,* 142–149.
Loewenstein, D. A., Arguelles, T., Arguelles, S., & Linn-Fuentes, P. (1994). Potential cultural bias in the neuropsychological assessment of the older adult. *Journal of Clinical and Experimental Neuropsychology, 16*(4), 623–629.
Loewenstein, D., Arguelles, T., Barker, W., & Duara, R. (1993). A comparative analysis of neuropsychological test performance of Spanish-speaking and English-speaking patients with Alzheimer's disease. *Journal of Gerontology, 48,* 142–149.
Loewenstein, D. A., & Rubert, M. P. (1992). The NINCDS-ADRDA neuropsychological criteria for the assessment of dementia: Limitations of current diagnostic guidelines. *Behavior, Health, and Aging, 2,* 113–121.
Loewenstein, D. A., Rubert, M., Arguelles, T., & Duara, R. (1995). Neuropsychological test performance and prediction of functional capacities among Spanish-speaking and English-speaking patients with dementia. *Archives of Clinical Neuropsychology, 10,* 75–88.
Loewenstein, D. A., Rubert, M. P., Zimmer, N. A., Guterman, A., Morgan, R., & Hayden, S. (1992). Neuropsychological test performance and prediction of functional capacities in dementia. *Behavior, Health, and Aging, 22,* 149–158.
Lopez, S. R., & Taussig, F. M. (1991). Cognitive-intellectual functioning of Spanish-speaking impaired and nonimpaired elderly: Implications for culturally sensitive assessment. *Psychological Assessment: A Journal of Consulting and Clinical Psychology, 3,* 448–454.

Magaziner, J., Bassett, S. S., & Hebel, J. R. (1987). Predicting performance on the Mini-Mental State Examination: Use of age- and education-specific equations. *Journal of the American Geriatric Society, 35,* 996–1000.

Magaziner, J., Simonsick, E. R., Kashner, T. M., & Hebel, J. R. (1988). Patient-proxy response comparability on measures of patient health and functional status. *Journal of Clinical Epidemiology, 4,* 1065–1074.

McKhann, G., Drachman, D., Folstein, M., Katzman, R., Price, D., & Stadlan, E. M. (1984). Clinical diagnosis of Alzheimer's disease: Report of the NINCDS-ADRDA work group under the auspices of Department of Health and Human Services Task Force on Alzheimer's Disease. *Neurology, 34,* 939–944.

Monsch, A. U., Bondi, M. W., Butters, N., Salmon, D. P., Katzman, R., & Thal, L. J. (1992). Comparisons of verbal fluency tasks in the detection of dementia of the Alzheimer type. *Archives of Neurology, 49,* 1253–1258.

Morris, J. C., & Fulling, K. (1988). Early Alzheimer's disease: Diagnostic considerations. *Archives of Neurology, 45,* 345–349.

Morris, J. C., Heyman, A., Mohs, R. C., Hughs, J. P., van Belle, G., Fillenbaum, G., Mellits, E. D., Clark, C., & the CERAD Investigators (1989). The Consortium to Establish a Registry for Alzheimer's Disease (CERAD). Pt. 1. Clinical and neuropsychological assessment of Alzheimer's disease. *Neurology, 39,* 1159–1165.

Mungas, D., Marshall, S. C., Weldon, M., Haan, M., & Reed, B. R. (1996). Age and education correction of Mini-Mental State Examination for English and Spanish-speaking elderly. *Neurology, 46,* 700–706.

Murden, R. A., McRae, T. D., Kaner, S., & Bucknam, M. E. (1991). Mini-Mental State Exam Scores Vary with Education in Blacks and Whites. *Journal of the American Geriatric Society, 39,* 149–155.

Prineas, R. J., Demirovic, J., Bean, J. A., Duara, R., Gomez-Marin, O., Loewenstein, D., Sevush, S., Stitt, F., & Szapocznik, J. (1995). South Florida Program on Aging and Health: Assessing the prevalence of Alzheimer's disease in three ethnic groups. *Journal of the Florida Medical Association, 82,* 805–810.

Rosen, W. G., Mohs, R. C., & David, K. L. (1984). A new rating scale for Alzheimer's disease. *American Journal of Psychiatry, 11,* 1356–1360.

Rubinstein, L., Schairer, C., Wieland, G., & Kane, R. (1984). Systematic biases is a functional status of elderly adults: Effects of different data sources. *Journal of Gerontology, 39,* 686–691.

Salmon, D. P., & Butters, N. M. (1992). Neuropsychological assessment of dementia in the elderly. In R. Katzman & J. W. Rowe (Eds.), *Principles of geriatric neurology* (pp. 144–163). Philadelphia: F. A. Davis.

Spreen, O., & Strauss, E. A compendium of neuropsychological tests: Administration, norms, and commentary. New York: Oxford University Press.

Storandt, M., Botwinick, J., Danziger, W. L., Berg, L., & Hughes, C. P. (1984). Psychometric differentiation of mild senile dementia of the Alzheimer type. *Archives of Neurology, 41,* 497–499.

Unverzagt, F. W., Hall, K. S., Torke, A. M., Rediger, J. D., Mercado, N., & Hendrie, H. C. (1994). *The CERAD neuropsychological test battery: Norms from an African-American sample.* Paper presented at the 22nd Annual Meeting of the International Neuropsychological Society, Cincinnati, OH.

Wechsler, D. (1968). *Escala de Inteligencia Wechsler para Adultos.* New York: Psychological Corporation.

Wechsler, D. (1981). *The Wechsler adult intelligence scale-revised.* New York: Psychological Corporation.

Wechsler, D., & Stone, C. (1945). *Wechsler Memory Scale.* New York: Psychological Corporation.

Weinberger, M., Samsa, G., Schmader, K., Greenberg, S., Carr, D., & Wildman, D. (1992). Comparing proxy and patients' perceptions of patients' functional status: Results from a geriatric outpatient clinic. *Journal of the American Geriatrics Society, 40,* 585–593.

Welsh, K. A., Butters, N., Hughes, J. P., Mohs, R., & Heyman, A. (1992). Detection of abnormal memory decline in mild cases of Alzheimer's disease using CERAD neuropsychological measures. *Archives of Neurology, 48,* 278–281.

Welsh, K. A., Fillenbaum, G., Wilkinson, W., Heyman, A., Mohs, R. C., Stern, Y., Harrell, L., Edland, S. D., & Beekly, D. (1995). Neuropsychological test performance in African-American and white patients with Alzheimer's disease. *Neurology, 45,* 2207–2211.

Zec, R. F. (1995). Neuropsychological functioning in Alzheimer's disease. In R. W. Parks, R. F. Zec, & R. S. Wilson (Eds.), *Neuropsychology of Alzheimer's disease and other dementias* (pp. 3–80). New York: Oxford University Press.

Zimmerman, S. I., & Magaziner, J. (1994). Methodological issues in measuring the functional status of cognitively impaired nursing home residents: The use of proxies and performance-based measures. *Alzheimer Disease and Associated Disorders, 8*(Suppl. 1), S281–S290.

CHAPTER 7

Uses of Neuroimaging Methods in the Diagnosis of Alzheimer's Disease Patients

Ranjan Duara

BACKGROUND

Alzheimer's disease (AD) is a degenerative disorder that presents insidiously with progressive alterations of memory and higher intellectual functions, along with the frequent development of a variety of psychiatric disorders. It is the classical example of a cortical dementia, although in the later stages of the disease, subcortical features also become evident (apathy and slowness of response), along with extrapyramidal signs (e.g., rigidity), gait apraxia, and incontinence. Neuropathologically, there are quantitative differences in Alzheimer's disease from what is seen in normal aging. These differences include marked neuronal loss, numerous senile plaques, and neurofibrillary tangles. These features, which are characteristic of AD, occur in the neocortex, the hippocampus and amygdala, and in many subcortical sites (Terry & Katzman, 1992).

The anatomical and functional effects of AD can be assessed qualitatively, as well as quantitatively, by neuroimaging methods. Imaging of the brain always should be considered an adjunct to the clinical evaluation of the patient and never a first-line method of evaluation. Used in their proper context, these methods can be valuable aids in the diagnosis of AD. Neuroimaging also has been important for furthering our understanding of the biology of AD.

The aims of this chapter are to present the salient contributions to clinical management and research in AD from four different neuroimaging methods, namely, computed X-ray tomography (CT), magnetic resonance imaging (MRI), positron emission tomography (PET), and single photon emission tomography (SPECT).

CT Studies in AD

At least 10 well-controlled CT scan studies have been done to evaluate morphological alterations affecting the ventricles and the sulci in Alzheimer's disease (see Table 7.1). These studies are consistent in demonstrating significant alterations, beyond those expected for age, in patients with even the early stages of AD. There is general agreement that for purposes of quantitation, linear measures are inferior to area or volumetric measures of ventricular enlargement. In assessing morphological changes of ventricle size and cortical atrophy, perceptual ratings by experienced observers have been shown to be sensitive and reliable (Le May et al., 1986). This last point is important from a clinical standpoint, as most neurologists or radiologists do not make detailed measurements routinely from CT scans. There is general agreement that CT scan linear measures of cortical atrophy, as assessed by increase in the subarachnoid space, are unreliable and insensitive to the changes in AD (De Carli, Kaye, Horwitz, & Rapoport, 1990; de Leon et al., 1980; Wu, Schenkenbert, Wing, & Osborn, 1981). Loss of gray-white matter discriminability in AD has been reported (George, de Leon, & Ferris, 1981) but has not yet been confirmed. CT measures of attenuation in Hounsfield or other units have not shown any consistent differences between AD and control subjects, although Albert, Naeser, Levine, and Garvey (1984) initially reported lower CT numbers in patients with senile dementia. A review of CT scan findings in aging and dementia reveals that volumetric analysis of the ventricle and subarachnoid space can achieve a sensitivity of 88% and a specificity of 90% in separating AD from control subjects (De Carli et al., 1990).

In spite of statistically significant greater ventricular and sulcal size in AD patients, compared to age-matched controls, the ability to discriminate

TABLE 7.1 CT Scan Studies of Alzheimer's Disease and Other Dementias

Author/Years[a]	Method of Measurement	Control N	Control xAge yrs.	Patient N	Patient xAge yrs.	Comments on Subjects[b]	Comments on Results[c]
Roberts & Caird, 1976	Maximum ventricular area and sulcal width measurement.	17	73 ±7	49	77 ±7	All patients considered to have degenerative dementia. Three grades of dementia.	Ventricular area enlarged in the demented but no difference in sulcal area. Correlation of $r = 0.49$ between maximum ventricular area and memory information test score.
Earnest et al., 1979	Width of sulci, linear ratios, and area of ventricles.	30	70 ±5	29	86 ±5	Not a true patient group; some were normals. Not a true control group; some were impaired.	Sulci and ventricles larger in the older and more impaired group. Correlation up to $r = 0.52$ between psychological measures and ventricular measures.

de Leon et al., 1980	Subjective ratings. Linear sulcal and ventricular measurements.	—	—	43	70 ±6	Detailed neurologic and psychiatric evaluation. All considered to have degenerative dementia.	65% of all correlations between ventricular rankings and psychiatric test scores were significant. Third ventricle width showed best correlations.	Subjective ranking or rating was superior to linear measurements.
Jacoby & Levy, 1980	Area of ventricle, Evan's ratio, and subjective rating of sulci.	50	73 ±6	40	79 ±7	All considered degenerative dementia (10 had cerebral infarcts on CT).	All measures showed highly significant differences between subject groups.	Highest correlations between ventricular area and memory. CT indices predicted group membership in 83% of cases.

(*continued*)

TABLE 7.1 (*continued*)

Author/Years[a]	Method of Measurement	Control N	Control xAge yrs.	Patient N	Patient xAge yrs.	Comments on Subjects[b]	Comments on Results[c]
Brinkman et al., 1981	Bifrontal and bicaudate ratios. Area of ventricles, distance from third ventricle to Sylvian Fissure (3V-SF), sulcal width measurement.	30	80 ±7	28	60 ±9	All considered degenerative dementia; (mild dementia: mean WAIS verbal IQ = 88.8). Patients significantly younger than controls.	No differences in bicaudate, bifrontal ratios. Age corrected ventricular area larger in the demented group; 3V-SF significantly less in demented group; sulcal width larger in controls.	Correlations between verbal and performance IQ and ventricular area/brain ratio was $r = 0.53$ and -0.65, respectively. 96% of demented patients and 41% of controls had abnormal findings for at least one measure.

| Ito et al., 1981 | Pixel counts of cranial volume, CSF volume and brain volume. | 130 | 20–79 | Although all subjects were described as normal, some demented patients were clearly included. Patients were not separated from controls. Significant increase in CSF volume and decrease in brain volume with age. Brain volume was correlated with a mental status score ($r = 0.43$) |

(continued)

TABLE 7.1 (*continued*)

Author/Years[a]	Method of Measurement	Control N	Control xAge yrs.	Patient N	Patient xAge yrs.	Comments on Subjects[b]	Comments on Results[c]
Wu et al., 1981	Linear measurements and subjective rating of ventricular and sulcal size.	31	50–77	24	50–77	Controls has neurological symptoms, were not demented, and had no focal lesions on CT. Patients were not separated in any of the analyses.	Highest correlation between CT and behavioral measures was that of orientation and bicaudate-index ($r = 0.52$). With the exception of the sulcal measurement, all other CT measures correlated significantly with at least one behavioral measures.
Gado et al., 1982	Pixel counts for ventricles, subarachnoid space, and cranial cavity. Linear indices and subjective ratings also obtained.	27	65–83	20	65–81	Controls described as healthy. Patients clinically diagnosed to have mild Alzheimer's disease.	Volumetric measures were clearly better than linear measures in separating demented patients from controls, though both gave significant results for ventricular and subarachnoid space. An unspecified degree of overlap was found between controls and patients using any of the CT measures.

176

| Wilson et al., 1982 | Linear and subjective ratings of ventricular sulcal size. CT density measures in 14 brain regions. | 38 | 69 | 42 | 69 | Controls were healthy. All patients were clinically diagnosed to have Alzheimer's disease. | On a composite score, patients had more atrophy than controls. High degree of overlap was noted between groups (not quantified). None of the CT density measures was different between groups. | Wechsler Memory Scale scores were correlated with atrophy ($r = 0.39$) only for the combined patient and control group. |

(continued)

TABLE 7.1 (*continued*)

Author/Years[a]	Method of Measurement	Control N	Control xAge yrs.	Patient N	Patient xAge yrs.	Comments on Subjects[b]	Comments on Results[c]
Le May et al., 1986 (41)	Perceptual ratings (0–4 scale) for atrophy in 13 regions by three neuroradiologists, and linear measurements.	22	65	24	67	Healthy controls. Patients were all diagnosed to have AD, but degree of dementia was not stated.	Perceptual rating, which was superior to linear measures, correctly classified over 80% of subjects. Specific temporal lobe atrophic changes discriminated up to 90% of subjects.	The size of the suprasellar cistern, the width of the interhemispheric fissure, and the Sylvian fissure were the best discriminators.

Note:
[a]References are included in the bibliography.
[b]Points to be emphasized regarding controls and patients.
[c]Points to be emphasized regarding the results.

between these two subject groups depends on the stage of the illness. In the early stage of AD, a great deal of overlap exists between normal and AD patients in the degree of brain atrophy. Many cognitively normal elderly subjects have enlargement of ventricles or relatively prominent cortical atrophy, and many patients with mild AD have unimpressive atrophic features. The history, examination, and assessment of the behavior of the patient remain the most important evidence in determining the presence of dementia. In spite of the poor separation of the findings in normal aging and AD, the CT scan is of great utility in excluding certain causes of dementia other than AD (e.g., multi-infarct dementia, cerebral tumor, subdural hematoma, normal pressure hydrocephalus). See Figures 7.1 and 7.2.

CT scan studies have demonstrated a gross overall relationship between quantitative measures of loss of brain tissue and behavioral deterioration.

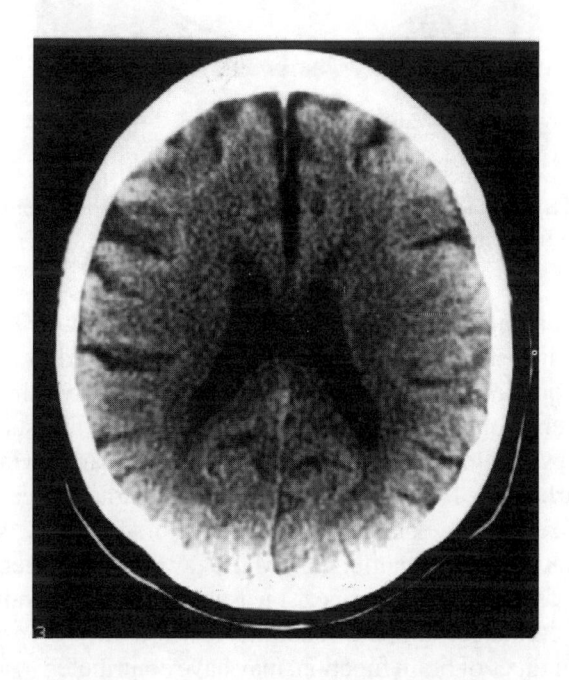

FIGURE 7.1 Alzheimer's disease: CT Scan at level of lateral ventricles, which are mildly enlarged. The sulci are moderately enlarged. There is no detectable periventricular leukomalacia (Note: Such a scan could be seen in normal elderly individuals).

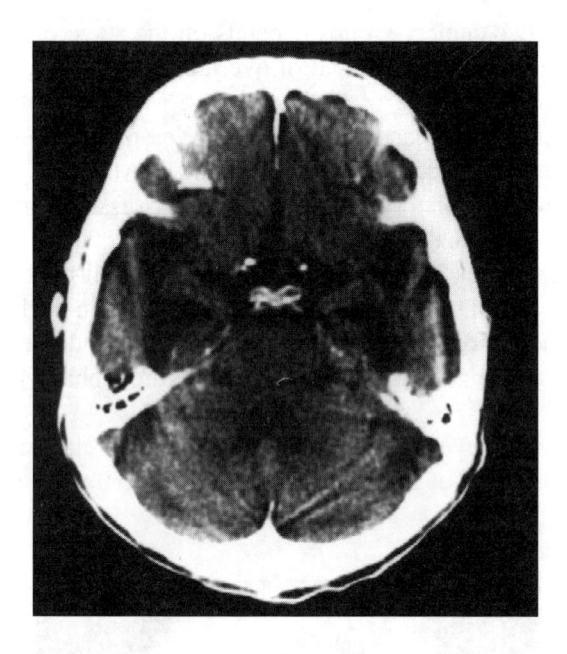

FIGURE 7.2 Alzheimer's disease: CT scan at level of inferior temporal lobe. Note enlarged Sylvian fissures, severely enlarged temporal horns of lateral ventricles, and prominent interuncal space.

However, brain atrophy does not explain more than 40% to 45% of the variance in behavioral measures. For example, studies of demented patients, or combined normal and demented patients, have shown correlation coefficients of 0.29 to 0.65 between CT scan measures of brain atrophy and psychological function (Brinkman, Sarwar, Levin, & Morris, 1981; De Carli et al., 1990; de Leon et al., 1980; Earnest, Heaton, Wilkinson, & Manke, 1979; Eslinger, Damasio, Graff-Radford, & Damasio, 1984; Ito, Hatazawa, Yamamura, & Matsuzawa, 1981). Methodological factors, such as the validity of linear measurements in the brain as indices of volumetric change, and the reliability and validity of psychological measures as indices of brain function, may have contributed to a weakening of these morphology-behavior correlations.

Longitudinal CT scan studies in AD patients have obtained consistent results (Burns, Jacoby, & Levy, 1991; de Leon et al., 1989; Luxenberg, Haxby, Creasey, Sundaram, & Rapoport, 1987). There is a significantly greater rate of increase of ventricular size over time in AD patients, compared to normal controls. In one study, the annual rate of change in ventricular volume was 9% in AD patients and 2% in controls (de Leon et al., 1989). The rate of change in ventricle size correlated with the rate of deterioration in neuropsychological scores. The initial size of the ventricles did not predict the subsequent rate of clinical deterioration in these patients (Burns et al., 1991; de Leon et al., 1989).

Behavioral heterogeneity in AD is well known (Botwinick, Storandt, & Berg, 1986; Mayeaux, Stern, & Spanton, 1985). Associations of behavioral subtypes of AD with the rate of progression of the disease or genetic forms of the disease have been described (Breitner & Folstein, 1984; Chui, Teng, Henderson, & Moy, 1985). The relationship of any of these behavioral subtypes to specific neuroimaging-neuroanatomical features would be of great interest, but remains to be defined. For example, asymmetry of ventricles and of cortical atrophy in AD has not been alluded to in any of the quantitative studies described in Table 7.1. In a review of CT changes in dementing diseases, LeMay et al. (1986) single out only Pick's disease as showing asymmetrical atrophy. In clinical practice and at autopsy, obvious asymmetry of ventricles and of cortical atrophy is observed in some patients with probable AD (Giannakapoulos, Hof, & Boures, 1994).

Comparing patients with AD to patients with vascular dementia, the CT scan findings that predicted vascular dementia were the presence of left subcortical infarcts, severe periventricular leukomalacia (PVL), and enlargement of the third ventricle (Charletta, Gorelick, Dollear, Freels, & Harris, 1995). However, in recent CT and MR scan studies, it has been emphasized that changes in periventricular white matter occur frequently in cases clinically diagnosed as having AD (Englund, Brun, & Persson, 1987; Erkinjuntti et al., 1987; Fazekas, Chawluk, Alavi, Hurtig, & Zimmerman, 1987; George et al., 1986; Goto, Ishii, & Fukasawa, 1981; Leys et al., 1990; Scheltens et al., 1992; Steingart et al., 1987). These periventricular lucencies in the white matter are more common in demented subjects than in age-matched controls (Englund & Brun, 1990; George et al., 1986; Scheltens et al., 1995). In CT scan studies, they occur in about 30% of AD patients and in 75% to 97% of vascular dementia patients (Stoppe, Staedt, & Bruhn, 1995). Patients with late age-of-onset AD more frequently have periventricular leukomalacia (76%) than patients with early age-of-onset AD (25%); patients with elevated systolic blood pressure also have more frequent PVLs (Blennow, Wallin, Uhlemann, &

Gottfries, 1991). Therefore, the presence of these lesions cannot be used to distinguish between AD and vascular dementia.

When patients with AD are classified on the basis of the occurrence of PVLs on CT scans, those with PVLs perform worse on cognitive tests than those without (Steingart et al., 1987). EEG abnormalities correlate with the presence of PVLs (Lopez, Brenner, et al., 1995). AD patients with CT determined PVLs also are more likely to have confusional symptoms, gait disorders, urinary incontinence, asymmetric neurological signs, and extensor plantar responses (Blennow et al., 1991; Lopez, Becker, 1995; Meguro et al., 1994). See Figure 7.3.

Many patients with clinical features of AD and with lucencies on CT have been found at autopsy to have AD (Englund et al., 1987; George et al., 1986; Leifer, Buonanno, & Richardson, 1990; Lotz, Ballinger, & Quisling, 1986; Meguro et al., 1994; Wade et al., 1987; Zahner, Lang, Englehardt, Theirauf, & Neundorfer, 1995). Corresponding to the white

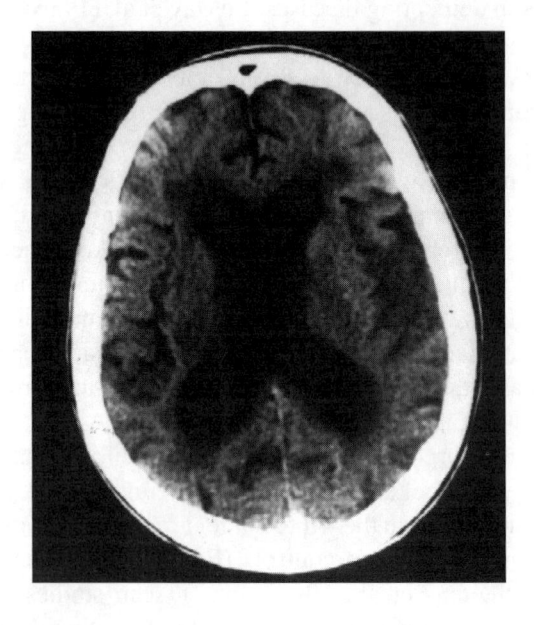

FIGURE 7.3 Alzheimer's disease: CT scan at level of the lateral ventricles, which are grossly enlarged. Sulci are also prominent. Periventricular lucency is evident in the region of the frontal and occipital horns of the lateral ventricles.

matter lucencies demonstrated on CT scans of AD patients, pathological abnormalities that have been described in these brain regions include demyelination, axonal loss, denudation of the ventricular lining, hyalinization and fibrous thickening of medullary arterioles and cystic degeneration (George et al., 1986; Leifer et al., 1990; Scheltens et al., 1995).

The blood-brain barrier permeability has been investigated in AD patients because of suspicions that the etiology of this disease may, in part, be related to disruption in this barrier (Glenner, 1985; Hardy, Mann, Webster, & Weinblad, 1986). In AD patients and age-matched controls, rapid, dynamic CT scanning of the brain, after injection of iodinated contrast material to investigate the blood-brain barrier, failed to reveal any significant differences in the washout curves in these two groups of subjects (Dysken, Nelson, Hoover, Kuskowski, & McGeachie, 1990). This study, therefore, failed to demonstrate any blood-brain barrier disruption in AD patients.

MRI Studies

MRI is more sensitive than CT to many AD-related changes (Erkinjuntti et al., 1987; George et al., 1986; Jack et al., 1987). The abnormalities that are especially amenable to definition by MRI are atrophic changes in specific neuroanatomical locations, as well as alterations in periventricular and subcortical white matter. Examples are atrophy of gray-matter structures, such as the hippocampus and amygdala, and enlargement of basal cisterns and the Sylvian fissure (Jack et al., 1987).

Volumetric studies of cerebro-spinal fluid (CSF) space, lateral and third ventricle size, and gray-matter volume have shown significant age-associated changes, especially in the caudate nucleus and anterior thalamus (Coffey et al., 1992; Jernigan, Salmon, Butters, & Hesselink, 1991; Murphy, DeCarli, Schapiro, Rapoport, & Horwitz, 1992). Comparisons of these volumes in age-matched controls and AD patients show significant atrophy of cortical and subcortical gray-matter structures, but not of the white matter in AD patients (Grundman, Corey-Bloom, Jernigan, Archibald, & Thal, 1996). However, the corpus callosum and its various subdivisions have been measured in AD patients, and a reduction in the area of the genu (Biegon, 1994) and the entire corpus callosum (Janowsky, Kaye, & Carper, 1996; Yoshii & Duara, 1989), compared to age-matched controls, has been found. This atrophy is correlated with cognitive deterioration (Janowsky et al.). See Figures 7.4, 7.5, and 7.6.

A number of studies have shown that the volume of the hippocampus is reduced in AD patients, compared to age-matched controls (Convit et al., 1995; Desmond et al., 1994; Deweer et al., 1995; Grundman et al., 1996; Jack, Petersen, O'Brien, & Tangalos, 1992; Killiany et al., 1993; Lehericy et al., 1994; Rusinek et al., 1991; Seab et al., 1988). In patients who are suspected of having incipient AD, but have insufficient cognitive impairment to meet the criteria for dementia, the hippocampal volume was found to be significantly less than in age-matched normal controls (de Leon et al., 1996; Parnetti et al., 1996).

A highly significant correlation, independent of age, gender, and generalized cerebral atrophy, was found between delayed memory performance and the size of the hippocampal formation in AD patients (Golomb et

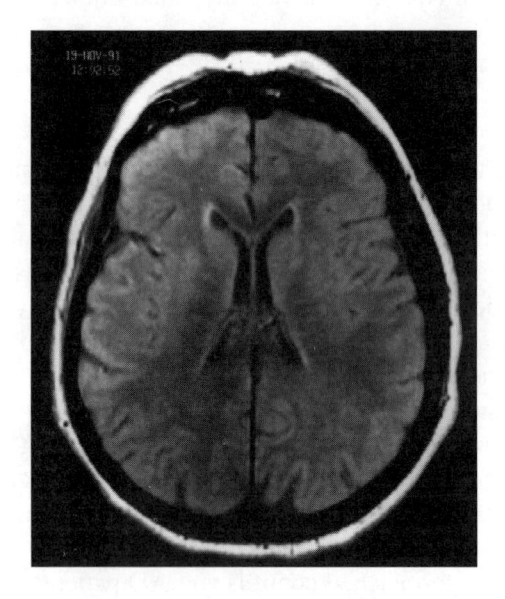

FIGURE 7.4 MRI of normal elderly individual (T_2 weighted proton density image at level of lateral ventricles). The sulci are narrow and the ventricles are small. Periventricular high signal intensity is seen capping the frontal horns.

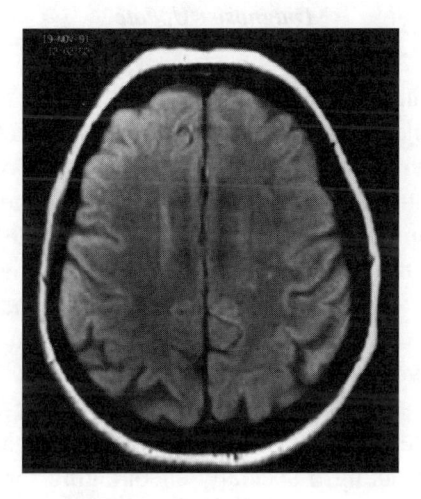

FIGURE 7.5 MRI of Alzheimer's disease patient (T$_2$ weighted proton density image at level above the lateral ventricles). The sulci are enlarged in the parietal-occipital region.

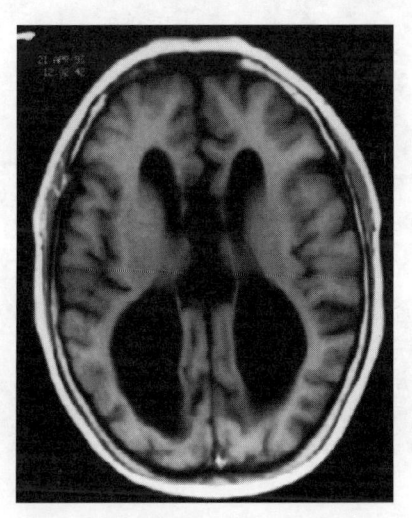

FIGURE 7.6 MRI of Alzheimer's disease patient (T$_1$ weighted image at level of lateral ventricles). There is severe enlargement of the occipital horns of the lateral ventricles. This patient presented with features of Balint's syndrome, including severe visual agnosia, as well as mild to moderate memory impairment.

al., 1994). A longitudinal study has shown that the size of the hippocampal formation at baseline, in normal elderly subjects, predicts change in memory scores at follow-up, approximately 4 years later (Golomb et al., 1996). Low body weight in AD patients also has been found to correlate with greater mesial temporal atrophy (Grundman et al., 1996).

The ε4 allele of the apolipoprotein E gene is associated with a heightened risk for AD. Soininen et al. (1995) reported that in nondemented elderly carrying the apolipoprotein E ε4 allele, the usual right larger than left hippocampal volume asymmetry was reduced, suggesting relative right hippocampal atrophy in this group. See Figures 7.7 to 7.10.

It should be noted that the measurement of hippocampal volumes is both tedious and exacting. Especially encouraging for the clinician who

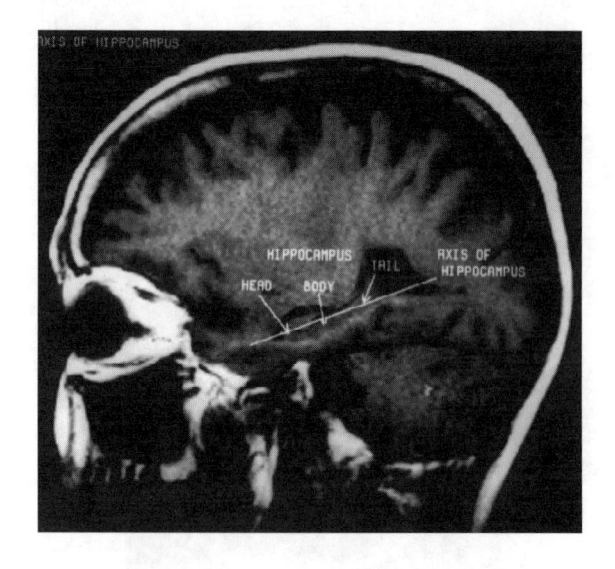

FIGURE 7.7* MRI of an Alzheimer's disease patient (T_1 weighted image in the sagittal plane). The image shows the medial temporal lobe and the anterior-posterior axis of the hippocampal formation.

*Courtesy of Brian Bowen, M.D., Ph.D., and Daniel Erdman, M.D., Department of Radiology, University of Miami School of Medicine, Miami, Florida.

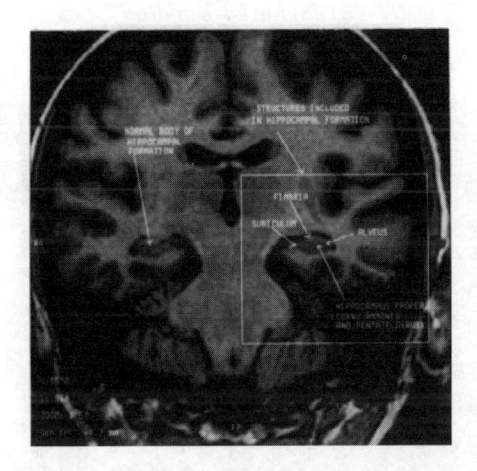

FIGURE 7.8* MRI in the coronal plane of a normal elderly individual (T_1 weighted image at level of middle cerebellar peduncle). The image shows normal hippocampal structures at the level of the body of the hippocampus.

*Courtesy of Brian Bowen, M.D., Ph.D., and Daniel Erdman, M.D., Department of Radiology, University of Miami School of Medicine, Miami, Florida.

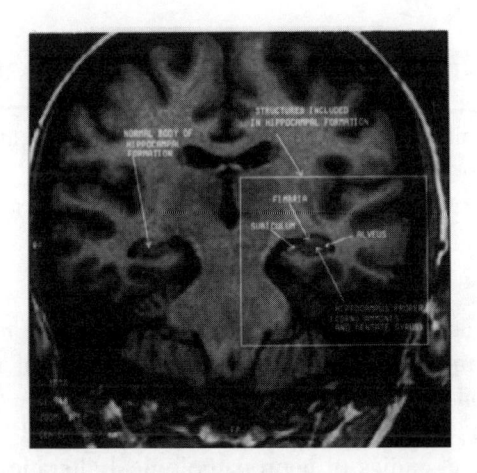

FIGURE 7.9* MRI in the coronal plane of an Alzheimer's disease patient (T_1 weighted image at level of the middle of cerebellar peduncle). The image shows generalized atrophy of the brain, including hippocampal atrophy. A region of interest (ROI) has been drawn around the body of the right hippocampus.

*Courtesy of Brian Bowen, M.D., Ph.D., and Daniel Erdman, M.D., Department of Radiology, University of Miami School of Medicine, Miami, Florida.

188 *Diagnosis: Update*

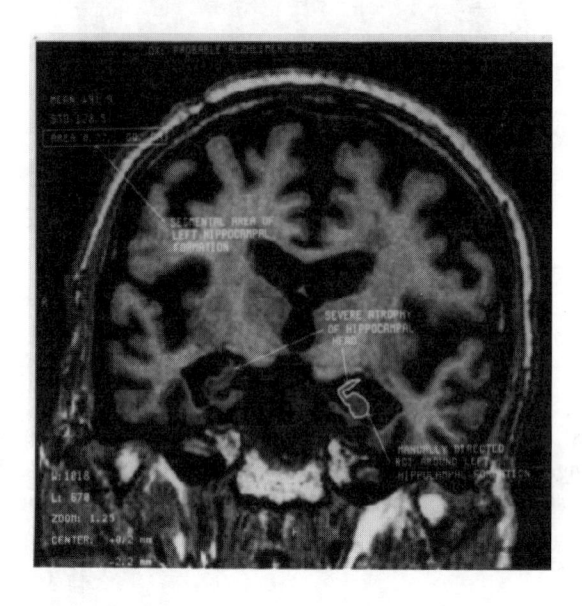

FIGURE 7.10* MRI in the coronal plane of an Alzheimer's disease patient (T_1 weighted image at the level of the hippocampus). There is severe generalized atrophy of the brain and severe atrophy of the head of the hippocampus, with an ROI drawn around the left hippocampal head.

*Courtesy of Brian Bowen, M.D., Ph.D. and Daniel Erdman, M.D., Department of Radiology, University of Miami School of Medicine, Miami, Florida.

has neither the access to the technology, nor the time to do volumetric studies, is the finding that simple visual assessment of mesial temporal structures demonstrated a sensitivity/specificity of 92%/93% for distinguishing AD patients from controls (Desmond et al., 1994).

Comprehensive studies of neuropathological alterations and postmortem MR relaxation times of white matter in patients with AD (Englund et al., 1987) have demonstrated that "incomplete white-matter infarction" is encountered in up to 60% of patients. This infarction is characterized by loss of myelin, axons, and oligodendrogial cells, mild reactive astrocytic gliosis, and hyaline fibrosis of arterioles in the deep white matter. These pathological changes gradually decrease in severity as the cortex is approached. In parallel to these pathological changes, prolongation of T_1

and T_2 relaxation times occurs. The MR imaging characteristics that would correspond to these T_1 and T_2 changes would be decreased signal intensity in T_1 weighted, and increased intensity in T_2, weighted images in a predominantly periventricular distribution. Erkinjuntti et al. (1987) noted that the MRI showed periventricular "white-matter changes" in about one third of their cases with AD, but did not report results in normal controls. It is not known, therefore, whether these periventricular changes were in excess of that expected for age. Bowen, Barker, Loewenstein, Sheldon, and Duara (1990) compared 87 patients with probable and possible Alzheimer's disease to 36 age-matched controls and showed a roughly twofold increase in periventricular lesions and a fivefold increase in subcortical white-matter lesions in AD subjects.

A study by Fazekas et al. (1987) described MRI findings in patients with clinically diagnosed probable Alzheimer's disease and compared them with patients diagnosed to have multi-infarct dementia. A "halo" of periventricular hyperintensity was found frequently in AD patients. This halo is characterized by a smooth margin and is significantly more extensive than the hyperintensity found in controls. See Figures 7.11 and 7.12.

Another type of lesion outside of the immediate periventricular area are punctate or partially confluent deep white-matter foci of hyperintensity, which are fairly frequently found in controls, AD, and MID patients. The existence of these foci, therefore, does not necessarily imply vascular dementia. On the other hand, in the study by Fazekas et al. (1987), extensive, irregular periventricular hyperintensity and widespread confluent areas of deep white-matter hyperintensity were found only in multi-infarct or mixed dementia. Since these patients were not confirmed to have AD or MID by pathological examination, the validity of these results is not clear.

Nevertheless, the MRI appearance of typical Binswanger's disease has been demonstrated in patients with pathological evidence of AD alone (Meguro et al., 1994; Zahner et al., 1995). Scheltens et al. (1992) found that periventricular, lobar white matter, and basal ganglia hyperintensities were more frequently found in senile-onset (onset at 65+ years), but not presenile-onset AD patients, than in age-matched normal control subjects. All the subjects in this study had been screened carefully for cerebrovascular risk factors. In a follow-up study by this group (Scheltens et al., 1995), the histopathologic correlates of postmortem MRI changes were investigated. The AD brains displayed significantly more white-matter

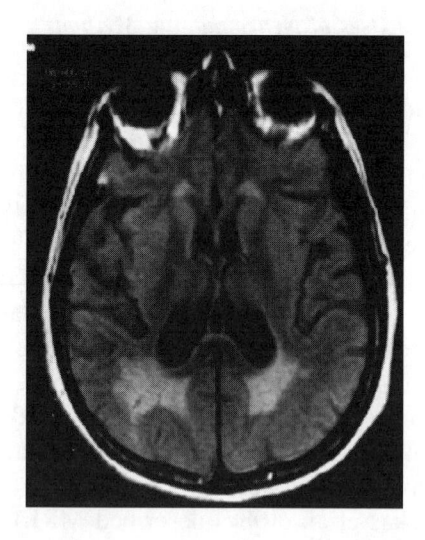

FIGURE 7.11 MRI of Alzheimer's disease patient (T_2 weighted proton density image). There is mild to moderate lateral ventricle and sulcal enlargement and prominent high signal intensity in the periventricular area adjacent to occipital horns.

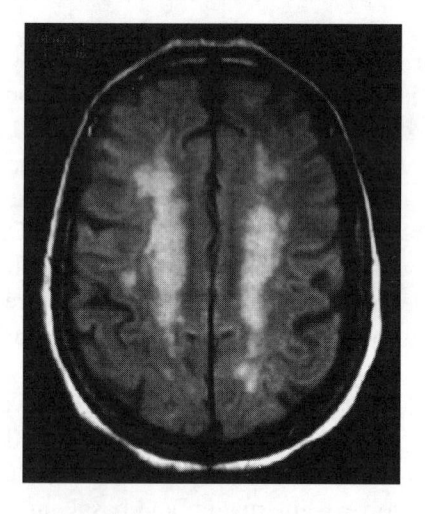

FIGURE 7.12 MRI of Alzheimer's disease patient (T_2 weighted proton density image at level above the lateral ventricles). The sulci are enlarged, and there is extensive high signal intensity in the centrum semiovale bilaterally.

hyperintensities on MRI than the controls. These hyperintensities correlated with loss of myelinated axons in the deep white matter, and denudation of the ventricular lining. Although these authors could find no evidence of arteriosclerosis, the mean thickness of the adventitia of the arteries of the deep white matter in AD patients was twice that in controls, suggesting a vascular element in the etiology of these MRI hyperintensities (Scheltens et al., 1995).

The high sensitivity of MRI for detecting changes in the white matter of the brain can lead to diagnostic confusion. The profusion of abnormalities seen on MRI often leaves the clinician unable to categorize a patient because the distinguishing MRI features between normal aging, Alzheimer's disease and multi-infarct dementia are not currently known. The additional information contributed by MRI studies in AD patients has resulted in enhanced sensitivity to pathology, but in a decreased specificity of diagnosis (Lopez, Becker, et al., 1995). Current studies suggest a continuum of white-matter signal abnormalities in AD and vascular dementia, without evidence of a bimodal distribution and with considerable overlap between the groups. The preceding reports show that the increase in the high signal intensity area in the vicinity of the ventricles can be associated with Alzheimer's disease alone, without any component of vascular dementia.

Both CT and MRI are used primarily for excluding other causes of dementia in the diagnosis of Alzheimer's disease. MRI is more sensitive, but CT is more specific for detecting vascular disease that may be causing dementia or contributing to the cause of dementia. Nevertheless, both CT and MRI should be used as adjuncts to clinical findings in making the diagnosis. With respect to visualizing some of the early atrophic changes that occur in AD, MRI is the most sensitive and specific tool available to the clinician at this time.

FUNCTIONAL MRI

MRI can be used to study the functioning brain in several ways:

1. Blood flow to the brain can be studied using a nonradioactive contrast agent with MRI indirectly, by measuring changes in regional cerebral blood volume, which correlates with blood flow.

2. The changes in regional cerebral volume of oxyhemoglobin in response to cognitive or other types of stimulation can be measured simply by utilizing the signal characteristics of oxyhemoglobin, which is distinct from that of deoxyhemoglobin. This technique has not yet been used to study AD.
3. Magnetic resonance spectroscopy can be used to study the concentration in the brain of several metabolically active or informative compounds.

Contrast MRI Studies

This technique has been used only recently to study AD. A relatively small study of AD and control subjects showed that the cerebral blood volume in the temporoparietal areas was reduced by 17% in AD patients (Harris et al., 1996).

Magnetic Resonance Spectroscopy Studies

MR proton (1H NMR) spectroscopic studies have been utilized to measure N-Acetyl L-aspartic acid (NAA) levels, myoinositol (MI), creatine, phosphocreatine, and choline levels in the brains of AD patients and age-matched controls. NAA is a neuronal marker and its levels decrease, whereas MI, which is a membrane phosphotidylinositol product, increases in the cortex of AD patients (Christiansen, Schlosser, & Henriksen, 1995; Klunk, Panchalingam, Moossy, McClure, & Pettegrew, 1992; Shonk et al., 1995). NAA also declines in other degenerative and vascular dementias, but MI increases seem to be more specific to AD (Shonk et al.). A recent study has demonstrated the regional effects of changes in NAA signal intensities in frontal, temporal, and parietal cortices, and of choline signal in the white matter (Tedeschi et al., 1996).

MR 31P spectroscopic studies have been used to study phosphomonoesters (PME), which are precursors, and phosphodiesters (PDE), which are breakdown products of membrane phospholipids. The low signal to noise ratio in all human 31P spectroscopic studies has resulted in studies with poor spatial resolution and, therefore, very restricted data about regional findings. Although the results from different laboratories are not consistent, PME levels appear to increase in the early stages of AD and Pick's disease, whereas in the late stages, PME levels decline and PDE and inorganic phosphorus levels increase (Cuenod et al., 1995; McClure,

Kanfer, Panchalingham, Klunk, & Pettegrew, 1994; Pettegrew, Panchalingham, Klunk, McClure, & Muenze, 1994; Smith, Gallenstein, Layton, Kryscio, Markesbery, 1993). Phosphocreatine/inorganic phosphorus ratios, also measured by 31P spectroscopy, give an index of the energy state of the brain. These studies also have given inconsistent results (Brown et al., 1989; Smith et al., 1995).

Functional MRI shows great promise as a diagnostic aid and a research tool for evaluating dementing diseases. Magnets with field strengths of 1.5 Tesla, or greater, can be used for functional MRI studies, provided that they are designed for three-dimensional acquisition of data, and have the software for obtaining the appropriate MRI sequences and data analyses. A major asset in MRI is the ability to acquire, within a few seconds or minutes, corresponding high-resolution anatomical information for the functional data that are obtained. In the next decade, MRI is likely to overtake all other diagnostic imaging modalities for studying both anatomy and function of the brain.

PET SCAN STUDIES

Although gross morphological changes in the brain in the early stages of Alzheimer's disease are subtle and variable, as judged by CT and MR scanning, alterations in function are more evident. Because a variety of functional alterations in the brain can be examined using PET and SPECT, these methods should be ideal in depicting abnormalities very early in the course of Alzheimer's disease. Moreover, function of the brain can be evaluated under a variety of behavioral and pharmacologic conditions. The optimal condition for depicting functional abnormalities in AD may vary according to the subtype or stage of the disease. For example, patients with subtle degrees of aphasia may need a verbal activation task to maximize functional imaging abnormalities.

Many studies have been done in the "resting state" to study Alzheimer's disease by PET (Alavi et al., 1986; Benson et al., 1983; Chase et al., 1984; Cutler et al., 1985; de Leon et al., 1983; Duara et al., 1986; Ferris et al., 1980; Foster et al., 1983; Frackowiak, Lenzi, Jones, & Heather, 1981; Friedland et al., 1983b; Friedland, Budinger, Brant-Zawadzki, & Jagust, 1984; Haxby et al., 1986; Haxby, Duara, Grady, Cutler, & Rapoport, 1985; Kuhl et al., 1985; Loewenstein et al., 1989; McGeer, Kamo, Harrop, et al., 1986a). With the exception of a study by Frackowiak et al. (1981), who used [0-15] labeled molecular oxygen and carbon dioxide to study cerebral blood flow, oxygen extraction ratio, and oxygen consumption, all the other studies have been done using [F-18] labeled fluorodeoxyglucose (FDG). The earlier studies (Benson et al., 1983; de Leon et al., 1983; de Leon et al., 1984; Ferris et al., 1980; Frackowiak et al., 1981) focused on alterations in absolute metabolic rate in AD patients, whereas in later studies, the regional pattern of change in metabolism has been examined (Duara et al., 1986; Duara, Barker, Loewenstein, Pascal, & Bowen, 1989; Foster et al., 1984; Friedland, Brun, & Budinger, 1985; Kumar, Schapiro, & Grady, 1991; McGeer, Kamo, McGeer, et al., 1986).

In general, an inverse correlation has been found between absolute metabolic rates and the severity of dementia; that is, the more severe the dementia, the lower the global glucose and oxygen metabolic rates and the cerebral blood flow. The extent of reduction in metabolic rate in severe dementia has been reported to be from 31% (Frackowiak et al., 1981) to 49% (Benson et al., 1983). In the mild and moderate stages of AD, however, often no significant reduction in global absolute metabolic rate has been found (Cutler et al., 1985; Duara et al., 1986; Haxby et al., 1986).

Many investigators have reported regional alterations in metabolic rate in AD. A pattern consistently found in AD is one of regional deficits in the association neocortices (e.g., parietotemporal, prefrontal) and relative sparing of primary sensory and motor cortices, such as peri-Rolandic and medial occipital, as well as the basal ganglia, thalamus, and cerebellar hemispheres (Duara et al., 1986; Kippenhan, Barker, Pascal, Nagel, & Duara, 1992; Kippenhan, Barker, Nagel, Grady, & Duara, 1994). Association cortex hypometabolism in AD has often been reported to affect parietotemporal regions to a greater extent and earlier in the course of the disease than frontal regions. However, many exceptions to this pattern have been found (Duara et al., 1989).

Although asymmetrical metabolic deficits could be expected to be a feature of multi-infarct dementia (Benson et al., 1983), metabolic asymmetry can appear early in the disease course in AD patients and predict the pattern of "neocortically mediated" neuropsychological deficits that will evolve (Haxby et al., 1986). Patients with predominant language deficits have been reported to manifest predominant left-sided metabolic deficits, whereas those with predominant visuoconstructive deficits, manifest predominant right-sided metabolic deficits (Chase et al., 1984; Foster et al., 1984; Haxby et al., 1985).

Several longitudinal PET studies of AD patients have been done. These have been summarized by Smith et al. (1992), who found in their own cohort of 14 AD patients that deficits seen initially, in temporoparietal regions, showed further deficits over a 2- to 3-year period. The reduction in regional glucose metabolism was greater than would be expected for the degree of atrophy that was seen on longitudinally performed CT scans by this group of investigators. Jagust, Haan, Eberling, Wolfe, and Reed (1996) reported that posterior temporal lobe and medial occipital lobe metabolism at initial evaluation best predicted the future rate of cognitive decline over a 2 1/2-year period.

In Down's syndrome patients, who are known invariably to have the neuropathology of AD by the age of 40 (Wisniewski, Wisniewski, & Wen, 1985), metabolic deficits similar to those described in AD have been found to occur (Shapiro et al., 1988). In other groups of patients who belong to families in which multiple members have been affected with AD, parietal metabolic deficits have been found in asymptomatic individuals who are known to be carrying two copies of the e4 allele of the apolipoprotein E gene. These metabolic deficits have been known to be present years before the subjects are at the age of onset of AD in that family (Reiman et al., 1996; Small et al., 1995).

The pathophysiology of the metabolic deficits in AD has been the source of some speculation. Pathology in the neocortical association areas in parietal, temporal, and frontal regions may give rise to the metabolic deficits in these same regions. Evidence in support of this hypothesis is that the distribution of neuronal loss in the neocortex of AD patients is similar to the distribution of metabolic deficits, particularly in the early stages of the disease (Brun & Englund, 1981; Friedland et al., 1985). Conversely, metabolic deficits in brain regions remote from those in which the major pathological abnormalities occur could be explained by transneuronal, functional, disconnection (diaschisis) effects. The lack of prominent metabolic deficits in the medial temporal cortex (Foster, Hansen, Siegel, & Kuhl, 1988; Jagust et al., 1993), where the pathology is known to be most severe in early AD, and the presence of the most prominent deficits in the association neocortex, supports this hypothesis. It has been reported that in 11 AD patients with very mild dementia, metabolism in the lateral temporal neocortex, but not in the medial temporal region, was lower than in controls; however, this pattern was variable, with more severely memory-impaired patients and older patients showing a trend toward greater medial temporal deficits (Jagust, 1994). Degeneration in basal forebrain nuclei or in amygdala-hippocampal regions, both of which are known to project heavily on the association neocortex, could result in disconnection of and hypometabolism in neocortical regions.

Another cause of regional hypometabolism, especially in cortical regions, is that regional brain atrophy can result in apparently reduced metabolism, because of what is known as the partial volume effect (Chawluk et al., 1987; Herscovitch, Auchua, Gado, Chi, & Raichle, 1986). Ideally, regional metabolic or blood flow values from individual scans should be corrected for the effects of regional atrophy. These partial volume effects have been found to be responsible for a substantial part (but not all) of the measured metabolic or blood flow reduction in AD patients (Alavi, Newberg, Souder, & Berlin, 1993; Schlageter, Carson, & Rapoport, 1987; Tanna et al., 1991). Labbé, Froment, Kennedy, Ashburner, and Cinotti (1996) have described a method for regional correction of brain glucose metabolic values for the effects of atrophy, using superimposed MRI scans, segmented into gray matter, white matter, and cerebrospinal fluid. They found that global cortical metabolism increased by 24% in controls and 65% in patients, after correction for atrophy; the difference between controls and AD patients decreased from 31% before correction to 17% after correction. Using similar methods, Meltzer et al. (1996) reported that correction for atrophy reduced the extent of metabolic deficits in AD patients, but significant hypometabolism persisted in frontal, posterior, temporal, and parietal regions and that correlation coefficients between neuropsychological and metabolic measures were reduced once atrophy correction had been done.

The accuracy by which PET data can be used to classify patients with AD as normal or abnormal has been investigated. Kippenhan et al. (1994) evaluated a high resolution camera (6 mm, full width at half maximum) to a low resolution camera (15 mm, full width at half maximum) and found, using a neural network classifier, that overall correct classification was 87% with the low resolution, and 95% with the high resolution camera. The profile that best discriminated AD subjects from controls was the findings of low parietal and temporal and high sensory-motor and occipital metabolism. Herholz et al. (1993) compared the diagnostic accuracy of PET studies for detecting AD in three different European centers, all using the same index of abnormality, namely, the ratio of the most affected region to the least affected region. The results across the centers were consistent, with an average accuracy of 96%. Minoshima, Frey, Koeppe, Foster, and Kuhl (1995) used three-dimensional stereotactic surface projections of high resolution PET data and were able to discriminate AD patients from normal controls with a sensitivity of 95% to 97%, and specificity of 100%.

Very few studies have reported on the correlation of antemortem metabolic deficits to postmortem neuropathological findings. McGeer, Kamo, and McGreer (1986b) reported on a single case of AD in which antemortem PET scan findings of glucose metabolism were correlated with postmortem neuropathological findings. On gross pathology, the left hemisphere, especially in the parietal regions, showed far greater atrophic changes than the right. Metabolism was also reduced asymmetrically with predominant left hemisphere hypometabolism. Reduced metabolism correlated best with severity of gliosis and least with the number of plaques in the brain area. In another study, it was reported that the density of neurofibrillary tangles, but not of senile plaques, correlated with regional glucose metabolic rates in AD patients (De Carli et al., 1992).

PET has been used to study the blood-brain barrier in AD. Friedland et al. (1983a) and Schlageter, Carson, et al. (1987) both studied the blood-brain barrier using PET methodology, but neither detected any evidence of disruption of the barrier by the methods used.

Behavioral activation studies in AD patients (Duara et al., 1987b; Miller et al., 1987) have not as yet yielded any results that have improved the diagnostic ability of PET scans to detect AD. These studies demonstrate that hypometabolic regions in the brain, in AD patients, are metabolically viable. Cerebral blood flow studies have also demonstrated a similar result (Berman & Weinberger, 1986). Increases in metabolic rates have been found to occur in areas of reduced metabolism in response to behavioral activation, with a tendency for these regions to normalize rather than appear more abnormal (Duara et al., 1992).

Receptor binding studies with PET, using a peripheral benzodiazepine receptor ligand that binds actively to microglia, has shown no increases in binding, suggesting that microgliosis in AD is undetectable with current technology (Groom, Junck, Foster, Frey, & Kuhl, 1995).

SPECT Studies

Several SPECT imaging studies have been reported thus far in Alzheimer's patients, with either I^{123} labeled iodoamphetamine or ^{99m}Tc labeled HMPAO used to obtain measures of cerebral blood flow. These studies have demonstrated the same distribution of deficits as are evident on PET studies of blood flow or glucose metabolism (Bonte, Ross, Chehabi, & Devous, 1986; Cohen et al., 1986; Eberling, Jagust, Reed, & Baker, 1992; Hellman & Collier, 1987; Jagust, 1994; Jagust, Budinger, & Reed, 1987;

Johnson et al., 1990; Johnson, Mueller, Walshe, English, & Holman, 1987; Neary et al., 1987; Perani et al., 1988; Sharp et al., 1986; Spampinato et al., 1991). See Figures 7.13–7.15, a–d.

Wolfe, Reed, Eberling, and Jagust (1995) also have found that temporal lobe perfusion patterns on SPECT predict the rate of cognitive decline on memory tests over the subsequent 1 to 4 years, whereas frontal lobe perfusion patterns predict the emergence of perseverative behaviors.

A recent in vivo receptor mapping study of cholinergic terminals in patients with AD has shown the utility of SPECT scanning with radiolabeled iodinated receptor ligands for demonstrating deficits in this disease (Kuhl et al., 1996). The D_2 receptor ligand ^{123}I-IBZM was used by Pizzolato et al. (1996) in SPECT studies to explore the basis of extrapyramidal symptoms in Alzheimer's disease. Mean-specific activity was reduced in striatal regions in AD patients compared to controls, showing that the parkinsonism of AD has a different pathophysiology than in Parkinson's disease and is related to postsynaptic dysfunction in the dopamine D_2 system rather than the presynaptic degeneration seen in Parkinson's disease.

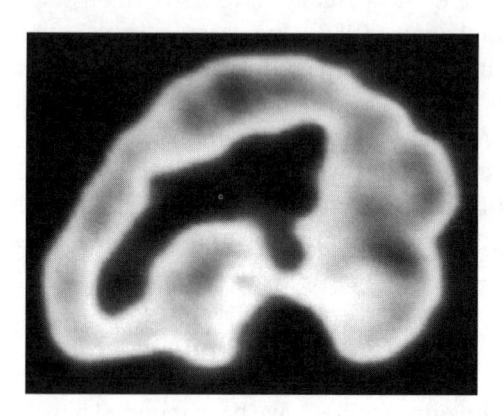

FIGURE 7.13 SPECT scan (using Tc^{99m} HMPAO) in the sagittal plane, in a normal elderly individual. Cerebral perfusion is color coded from highest perfusion to lowest perfusion as follows: red, yellow, green, blue.

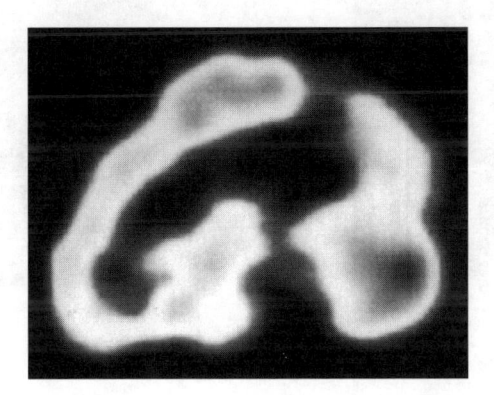

FIGURE 7.14 SPECT scan (using Tc^{99m} HMPAO) in the sagittal plane in an Alzheimer's disease patient. There is interruption of cortical gray-matter perfusion pattern in the superior parietal lobe.

The greater availability of SPECT cameras and the lack of the necessity for a local cyclotron to produce the isotopes needed for SPECT studies, makes SPECT an attractive alternative to PET for assessment of the functional disturbances in dementia. However, the poorer spatial resolution and lack of true quantitation of data remain disadvantages. SPECT studies, because of their general availability, are valuable in the mildly or questionably demented individual, especially where other factors such as depression, medication effects, or educational/cultural factors cast doubt on the diagnosis of anorganic dementia. A clearly abnormal SPECT study in this situation indicates organicity. The poorer resolution of SPECT, compared to PET, negatively affects the sensitivity for detecting abnormalities. Distinctions between the various causes of the organic brain disorder are less than optimal by both SPECT and PET.

CONCLUSIONS

Brain imaging techniques are in wide use to diagnose and understand Alzheimer's disease. Accordingly, they have become a standard part of the evaluation of the patient presenting with dementia. Anatomical imaging

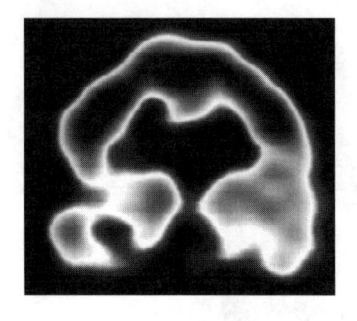

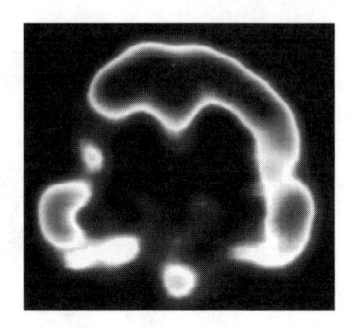

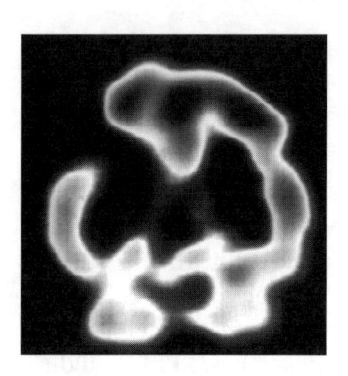

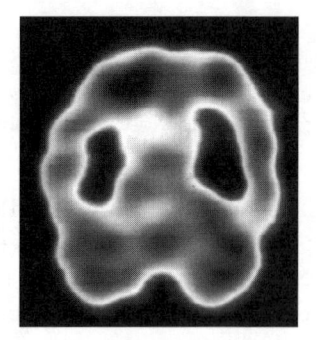

FIGURE 7.15, a, b, c, d. Serial SPECT scans (using Tc^{99m} HMPAO) in the coronal plane from anterior (a) to posterior (d) in an Alzheimer's disease patient, showing a mild perfusion deficit in the right inferior frontal region (15a), moderate to severe deficit in the right inferior parietal region (15b), severe deficit in the right superior parietal region (15c), and normal occipital perfusion (15d).

by CT or MRI, though not required by commonly used criteria for diagnosing AD, is desirable, primarily to exclude other dementing diseases that have distinct imaging features. The diagnosis of AD can be enhanced by demonstrating atrophy of specific brain regions, especially the hippocampus, which is best visualized in coronally oriented MRI slices. Whitematter abnormalities, which are seen frequently in CT and, especially in MRI scans in AD patients, do not help to distinguish vascular from degenerative dementia, in the absence of definitive evidence of cortical and/or subcortical infarction. Functional imaging can be performed by PET, SPECT and, most recently, MRI scanning. The diagnostic utility of functional imaging is in distinguishing the early stages of a degenerative disease, such as AD, from a nonorganic brain disorder, such as depression or anxiety disorder, which can sometimes present as a pseudodementia. Recent studies suggest that patients with even mild degenerative dementia can be distinguished from normal controls by PET, in 95% of cases. Patients with a genetic susceptibility to AD may show regional functional deficits years before the appearance of any symptoms. Functional imaging is less useful in determining the different organic causes of dementia, because there are overlapping patterns, even though the pattern of parietal-temporal deficits in blood flow or metabolism are common in AD. The future in functional imaging with MRI is especially promising, because of the ease with which both anatomical and functional data can be combined when using this method. Functional imaging may elucidate many aspects of the biology of AD through studies of receptor concentrations and binding, as well as the concentrations of many metabolically active compounds in the brain. Functional imaging may have important applications in monitoring the effects of different treatments for AD.

REFERENCES

Alavi, A., Dann, R., Chawluk, J., Alavi, J., Kushner, M., & Reivich, M. (1986). Positron emission tomography imaging of regional cerebral glucose metabolism. *Seminars in Nuclear Medicine (New York), 16*, 2–34.

Alavi, A., Newberg, A. B., Souder, E., & Berlin, J. A. (1993). Quantitative analysis of PET and MRI data in normal aging and Alzheimer's disease: Atrophy-weighted total brain metabolism and absolute whole brain metabolism as reliable discriminators. *Journal of Nuclear Medicine, 34*, 1681–1687.

Albert, M., Naeser, M. A., Levine, H. L., & Garvey, A. J. (1984). Ventricular size in patients with presenile dementia of the Alzheimer's type. *Archives of Neurology, 41*, 1258–1263.

Benson, D. F., Kuhl, D. E., Hawkins, R. A., Phelps, M. E., Cummings, J. L., & Tsai, S. Y. (1983). The fluorodeoxyglucose ^{18}F scan in Alzheimer's disease and multi-infarct dementia. *Archives of Neurology, 40*, 711–714.

Berman, K. F., & Weinberger, D. R. (1986). Cortical physiological activation in Alzheimer's disease: rCBF studies during resting and cognitive states [Abstract]. *Society of Neuroscience Abstracts, 12*, 1160.

Biegon, A., Eberling, J. L., Richardson, B. C., Roos, M. S., Wong, S. T., Reed, B. R., & Jagust, W. J. (1994). Human corpus callosum in aging and Alzheimer's disease: A magnetic resonance imaging study. *Neurobiology of Aging, 15*, 393–397.

Blennow, K., Wallin, A., Uhlemann, C., &. Gottfries, C. G. (1991). White-matter lesions on CT in Alzheimer patients: Relation to clinical symptomatology and vascular factors. *Acta Neurologica Scandinavica (Copenhagen), 83*, 187–193.

Bonte, F. J., Ross, E. D., Chehabi, H. H., & Devous, M. D. (1986). SPECT study of regional cerebral blood flow in Alzheimer disease. *Journal of Computer Assisted Tomography, 10*, 579–583.

Botwinick, J., Storandt, M., & Berg, L. (1986) A longitudinal, behavioral study of senile dementia of the Alzheimer's type. *Archives of Neurology, 43*, 1124–1127.

Bowen, B. C., Barker, W. W., Loewenstein, D. A., Sheldon, J., & Duara, R. (1990). MR signal abnormalities in memory disorder and dementia. *American Journal of Neuroradiology, 11*, 283–290.

Breitner, J. C. S., & Folstein, M. F. (1984). Familial Alzheimer's dementia: A prevalent disorder with specific clinical features. *Psychological Medicine, 14*, 3–80.

Brinkman, S. D., Sarwar, M., Levin, H. S., & Morris, H. H., III. (1981). Quantitative indexes of computed tomography in dementia and normal aging. *Radiology, 138*, 89–92.

Brown, G. G., Levine, S. R., Gorell, J. M., Pettegrew, J. W., Gdowski, J. W., Bueri, J. A., Helpern, J. A., & Welch, K. M. A. (1989). In vivo 31P NMR profiles of Alzheimer's disease and multiple subcortical infarct dementia. *Neurology, 39*, 1423–1427.

Brun, A., & Englund, E. (1981). The pattern of degeneration in Alzheimer's disease: Neuronal loss and histopathological grading. *Histopathology, 5*, 549–564.

Burns, A., Jacoby, R., & Levy, R. (1991). Computed tomography in Alzheimer's disease: A longitudinal study. *Biological Psychiatry, 29*, 383–390.

Charletta, D., Gorelick, P. B., Dollear, T. J., Freels, S., & Harris, Y. (1995). CT and MRI findings among African-Americans with Alzheimer's disease, vascular dementia, and stroke without dementia. *Neurology, 8*, 1456–1461.

Chase, T. N., Fedio, P., Foster, N. L., Brooks, R., Di Chiro, G., & Mansi, L. (1984). Wechsler Adult Intelligence Scale performance. Cortical localization by fluorodeoxyglucose F18-positron emission tomography. *Archives of Neurology, 41,* 1244–1247.

Chawluk, J. B., Alavi, A., Dann, R., Hurtig, H. I., Bias, S., Kushner, M. J., Zimmerman, R. A., & Reivich, M. (1987). Positron emission tomography in aging and dementia: Effect of cerebral atrophy. *Journal of Nuclear Medicine, 28,* 431–437.

Chiu, H. C., Teng, E. L., Henderson, V. W., & Moy, A. C. (1985). Clinical subtypes of dementia of the Alzheimer's type. *Neurology, 35*(11), 1544–1550.

Christiansen, P., Schlosser, A., & Henriksen, O. (1995). Reduced N-acetylaspartate content in the frontal part of the brain in patients with probable Alzheimer's disease. *Magnetic Resonance Imaging, 13,* 457–462.

Coffey, C. E., Wilkinson, W. E., Parashos, I. A., Soady, S. A. R., Sullivan, R. J., Patterson, L. J., Figiel, G. S., Webb, M. C., Spritzer, C. E., & Djang, W. T. (1992). Quantitative cerebral anatomy of the aging human brain: A cross-sectional study using magnetic resonance imaging. *Neurology, 42,* 527–536.

Cohen, M. B., Graham, L. S., Lake, R., Metter, E. J., Fitten, J., Kulkarni, M. K., Sevrin, R., Yamada, L., Chang, C. C., Woodruff, N., & Kling, A. S. (1986). Diagnosis of Alzheimer's disease and multiple infarct dementia by tomographic imaging of Iodine-123 IMP. *Journal of Nuclear Medicine, 27,* 769–774.

Convit, A., de Leon, M. J., Tarshish, C., De Santi, S., Rusinek, H., & George, A. E. (1995). Hippocampal atrophy and cognitive impairment. *Lancet, 345,* 992.

Cuenod, C. A., Kaplan, D. B., Michot, J. L., Jehenson, P., Leroy-Willig, A., Forette, F., Syrota, A., & Boller, F. (1995). Phospholipid abnormalities in early Alzheimer's disease. In vivo phosphorus 31 magnetic resonance spectroscopy. *Archives of Neurology, 52,* 89–94.

Cutler, N. R., Haxby, J. V., Duara, R., Grady, C. L., Moore, A. M., Parisi, J. E., White, J., Heston, L., Margolin, R. M., & Rapoport, S. I. (1985). Brain metabolism as measured with positron emission tomography: Serial assessment in a patient with familial Alzheimer's disease. *Neurology, 35,* 1556–1561.

De Carli, C., Atack, J. R., Ball, M. J., Kay, J. A., Grady, C. L., Fewster, P., Pettigrew, K. D., Rapoport, S. I., & Shaprio, M. B. (1992). Post-mortem regional neurofibrillary tangle densities but not senile plaque densities are related to regional cerebral metabolic rates for glucose during life in Alzheimer's disease patients. *Neurodegeneration, 1,* 113–121.

De Carli, D., Kaye, J. A., Horwitz, B., & Rapoport, S. I. (1990). Critical analysis of the use of computer-assisted transverse axial tomography to study human brain in aging and dementia of the Alzheimer type. *Neurology, 40,* 872–883.

de Leon, M. J., Convit, A., George, A. E., Golomb, J., de Santi, S., Tarshish, C., Rusinek, H., Bobinski, M., Ince, C., Miller, D., & Wisniewski, H. (1996).

In vivo structural studies of the hippocampus in normal aging and in incipient Alzheimer's disease. *Annals of the New York Academy of Science, 777*, 1–13.
de Leon, M. J., Ferris, S. H., George, A. E., Christman, D. R., Fowler, J. S., Gentes, C. I., Reisberg, B., Gee, B., Kricheff, I. I., Emmerich, M., Yonekura, Y., Brodie, J., Kricheff, I. I., & Wolf, A. P. (1983). Positron emission tomography studies of aging and Alzheimer disease. *American Journal of Neuroradiology, 4*, 568–571.
de Leon, M. J., Ferris, S. H., George, A. E., Reisberg, B., Kricheff, I. I., & Gershon, S. (1980). Computed tomography evaluations of brain-behavior relationships in senile dementia of the Alzheimer's type. *Neurobiology of Aging, 1*, 9–79.
de Leon, M. J., George, A. E., Ferris, S. H., Christman, D. R., Fowler, J. S., Gentes, C., Brodie, J., Resiberg, B., & Wolf, A. P. (1984). Positron emission tomography and computerized tomography of the aging brain. *Journal of Computer Assisted Tomography, 8*, 88–94.
de Leon, M. J., George, A. E., Reisberg, B., Ferris, S. H., Kluger, A., Stylopoulos, L. A., Miller, J. D., La Regina, M. E., Chen, C., & Cohen, J. (1989). Alzheimer's disease: Longitudinal CT studies of ventricular change. *American Journal of Neuroradiology, 10*, 371–376.
Desmond, P. M., O'Brien, J. T., Tress, B. M., Ames, D. J., Clement, J. G., Clement, P., Schweitzer, I., Tuckwell, V., & Robinson, G. S. (1994). Volumetric and visual assessment of the mesial temporal structures in Alzheimer's disease. *Australian and New Zealand Journal of Medicine, 24*, 547–553.
Deweer, B., Lehericy, S., Pillon, B., Baulac, M., Chiras, J., Marsault, C., Agid, Y., & Dubois, B. (1995). Memory disorders in probable Alzheimer's disease: The role of hippocampal atrophy as shown with MRI. *Journal of Neurology, Neurosurgery, and Psychiatry, 58*, 590–597.
Duara, R., Barker, W. W., Chang, J. Y., Yoshii, F., Loewenstein, D. A., & Pascal, S. (1992). Viability of neocortical function shown in behavioral activation state PET studies in Alzheimer's disease. *Journal of Cerebral Blood Flow and Metabolism, 12*, 927–934.
Duara, R. D., Barker, W. W., Loewenstein, D. A., Pascal, S., & Bowen, B. (1989). Sensitivity and specificity of PET and MRI studies in Alzheimer's disease and multi-infarct dementia. *European Neurology, 29*(Suppl. 3), 9–15.
Duara, R., Grady, C., Haxby, J., Sundaram, M., Cutler, N. R., Heston, L., Moore, A., Schlageter, N., Larson, S., & Rapoport, S. I. (1986). Positron emission tomography in Alzheimer's disease. *Neurology, 36*, 879–887.
Duara, R., Gross-Glenn, K., Barker, W. W., Chang, J. Y., Apicella, A., Loewenstein, D. A., & Boothe, T. (1987b). Behavioral activation and the variability of cerebral glucose metabolic measurements. *Journal of Cerebral Blood Flow and Metabolism, 7*, 266–271.
Dysken, M. W., Nelson, M. J., Hoover, K. M., Kuskowski, M., & McGeachie, R. (1990). Rapid dynamic CT scanning in primary degenerative dementia and age-matched controls. *Biological Psychiatry, 28*, 425–434.

Earnest, M. P., Heaton, R. K., Wilkinson, W. E., & Manke, W. F. (1979). Cortical atrophy, ventricular enlargement and intellectual impairment in the aged. *Neurology, 29*, 1138–1143.
Eberling, J. L., Jagust, W. J., Reed, B. R., & Baker, M. G. (1992). Reduced temporal lobe blood flow in Alzheimer's disease. *Neurobiology of Aging, 13*, 483–491.
Englund, E., & Brun, A. (1990). White matter changes in dementia of Alzheimer's type: The difference in vulnerability between cell compartments. *Histopathology, 16*, 433–439.
Englund, E., Brun, A., & Persson, B. (1987). Correlations between histopathologic white matter changes and proton MR relaxation times in dementia. *Alzheimer Disease and Related Disorders, 1*(3), 156–170.
Erkinjuntti, T., Ketonen, L., Sulkava, R., Sipponen, N., Vuorialho, M., & Iivanainen, M. (1987). Do white matter changes on MRI and CT differentiate vascular dementia from Alzheimer's disease? *Journal of Neurology, Neurosurgery, and Psychiatry, 50*, 37–42.
Eslinger, P. J., Damasio, H., Graff-Radford, N., & Damasio, A. R. (1984). Examining the relationship between computed tomography and neuropsychological measures in normal and demented elderly. *Journal of Neurology, Neurosurgery, and Psychiatry, 47*, 1319–1325.
Fazekas, F., Chawluk, J. B., Alavi, A., Hurtig, H. I., & Zimmerman, R. A. (1987). MR signal abnormalities at 1.5 T in Alzheimer's dementia and normal aging. *American Journal of Neuroradiology, 8*, 421–426.
Ferris, S. H., de Leon, M. J., Wolf, A. P., Farkas, T., Christman, D. R., Reisberg, B., Fowler, J. R., MacGregor, R., Goldman, A., George, A. E., & Rampal, S. (1980). Positron emission tomography in the study of aging and senile dementia. *Neurobiology of Aging, 1*, 127–131.
Foster, N. L., Chase, T. N., Fedio, P., Patronas, N. J., Brooks, R. A., & DiChiro, G. (1983). Alzheimer's disease: Focal cortical changes shown by positron emission tomography. *Neurology, 33*, 961–965.
Foster, N. L., Chase, T. N., Mausi, L., Brooks, R., Patrona, N. J., & DeChiro, G. (1984). Cortical abnormalities in Alzheimer's disease. *Annals of Neurology, 16*, 649–654.
Foster, N. L., Hansen, M. S., Siegel, G. J., & Kuhl, D. E. (1988). Medial and lateral temporal glucose metabolism in aging and Alzheimer's disease studied by PET [Abstract]. *Neurology, 38*(Suppl. 1), 133.
Frackowiack, R. S. J., Lenzi, G. L., Jones, T., & Heather, J. D. (1980). Quantitative measurement of regional cerebral blood flow and oxygen metabolism in man using [15]O and positron emission tomography: Theory, procedure, and normal values. *Journal of Computer Assisted Tomography, 4*, 727–736.
Frackowiak, R. S. J., Pozzilli, C., Legg, N. J., Du Boulay, G. H., Marshall, J., Lenzi, G. L., & Jones, T. (1981). Regional cerebral oxygen supply and utilization in dementia: A clinical and physiological study with oxygen-15 and positron tomography. *Brain, 104*, 753–778.

Friedland, R. P., Budinger, T. F., Brant-Zawadzki, M., & Jagust, W. J. (1984). The diagnosis of Alzheimer-type dementia. *Journal of the American Medical Association, 252,* 2750–2752.

Friedland, R. P., Budinger, T. F., Ganz, E., Yano, Y., Mathid, C. A., Koss, B., Ober, B. A., Huesman, R. H., & Derenzo, S. E. (1983b). Regional cerebral metabolic alterations in dementia of the Alzheimer type: Positron emission tomography with [^{18}F]fluorodeoxy-glucose. *Journal of Computer Assisted Tomography, 7,* 590–598.

Friedland, R. P., Brun, A., & Budinger, T. F. (1985). Pathologic and positron emission tomographic correlations in Alzheimer's disease. *Lancet, 1,* 228.

Friedland, R. P., Yano, Y., Budinger, T. F., Ganz, E., Huesman, R. H., Derenzo, S. E., & Knittel, B. (1983a). Quantitative evaluation of blood brain barrier integrity in Alzheimer-type dementia: Positron emission tomographic studies with Rubidium-82. *European Neurology, 22*(Suppl. 2), 19–20.

Gado, M., Hughes, C. P., Danziger, W., Chi, D., Jost, G., & Berg, L. (1982). Volumetric measures of the cerebrospinal fluid spaces in demented subjects and controls. *Radiology, 144,* 535–538.

George, A. E., de Leon, M. J., & Ferris, S. H. (1981). Parenchymal CT correlates of senile dementia: Loss of gray-white discriminability. *American Journal of Neuroradiology, 2,* 205–213.

George, A. E., de Leon, M. J., Gentes, C. I., Miller, J., London, E., Budzilovich, G. N., Ferris, S., & Chase, N. (1986). Leukoencephalopathy in normal and pathologic aging. Pt. 1. CT of brain lucencies. *American Journal of Neuroradiology, 7,* 561–566.

Giannakapoulos, P., Hof, P. R., & Boures, C. (1994). Alzheimer's disease with asymmetrical atrophy of the cerebral hemispheres: Morphometric analysis of four cases. *Acta Neuropathologica, 88*(5), 440–447.

Glenner, G. G. (1985). On causative theories in Alzheimer's disease. *Human Pathology, 16,* 433–435.

Golomb, J., Kluger, A., de Leon, M. J., Ferris, S. H., Convit, A., Mittelman, M. S., Cohen, J., Rusinek, H., De Santi, S., & George, A. E. (1994). Hippocampal formation size in normal human aging: A correlate of delayed secondary memory performance. *Learning and Memory, 1,* 45–54.

Golomb, J., Kluger, A., de Leon, M. J., Ferris, S. H., Mittelman, M., Cohen, J., & George, A. E. (1996). Hippocampal formation size predicts declining memory performance in normal aging. *Neurology, 47,* 810–813.

Goto, K., Ishii, N., & Fukasawa, H. (1981). Diffuse white-matter disease in the geriatric population. *Radiology, 141,* 687–695.

Groom, G. N., Junck, L., Foster, N. L., Frey, K. A., & Kuhl, D. E. (1995). PET of peripheral benzodiazepine binding sites in the microgliosis of Alzheimer's disease. *Journal of Nuclear Medicine, 36,* 2207–2210.

Grundman, M., Corey-Bloom, J., Jernigan, T., Archibald, M. A., & Thal, L. J. (1996). Low body weight in Alzheimer's disease is associated with mesial temporal cortex atrophy. *Neurology, 46,* 1585–1591.

Hardy, J. A., Mann, D. M. A., Webster, P., & Weinblad, B. (1986). An integrative hypothesis concerning the pathogenesis and progression of Alzheimer's disease. *Neurobiology of Aging, 7*, 489–502.

Harris, G. J., Lewis, R. F., Satlin, A., English, C. D., Scott, T. M., Yurgelun-Todd, D. A., & Renshar, P. F. (1996). Dynamic susceptibility contrast MRI of regional cerebral blood volume in Azlheimer's disease. *American Journal of Psychiatry, 153*, 721–724.

Haxby, J. V., Duara, R., Grady, C. L., Cutler, N. R., & Rapoport, S. I. (1985). Relations between neuropsychological and cerebral metabolic asymmetries in early Alzheimer's disease. *Journal of Cerebral Blood Flow and Metaboliam, 5*, 193–200.

Haxby, J. V., Grady, C. L., Duara, R., Schlageter, N., Berg, G., & Rapoport, S. I. (1986). Neocortical metabolic abnormalities precede nonmemory cognitive defects in early Alzheimer's-type dementia. *Archives of Neurology, 43*, 882–885.

Hellman, R. S., & Collier, B. D. (1987). Single photon emission computed tomography: A clinical experience. In L. M. Freeman & H. S. Weissmann (Eds.), *Nuclear medicine annual* (p. 51). New York: Raven Press.

Herholz, K., Perani, D., Salomon, E., Franck, G., Fazio, F., Heiss, W. D., & Comar, D. (1993). Comparability of FDG PET studies in probable Alzheimer's disease. *Journal of Nuclear Medicine, 34*, 1460–1466.

Herscovitch, P., Auchua, A., Gado, M., Chi, D., & Raichle, M. (1986). Correction of positron emission tomography data for cerebral atrophy. *Journal of Cerebral Blood Flow and Metabolism, 6*, 120–124.

Ito, B., Hatazawa, J., Yamaura, H., & Matsuzawa, T. (1981). Age-related brain atrophy and mental deterioration: A study with computed tomography. *British Journal of Radiology, 54*, 384–390.

Jack, C. R., Jr., Mokri, B., Laws, E. R., Houser, O. W., Baker, H. L., Jr., & Petersen, C. (1987). MR findings in normal-pressure hydrocephalus: Significance and comparison with other forms of dementia. *Journal of Computer Assisted Tomography, 11*, 923–931.

Jack, C. R., Petersen, R. C., O'Brien, P. C., & Tangalos, E. G. (1992). MRI-based hippocampal volumetry in the diagnosis of Alzheimer's disease. *Neurology, 42*, 183–188.

Jacoby, R. J., & Levy, R. (1980). Computed tomography in the Elderly. Pt. 2. Senile dementia: Diagnosis and functional impairment. *British Journal of Psychiatry, 136*, 256–269.

Jagust, W. (1994). Cerebral blood flow and metabolism in dementia: Regional patterns and the biology of Alzheimer's disease. *Developmental Brain Dysfunction, 7*, 302–310.

Jagust, W. J., Budinger, T. F., & Reed, B. R. (1987). The diagnosis of dementia with single photon emission computed tomography. *Archives of Neurology, 44*, 259–262.

Jagust, W. J., Eberling, J. L., Richardson, B. C., Reed, B. R., Baker, M. G., Nordahl, T. E., & Budinger, T. F. (1993). The cortical topography of temporal lobe hypometabolism in early Alzheimer's disease. *Brain Research, 629,* 189–198.

Jagust, W. J., Haan, M. N., Eberling, J. L., Wolfe, N., & Reed, B. R. (1996). Functional imaging predicts cognitive decline in Alzheimer's disease. *Journal of Neuroimaging, 6,* 156–160.

Janowsky, J. S., Kaye, J. A., & Carper, R. A. (1996). Atrophy of the corpus callosum in Alzheimer's disease versus healthy aging. *Journal of the American Geriatric Society, 44,* 798–803.

Jernigan, T. L., Salmon, D. P., Butters, N., & Hesselink, J. R. (1991). Cerebral structure on MRI. Pt. 2. Specific changes in Alzheimer's and Huntington's disease. *Biological Psychiatry, 29,* 68–81.

Johnson, K. A., Holman, B. L., Rosen, T. J., Nagle, J. S., English, R. J., & Growdon, J. H. (1990). Iofetamine I 123 single photon emission computed tomography is accurate in the diagnosis of Alzheimer's disease. *Archives of Internal Medicine, 150,* 752–756.

Johnson, K. A., Mueller, S. T., Walshe, M., English, R. J., & Holman, B. L. (1987). Cerebral perfusion imaging in Alzheimer's disease. *Archives of Neurology, 44,* 165–168.

Killiany, R. J., Moss, M. B., Albert, M. S., Sandor, R., Tieman, J., & Jolesz, F. (1993). Temporal lobe regions on magnetic resonance imaging identify patients with early Alzheimer's disease. *Archives of Neurology, 50,* 949–954.

Kippenhan, J. S., Barker, W. W., Nagel, J., Grady, C., & Duara, R. (1994). Neural-network classification of normal and Alzheimer's disease subjects using high and low resolution PET cameras. *Journal of Nuclear Medicine, 35,* 7–15.

Kippenhan, J. S., Barker, W. W., Pascal, S., Nagel, J., & Duara, R. (1992). Evaluation of a neural-network classifier of PET scans of normal and Alzheimer disease subjects. *Journal of Nuclear Medicine, 33,* 1459–1467.

Klunk, W. E., Panchalingam, K., Moossy, J., McClure, R. J., & Pettegrew, J. W. (1992). N-acetyl-L-aspartate and other amino acid metabolites in Alzheimer's disease brain: A preliminary proton nuclear magnetic resonance study. *Neurology, 42,* 1578–1585.

Kuhl, D. E., Metter, E. J., Benson, F., Ashford, J. W., Riege, W. H., Fujikawa, D. G., Markham, C. H., Mazziotta, J. C., Maltese, A., & Dorsey, D. A. (1985). Similarities of cerebral glucose metabolism in Alzheimer's and Parkinson's dementia. *Journal of Cerebral Blood Flow and Metabolism, 5*(Suppl. 1), S169–S170.

Kuhl, D. E., Minoshima, S., Fessler, J. A., Frey, K. A., Foster, N. L., Ficaro, E. P., Wieland, D. M., & Koeppe, R. A. (1996). In vivo mapping of cholinergic terminals in normal aging, Alzheimer's disease, and Parkinson's disease. *Annals of Neurology, 40,* 399–410.

Kumar, A., Schapiro, M., & Grady, C. (1991). High resolution PET studies in Alzheimer's disease. *Neuropsychopharmacology, 4*, 35–46.

Labbé, C., Froment, J. C., Kennedy, A., Ashburner, J., & Cinotti, L. (1996). Positron emission tomography metabolic data corrected for cortical atrophy using magnetic resonance imaging. *Alzheimer Disease and Associated Disorders, 10*, 141–170.

Lehericy, S., Baulac, M., Chiras, J., Pierto, L., Martin, N., Pillon, B., Deweer, B., Dubois, B., & Marsault, C. (1994). *American Journal of Neuroradiology, 15*, 929–937.

Leifer, D., Buonanno, F. S., & Richardson, E. P., Jr. (1990). Clinicopathologic correlations of cranial magnetic resonance imaging of periventricular white matter. *Neurology, 40*, 911–198.

LeMay, M. (1986). CT changes in dementing diseases: A review. *American Journal of Neuroradiology, 7*, 841–853.

LeMay, M., Stafford, J. L., Sandor, T., Albert, M., Haykal, H., & Samani, A. (1986). Statistical assessment of perceptual CT scan ratings in patients with Alzheimer type dementia. *Journal of Computer Assisted Tomography, 10*, 802–809.

Ley, D., Soetaert, G., Petit, H., Fauquette, A., Pruvo, J.-P., & Steinling, M. (1990). Periventricular and white matter magnetic resonance imaging hyperintensities do not differ between Alzheimer's disease and normal aging. *Archives of Neurology, 47*, 524–527.

Loewenstein, D. A., Yoshii, F., Barker, W. W., Apicella, A., Emran, A., Chang, J. Y., & Duara, R. (1989). Predominant left hemisphere metabolic dysfunction in dementia. *Archives of Neurology, 46*, 146–152.

Lopez, O. L., Becker, J. T., Jungreis, C. A., Rezek, D., Estol, C., Boller, F., & DeKosky, S. T. (1995). Computed tomography—but not magnetic resonance imaging—identified periventricular white-matter lesions predict symptomatic cerebrovascular disease in probable Alzheimer's disease. *Archives of Neurology, 52*, 659–664.

Lopez, O. L., Brenner, R. P., Becker, J. T., Jungrei, C. A., Rezek, D., & DeKosky, S. T. (1995). Electroencephalographic correlates of periventricular white matter lesions in probable Alzheimer's disease. *Dementia, 6*, 343–347.

Lotz, P. R., Ballinger, W. E., Jr., & Quisling, R. G. (1986). Subcortical arteriosclerotic encephalopathy: CT spectrum and pathologic correlation. *American Journal of Neuroradiology, 7*, 817–822.

Luxenberg, J. S., Haxby, J. V., Creasey, H., Sundaram, M., & Rapoport, S. I. (1987). Rate of ventricular enlargement in dementia of the Alzheimer type correlates with rate of neuropsychological deterioration. *Neurology, 37*, 1135–1140.

Mayeaux, R., Stern, Y., & Spanton, S. (1985). Heterogeneity in dementia of the Alzheimer type: Evidence of subgroups. *Neurology, 35*, 453–461.

McClure, R. J., Kanfer, J. N., Panchalingham, K., Klunk, W. E., & Pettegrew, J. W. (1994). Alzheimer's disease: Membrance-associated metabolic changes. *Annals of the New York Academy of Sciences, 747*, 110–124.

McGeer, P. L., Kamo, H., Harrop, R., Li, D. K. B., Tuokko, H., McGeer, E. G., Adam, M. J., Ammann, W., Beattie, B. L., Calne, D. B., Martin, W. R. W., Pate, B. D., Rogers, J. G., Ruth, T. J., Sayre, C. I., & Stoessel, A. J. (1986a). Positron emission tomography in patients with clinically diagnosed Alzheimer's disease. *Canadian Medical Association Journal, 134*, 597–607.

McGeer, P. L., Kamo, H., McGeer, E. G., Martin, W. R. W., Pate, B. D., & Li, D. K. B. (1986b). Comparison of PET, MRI and CT with pathology in a proven case of Alzheimer's disease. *Neurology, 36*, 1569–1574.

Meguro, K., Marsushita, M., Yoshida, R., Otomo, E., Yamaguchi, S., Nakagawa, T., & Sasaki, H. (1994). A clinicopathological study of senile dementia of Alzheimer's type (SDAT) and white matter lesions of Binswanger's type. *Nippon Ronen Igakkai Zasshi [Japanese Journal of Geriatrics], 31*, 226–231.

Meltzer, C. C., Zubieta, J. K., Brandt, J., Tune, L. E., Mayberg, H. S., & Frost, J. J. (1996). Regional hypometabolism in Alzheimer's disease as measured by positron emission tomography after correction for effects of partial volume averaging. *Neurology, 47*, 454–461.

Miller, J. D., de Leon, M. J., Ferris, S. H., Kluger, A., George, A. E., Reisberg, B., Sachs, S. J., & Wolf, A. P. (1987). Abnormal temporal lobe response in Alzheimer's disease during cognitive processing as measured by ^{11}C-2-deoxy-d-glucose and PET. *Journal of Cerebral Blood and Flow Metabolism, 7*, 248–251.

Minoshima, S., Frey, K. A., Koeppe, R. A., Foster, N. L., & Kuhl, D. E. (1995). A new diagnostic approach in Alzheimer's disease using three-dimensional stereotactic surface projections of [^{18}F] FDG. *Journal of Nuclear Medicine, 36*, 1238–1248.

Murphy, D. G., DeCarli, C., Schapiro, M. B., Rapoport, S. I., & Horwitz, B. (1992). Age-related differences in volumes of subcortical nuclei, brain matter, and cerebrospinal fluid in healthy men as measured with magnetic resonance imaging. *Archives of Neurology, 49*, 839–846.

Neary, D., Snowden, J. S., Shields, R. A., Burjan, A. W. I., Northen, B., MacDermott, N., Prescott, M. C., & Testa, H. J. (1987). Single photon emission tomography using ^{99m}Tc-HM-PAO in the investigation of dementia. *Journal of Neurology, Neurosurgery Psychiatry, 50*, 1101–1109.

Parnetti, L., Lowenthal, D. T., Presciutti, O., Pelliccioli, G. P., Palumbo, R., Gobbi, C., Chiarini, P., Palumbo, B., Tarducci, R., & Senin, U. (1996). 1H-MRS, MRI-based hippocampal volumetry, and 99mTc-HMPAO-SPECT in normal aging, age-associated memory impairment, and probable Alzheimer's disease. *Journal of the American Geriatrics Society, 44*, 133–138.

Perani, D., Di Piero, V., Vallar, G., Cappa, S., Messa, C., Bottini, G., Berti, A., Passafiume, D., Scarlato, G., Gerundini, P., Lenzi, G. L., & Fazio, F. (1988).

Technetium-99m HM-PAO-SPECT study of regional cerebral perfusion in early Alzheimer's disease. *Journal of Nuclear Medicine, 29*, 1507–1514.
Pettegrew, J. W., Panchalingam, K., Klunk, W. E., Mc Clure, R. J., & Muenz, L. R. (1994). Alterations of cerebral metabolism in probable Alzheimer's disease: A preliminary study. *Neurobiology of Aging, 15*, 117–132.
Pizzolato, G., Chierichetti, F., Fabbri, M., Cagnin, A., Dam, M., Ferlin, G., & Battistin, L. (1996). Reduced striatal dopamine receptors in Alzheimer's disease: Single photon emission tomography study with the D_2 tracer [^{123}I]-IBZM. *Neurology, 47*, 1065–1068.
Reiman, E. M., Caselli, R. J., Yun, L. S., Chen, K., Bandy, D., Minoshima, S., Thibodeau, S. N., & Osborne, D. (1996). Preclinical evidence of Alzheimer's disease in persons homozygous for the ε 4 allele for apolipoprotein E. *New England Journal of Medicine, 334*, 752–758.
Roberts, M. A., & Caird, F. I. (1976). Computerized tomography and intellectual impairment in the elderly. *Journal of Neurology, Neurosurgery, & Psychiatry, 39*, 986–989.
Rusinek, H., DeLeon, M. J., George, A. E., Stylopoulos, L. A., Chandra, R., Smith, G., Rand, T., Mourino, M., & Kowalski, H. (1991). Alzheimer disease: Measuring loss of cerebral gray-matter with MR imaging. *Neuroradiology, 178*, 109–114.
Scheltens, P., Barkhof, F., Leys, D., Wolters, E. C., Ravid, R., & Kamphporst, W. (1995). Histopathologic correlates of white matter changes on MRI in Alzheimer's disease and normal aging. *Neurology, 45*, 883–888.
Scheltens, P., Barkhof, F., Valk, J., Algra, P. R., van der Hoop, R. G., Nauta, J., & Wolters, E. C. (1992). White matter lesions on magnetic resonance imaging in clinically diagnosed Alzheimer's disease. Evidence for heterogeneity. *Brain, 115*, 735–748.
Schlageter, N. L., Carson, R. E., & Rapoport, S. I. (1987). Examination of blood-brain barrier permeability in dementia of the Alzheimer type with [^{68}Ga]EDTA and positron emission tomography. *Journal of Cerebral Blood Flow and Metabolism, 67*, 1–8.
Schlageter, N. L., Horwitz, B., Creasey, H., Carson, R., Duara, R., Berg, G. W., & Rapoport, S. I. (1987). Relation of measured brain glucose utilization and cerebral atrophy in man. *Journal of Neurology, Neurosurgery and Psychiatry, 50*, 779–785.
Seab, J. P., Jagust, W. J., Wong, S. T. S., Roos, M. S., Reed, B. R., & Budinger, T. F. (1988). Quantitative NMR measurements of hippocampal atrophy in Alzheimer's disease. *Magnetic Resonance in Medicine, 8*, 200–208.
Shapiro, M. B., Ball, M. J., Grady, C. L., Haxby, J. V., Kaye, J. A., & Rapoport, S. I. (1988). Dementia in Down's syndrome: Cerebral glucose utilization, neuropsychological assessment, and neuropathology. *Neurology, 38*, 938–942.

Sharp, P., Gemmell, H., Cherryman, G., Besson, J., Crawford, J., & Smith, F. (1986). Application of Iodine-123-labeled Isopropylamphetamine imaging to the study of dementia. *Journal of Nuclear Medicine, 27*, 761–768.

Shonk, T. K., Moats, R. A., Gifford P., Michaelis, T., Mandigo, J. C., Izumi, J., & Ross, B. D. (1995). Probable Alzheimer disease: Diagnosis with MR spectroscopy. *Radiology, 195*, 65–72.

Small, G. W., Mazziotta, J. C., Collins, M. T., Baxter, L. R., Phelps, M. E., Mandelkern, M. A., Kaplan, A., La Rue, A., Adamson, C. F., Chang, Guze, B. H., Corder, E. H., Saunders, A. M., Haines, J. L., Pericak-Vance, M. A., & Roses, A. (1995). Apolipoprotein E type 4 allele and cerebral glucose metabolism in relatives at risk for familial Alzheimer disease. *Journal of the American Medical Association, 273*, 942–947.

Smith, G. W., de Leon, M. J., George, A. E., Kluger, A., Volkow, N. D., McRae, T., Golomb, J., Ferris, S. H., Resiberg, B., Ciaravino, J., & La Regina, M. E. (1992). Topography of cross-sectional and longitudinal glucose metabolic deficits in Alzheimer's disease. *Archives of Neurology, 49*, 1142–1150.

Smith, C. D., Gallenstein, L. G., Layton, W. J., Kryscio, R. J., & Markesbery, W. R. (1993). 31P magnetic resonance spectroscopy in Alzheimer's and Pick's disease. *Neurobiology of Aging, 14*, 85–92.

Smith, C. D., Pettigrew, L. C., Avison, M. J., Kirsch, J. E., Tinkhtman, A. J., Schmitt, F. A., Wermeling, D. P., Wekstein, D. R., & Markesberry, W. R. (1995). Frontal lobe phosphorus metabolism and neuropsychological function in aging and in Alzheimer's disease. *Annals of Neurology, 38*, 194–201.

Soininen, H., Partanen, K., Pittkänen, A., Hallikainen, M., Hänninen, T., Helisalmi, S., Mannermaa, A., Ryynänen, M., Koivisto, K., & Reikkinen, P. (1995). Decreased hippocampal volume asymmetry on MRIs in nondemented elderly subjects carrying the apolipoprotein E e4 allele. *Neurology, 45*, 391–392.

Spampinato, U., Habert, M. O., Mas, J. L., Bourdel, M. C., Ziegler, M., de Recondo, J. Askienazy, S., & Rondot, P. (1991). ^{99m}Tc-HM-PAO SPECT and cognitive impairment in Parkinson's disease: A comparison with dementia of the Alzheimer type. *Journal of Neurology, Neurosurgery, and Psychiatry, 54*, 787–792.

Steingart, A., Hachinski, V., Lau, C., Fox, A., Diaz, F., Cape, R., Lee, D., Initari, D., & Merskey, H. (1987). Cognitive and neurologic findings in subjects with diffuse white matter lucencies on computed tomographic scan (leukoaraisosis). *Archives of Neurology, 44*, 32–35.

Stoppe, G., Staedt, J., & Bruhn, H. (1995). Patchy changes in white matter in cranial computerized and magnetic resonance tomography—significance for (differential) diagnosis of dementia of the Alzheimer type and vascular dementia. *Fortschritte der Neurologie-Psychiatrie [Progress in Neurology & Psychiatry], 63*, 425–440.

Tanna, N. K., Kohn, M. I., Horwich, D. N., Jolles, P. R., Zimmerman, R. A., Alves, W. M., & Alavi, A. (1991). Analysis of brain and cerebrospinal fluid volumes with MR imaging: Impact on PET data correction for atrophy. Pt. 2. Aging and Alzheimer dementia. *Radiology, 178*, 123–130.

Tedeschi, G., Bertolino, A., Lundbom, N., Bonavita, S., Patronas, N. J., Duyn, J. H., Metman, L. V., Chase, T. N., & Di Chiro, G. (1996). Cortical and subcortical chemical pathology in Alzheimer's disease as assessed by multislice proton magnetic resonance spectroscopic imaging. *Neurology, 47*, 696–704.

Terry, R., & Katzman, R. (1992). Alzheimer's disease and cognitive loss. In R. Katzman & J. W. Rowe (Eds.), *Principles of geriatric neurology* (pp. 207–265). Philadelphia, PA: F. A. Davis.

Wade, J. P. H., Mirsen, T. R., Hachinski, V. C., Fisman, M., Lau, C., & Merskey, H. (1987). The clinical diagnosis of Alzheimer's disease. *Archives of Neurology, 44*, 24–29.

Wilson, R. S., Fox, J. H., Huckman, M. S., Bacon, L. D., & Lobick, J. J. (1982). Computed tomography in dementia. *Neurology, 32*, 1054–1057.

Wisniewski, K. E., Wisniewski, H. M., & Wen, G. Y. (1985). Occurrence of neuropathological changes and dementia of Alzheimer's disease in Down's syndrome. *Annals of Neurology, 17*, 278–282.

Wolfe, N., Reed, B. R., Eberling, J. L., & Jagust, W. J. (1995). Temporal lobe perfusion on single photon emission computed tomography predicts the rate of decline in Alzheimer's disease. *Archives of Neurology, 52*, 257–262.

Wu, S., Schenkenbert, T., Wing, S. D., & Osborn, A. G. (1981). Cognitive correlates of diffuse cerebral atrophy determined by computed tomography. *Neurology, 31*, 1180–1184.

Yoshii, F., & Duara, R. (1989). Size of corpus callosum in normal subjects and patients with Alzheimer's disease: Magnetic resonance imaging study. *Clinical Neurology [Journal of the Japanese Neurological Association], 29*, 1–7.

Zahner, B., Lang, C. J., Englehardt, A., Thierauf, P., & Neundorfer, B. (1995). A case of Alzheimer's disease with extensive focal white matter changes. *Dementia, 6*, 294–300.

CHAPTER 8

Biological Test to Confirm the Diagnosis of Alzheimer's Disease in Cognitively Impaired Patients. A Fact or Fiction?

**P. D. Mehta, T. Pirtillä
H. M. Wisniewski**

At present, there is no specific laboratory test for the diagnosis of Alzheimer's disease (AD), and the diagnosis is generally made by clinical evaluations and exclusion of other causes of dementia. Without histopathologic confirmation of the autopsy brain tissue, the diagnosis can not be made with certainty. Although there is no noninvasive laboratory test to confirm the diagnosis of AD in living patients, studies of histopathologic correlation have shown accuracies of greater than 88%

This study was supported by the New York State Office of Mental Retardation and Developmental Disabilities and a grant from the National Institutes of Health, National Institute on Aging, No. PO1 AG 04220.

(Galasko et al., 1994), based on NINCDS-ADRDA Work Group guidelines (McKhann et al., 1984). A biological marker confirms the presence or the absence of a given disease or identifies presymptomatic individuals at high risk of developing a disease. A marker may reflect the primary pathogenesis of the disease or secondary processes involved in the progression of the disease, or it may be epiphenomenon.

Blood, cerebrospinal fluid (CSF), and peripheral tissues have been examined to find a biochemical marker for the diagnosis of AD in living patients. In this chapter, we have discussed measurements of blood or CSF constituents. Our focus is on the measurements of amyloid proteins, amyloid-associated proteins, tau protein and neurotransmitters in blood or CSF, because of their putative role in the pathogenesis of AD. In addition, we have included unpublished observations from our current research.

NEUROPATHOLOGICAL CHANGES IN AD

Accumulation of intraneuronal neurofibrillary tangles (NFT) and extracellular amyloid plaques in the limbic and cerebral cortices and in walls of leptomeningeal and parenchymal vessels are characteristic neuropathological lesions in AD brains (Wisniewski & Wegiel, 1995). The core protein of the amyloid plaque is a 4-kDa peptide, Aβ protein, which is proteolytically derived from a larger, transmembrane glycoprotein, β-amyloid precursor protein (βAPP) (Selkoe, 1994). Amorphous, mainly nonfibrillar Aβ deposits, are referred to as diffuse plaques, and their numbers increase with age in brains of nondemented individuals (Tagliavini et al., 1988). They also are abundant in brains from patients with AD and Down's syndrome (Wisniewski et al., 1994; Wisniewski & Wegiel, 1995). Neuritic plaques or senile plaques consist of deposits of fibrillar Aβ protein and dystrophic neurites, as well as amyloid-associated proteins, including apolipoprotein E (Apo E), sulfated glycosaminoglycans, serum amyloid component P, cytokines, and acute phase proteins such as $\propto$1-antichymotrypsin ($\propto$1-ACT), $\propto$2-macroglobulin ($\propto$2-MG), $\propto$1-antitrypsin ($\propto$1-AT), and complement components (Kalaria, 1993).

The major constituents of NFT are paired helical filaments (PHF). Immunocytochemical and biochemical studies show that the major components of PHF are the microtubule-associated protein tau in a highly phosphorylated state, and ubiquitin. Although ubiquitin is involved extensively in protein degradation, its function in PHF is unknown. However, it may be that phosphorylated forms of tau are linked to ubiquitin in PHF.

RELATIONSHIP BETWEEN BRAIN AND CSF

About 70%–80% of CSF is produced in the choroid plexus of the brain ventricles and additional CSF is formed from the brain extracellular fluid (ECF) (Segal, 1993). Brain ECF is in direct contact with CSF via patent ependymal and pial surfaces along the ventriculo-subarachnoid space, and the molecules entering brain ECF eventually will diffuse into the CSF. Both CSF and ECF maintain homeostasis by removing brain metabolic waste products and by preserving a stable chemical microenvironment for brain cells. They also serve as an intracerebral transport mechanism to permit diffusion of substances released by neurons and glia. The protein composition of CSF is likely to reflect that of the brain intercellular spaces, and, therefore, the CSF examination is a way to sample the microenvironment of the brain.

βAPP DERIVATIVES IN PLASMA AND CSF

There are at least six forms of secreted βAPP that are translated from alternatively spliced mRNAs (Selkoe, 1994). Of three major forms of βAPP (APP 770, APP 751, and APP 695), APP 770 and APP 751 contain a domain homologous to Kunitz-type serine protease inhibitors. APP 770 and APP 751 are expressed widely in different tissues, whereas APP 695 is brain specific. Secreted βAPPs are normally present in blood and CSF. Investigators show qualitative differences in βAPP in plasma and CSF with age (Palmert et al., 1990) and in AD (Bush et al., 1992). Carroll, Lust, Kim, Doyle, and Emmerling (1995) showed that CSF βPP levels remain unchanged with age in nondemented controls. Comparisons of different APP isoforms in CSF from AD patients and controls have shown conflicting results (see Table 8.1). Some studies demonstrate a decrease of CSF βPP in AD patients compared to controls (Henriksson et al., 1991; Van Nostrand et al., 1992), whereas others show that the levels are either similar (Chong, Miller, & Ghanbari, 1990; Henriksson et al., 1991; Nakamura et al., 1994) or increased (Kitaguchi et al., 1990) in AD patients.

TABLE 8.1 CSF βAPP in AD, Patients with Other Neurological Diseases (OND), and Controls (CO)

	N	Group	Age	(mean)	Method	Ab	Results
Chong et al., 1990	27	AD	60–86	(73)	Immunoblot	P	No change of 105 kDa and 90 kDa bands
	30	CO	28–80	(57)			↑ Significant increase with age of both bands
Kitaguchi et al., 1990	12	AD	46–74	(59)	trypsin-ELISA	P	↑ Increase compared to VD and CO
	4	VD	50–77	(65)			No change compared to CO
	7	CO	51–69	(60)			
Henriksson et al., 1991							
Set 1	20	AD	NA	(72)	CI-ELISA	M	↓ Decrease compared to CO
	10	PD	NA	(70)			↓ Decrease compared to CO
	9	CO	NA	(59)			↓ Decrease with age
Set 2	20	AD	NA	(80)			No change compared to CO
	7	CO	NA	(67)			
Van Nostrand et al., 1992	13	AD	53–85	(69)	ELISA	M	↓ Decrease compared to VD and CO
	18	D	59–78	(69)			No change compared to CO
	16	CO	29–82	(62)			
Pirttilä et al., 1994b	72	AD	51–81	(68)	CI-ELISA	P	↓ Decrease compared to CO
	72	CO	50–84	(64)			
Nakamura et al., 1994	14	e-AD	40–71	(59)	Immunoblot	M	No change compared to CO
	24	l-AD	68–94	(79)			No change compared to CO
	32	OND	22–81	(54)			
	25	CO	16–75	(43)			
Carroll et al., 1995	34	OND	0–82	(NA)	Immunoblot	M	No change with age
	76	CO	0–82	(NA)			No change with age
							No change with age

Note: βAPP = β-amyloid precursor protein; Aβ = amyloid-β protein; Ab = antibody; P = polyclonal; M = monoclonal; AD = Alzheimer's disease (e-AD = early-onset AD; l-AD = late-onset AD); CO = controls; OND = other neurological diseases; PD = Parkinson's disease; VD = vascular dementia.

Recently, we measured APP levels in CSF from 72 patients with probable AD and 72 non-demented controls, using a polyclonal antibody raised against N-terminal 45-62 amino acids of APP in a competitive inhibition enzyme-linked immunosorbent assay (ELISA) (Pirttilä et al., 1994c). CSF APP levels were lower in patients with probable AD than those in controls, but there was a considerable overlap between the groups.

Soluble Aβ is secreted during normal cell metabolism and is found in plasma and CSF (Mehta, Kim, & Wisniewski, 1991; Seubert et al., 1992). The influence of age on CSF sAβ levels is unclear (Table 8.1). Investigators have shown that CSF sAβ concentrations may increase (Van Gool, Schenk, & Bolhuis, 1994), decrease (Nakamura et al., 1994), or remain unchanged with age (Carroll et al., 1995; Pirttilä, Kim, Mehta, Frey, & Wisniewski, 1994b). Thus comparisons of sAβ concentrations in CSF from AD patients and controls have shown conflicting results (see Table 8.2). For example, Nakamura et al. (1994) showed a significant elevation of CSF sAβ levels in patients with early-onset AD compared to those in controls. However, Van Gool, Kuiper, Walstra, Wolters, and Bolhuis (1995) found no differences in CSF sAβ levels between patients with probable AD, Parkinson's disease, and controls. We measured sAβ levels in CSF from 25 patients with probable early-onset AD, 42 patients with probable late-onset AD, 23 patients with VD, and 76 controls using two mouse monoclonal antibodies against Aβ (6E10 and 4G8) and sandwich ELISA (Pirttilä et al., 1994b). Although patients with early-onset and late-onset AD had significantly lower CSF sAβ levels than controls, there was a considerable overlap between the groups (see Fig. 8.1). The changes in CSF sAβ levels were, however, not specific for AD since patients with VD also had lower CSF sAβ levels than controls. Moreover, we found that sAβ levels in CSF from controls with the Apo E4 allele were significantly lower than those in controls without Apo E4 (see Fig. 8.2) (Pirttilä et al., 1994c). No such effect was found in AD patients. Recently, Nitsch et al. (1995) confirmed our data showing that Apo E genotype did not influence sAβ levels in CSF from AD patients.

The source of sAβ in CSF and the relationship between CSF sAβ and accumulation of Aβ in the brain are not known. Tabaton et al. (1994) did not detect sAβ in brains from controls, although it was present in the CSF. Our recent studies indicated that CSF sAβ reflect amyloid deposition in the brain. We measured sAβ in CSF and brain extracts from 19 AD patients, and examined the relationship of Aβ in the brain and CSF (Pirttilä et al., 1996). We showed that CSF sAβ concentrations correlate with

TABLE 8.2 CSF sAβ in AD Patients with Other Neurological Diseases (OND) and Controls (CO)

	N	Group	Age	(mean)	Method	Ab	Results
Pirttilä et al., 1994b	25	e-AD	51–66	(60)	ELISA	M	↓ Decrease compared to age-matched CO
	42	l-AD	65–81	(73)			↓ Decrease compared to age-matched CO
	23	VD	58–87	(72)			↓ Decrease compared to L-AD and CO
	76	CO	43–84	(62)			No change with age
Pirttilä et al., 1994c	72	AD	51–81	(68)	ELISA	M	↓ Decrease compared to CO
							No correlation with Apo E phenotype
	72	CO	50–84	(64)			Significant correlation with Apo E phenotype
Nakamura et al., 1994	14	e-AD	40–71	(59)	Immunoblot	P+M	↑ Increase compared to CO
	24	l-AD	68–94	(79)			No change compared to CO
	32	OND	22–81	(54)			
	25	CO	16–75	(43)			↓ Decrease with age
Van Gool et al., 1994	18	OND	22–84	(NA)	ELISA	M	↑ Increase with age
Van Gool et al., 1995	18	AD	60–87	(74)	ELISA	M	No change
	28	PD	57–84	(68)			No change
	10	OND	59–84	(72)			
Carroll et al., 1995	34	OND	0–82	(NA)	ELISA	M	No change with age
	76	CO	0–82	(NA)			No change with age
Nitsch et al., 1995	19	AD	55–80	(68)	ELISA	M	No change compared to CO
							Negative correlation with severity of dementia
	10	CO	51–77	(71)			No correlation with Apo E genotype

Abbreviations: see Table 8.1.

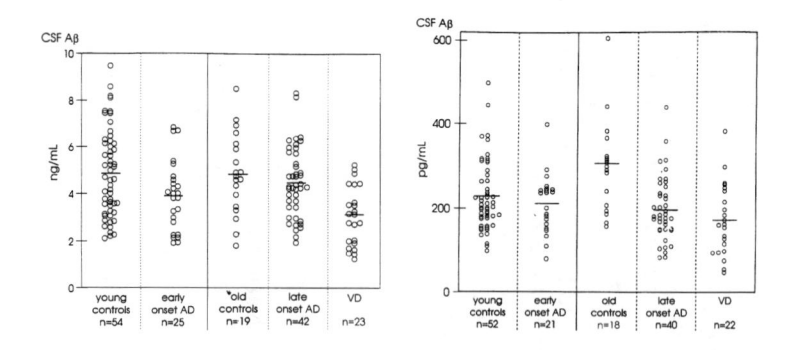

FIGURE 8.1 CSF Aβ concentrations in young and old controls, in early-onset and late-onset AD patients and VD patients measured in ELISA I(A) or in ELISA II (B).

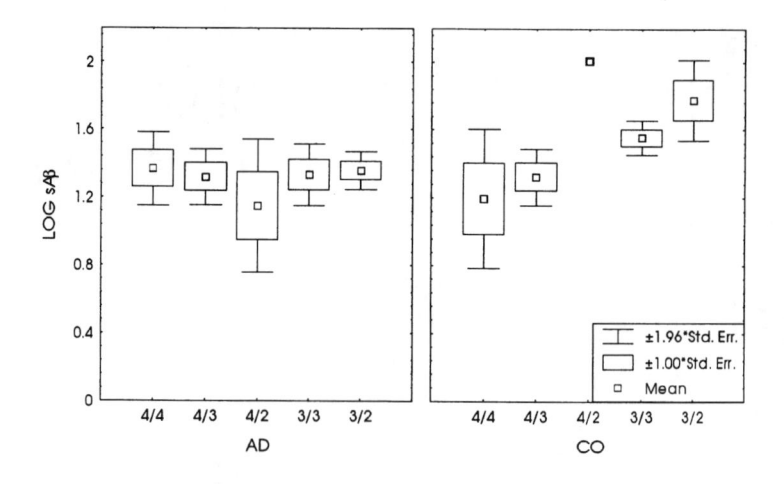

FIGURE 8.2 sAβ in CSF from AD patients and nondemented controls as a function of Apo E phenotype.

amyloid load in cerebral blood vessels and, to a lesser extent, with the amount of Aβ in the frontal cortex from AD patients.

Nitsch et al. (1995) showed that sAβ levels in CSF correlated inversely with the cognitive and functional measures of dementia severity. There are, however, no published longitudinal studies of CSF sAβ in AD. We recently measured sAβ levels in serial CSF collected at intervals during a 3-year period from 25 patients with probable AD. Our preliminary results showed that CSF sAβ levels decrease in AD patients with time, and there is a significant correlation between CSF sAβ levels and the progression of dementia.

AMYLOID-ASSOCIATED PROTEINS IN BLOOD AND CSF

Apo E has been of special interest in research of AD since investigators showed that the presence of the Apo E4 allele is the strongest known risk factor for the development of late-onset AD (Saunders et al., 1993). We measured CSF Apo E concentrations, using ELISA, and showed that CSF Apo E levels were lower in patients with probable AD than those in age-matched, non-demented controls, although there was significant overlap between the groups (Pirttilä et al., 1994c). CSF Apo E concentrations correlated with CSF sAβ levels. Our preliminary results showed that CSF Apo E levels decrease with time in patients with probable AD, and changes of Apo E levels correlate with changes of sAβ levels in CSF.

The presence of acute phase reaction in AD brains is well established. However, data on inflammatory mediators in blood or CSF in AD are fragmentary and controversial. Many investigators have examined serum or CSF $\propto$1-ACT levels. Several studies (Brugge, Katzman, Hill, Hansen, & Saitoh, 1992; Matsubara et al., 1990) have shown an increase of $\propto$1-ACT levels in blood or CSF in patients with AD compared to those in nondemented controls or patients with VD. However, others (Delamarche, Berger, Gallard, & Pouplard-Barthelaix, 1991; Pirttilä, Mehta, Frey, & Wisniewski, 1994a) reported no difference in the levels between AD and controls. We measured concentrations of several acute phase reactants, including $\propto$1-AT, $\propto$2-MG, C-reactive protein, and serum amyloid component P in paired serum, as well as CSF from patients with probable AD and nondemented controls using ELISA (Mehta, Pirttilä, Mehta, Dalton, & Wisniewski, 1995). Serum or CSF concentrations of these acute phase reactants were similar in patients with probable AD, definite AD, and in nondemented controls.

Although Cacabelos, Barquero, Garcia, Alvarez, and Varela-Deseijas (1991) showed an increase of CSF IL-1β levels in a small number of AD patients, we were not able to confirm their findings. Licastro, Morini, Polazzi, and Davis (1995) showed a marginal increase of serum IL-6 levels in patients with AD compared to controls, whereas Van Duijn, Hofman, and Nagelkerken (1990) found similar levels between AD and controls. We found an increase in serum IL-6 in patients with AD (Mehta et al., 1995); however, CSF IL-6 levels were below the detection limit, using the commercial ELISA kits.

NFT-RELATED PROTEINS IN CSF

Several studies suggested that the microtubule-associated protein tau, shown to be part of the PHF, might be present in CSF. Based on this information, we developed an ELISA to measure a soluble PHF protein in the CSF, which is in a ubiquitinated form. We examined the presence of PHF antigen in the CSF from AD and control patients, using a monoclonal antibody to PHF in ELISA (Mehta, Thal, Wisniewski, Grundke-Iqbal, & Iqbal, 1985). Our data showed that the mean concentrations of PHF antigen were significantly higher in CSF from AD compared to the control group. However, some degree of overlap was observed between the groups. Wolozin and Davies (1987) showed the presence of a modified form of tau, that is, PHF-tau, in CSF from AD patients. Recent studies showed that the levels of the tau protein in CSF from patients with probable AD were significantly higher than those in nondemented controls (Munroe et al., 1995; Vandermeeren et al., 1993; Vigo-Pelfrey et al., 1995). Although there was a good discrimination between the levels of tau in CSF of AD patients and controls, there was a significant overlap in the levels between patients with AD and those with other neurological diseases. The higher range of tau values in the AD group may serve as a useful adjunct to the diagnosis and therapeutic response when combined with appropriate neurological and neuropsychological evaluations.

NEUROTRANSMITTERS

Selective neuronal groups with specific neurotransmitter characteristics are affected in the AD brain. One of the earliest lesions is a loss of the large cholinergic neurons in the basal nucleus of the forebrain that leads to a loss of the cholinergic markers choline acetyltransferase and acetylcholinesterase (AChE) in the cerebral neocortex and hippocampus (Katzman & Jackson, 1991). Due to an extensive cholinergic deficit in the AD brain, cholinergic markers in CSF have been studied extensively. Data on neurotransmitter changes in CSF from AD patients are controversial.

Investigators have shown qualitative and quantitative differences in CSF AChE in patients with AD compared to the control group. Navaratnam et al. (1991), using the isoelectric focusing method, showed an additional band that indicated an anomalous form of AChE in CSF of a majority of histopathologically confirmed AD patients, but the band was absent in CSF from nondemented controls. Many studies have shown that AChE activity in CSF obtained by lumbar puncture is lower in patients with AD than nondemented controls (Appleyard & McDonald, 1992; Kumar, Giacobini, & Markwell, 1989; Malm, Kristensen, Ekstedt, Adolfsson, & Wester, 1991; Soininen, Jolkkonen, Reinikainen, Halonen, & Riekkinen, 1984). The results showed, however, a considerable overlap between the groups, and thus the diagnostic utility of this measurement is of limited value. Lumbar CSF AChE activity correlated significantly with the severity of dementia in one study (Soininen et al.), but it was not found by others (Kumar et al.).

PROBLEMS AND LIMITATIONS IN SEARCH OF A DIAGNOSTIC MARKER

To support the clinical diagnosis of AD, a diagnostic test should be relatively simple to perform, reproducible, cost-effective, and have a high degree of sensitivity and specificity. Data on blood or CSF constituents in AD are controversial. The reasons may be: (a) patient material, (b) handling of blood and CSF samples, (c) type of test, and (d) the significance of the putative marker in the pathogenesis of the disease.

The size and type of patient material vary in different studies (Table 8.1). In general, most studies have included a small number of AD patients and nondemented controls, and lacked appropriate controls such as patients with other types of dementia. Because the studies have been conducted using living patients with probable AD, the classification of the patients is important. Although the diagnosis of probable AD can be made accurately in over 88% of the cases using the NINCDS-ADRDA criteria

(Galasko et al., 1994; McKhann et al., 1984), it is difficult to rule out the presence of neuropathological changes of AD in elderly control subjects. Also, patients with dementia and significant cerebrovascular disease often have simultaneous changes in AD neuropathology. The type of AD patients included in the studies may influence the results. For example, patients with severe dementia may have elevated levels of acute phase reactants secondary to end-stage illness or due to subclinical infections. The latter are common in institutionalized patients.

Although blood is easy to obtain, it is unclear if systemic changes are specific to AD, and to what extent they reflect pathological changes in the brain. CSF may be a better representative of brain pathology than blood, but lumbar puncture is an invasive procedure and generally carried out in the hospital. CSF from healthy individuals is difficult to obtain, and normal values as well as the information regarding the influence of aging on many previously mentioned putative markers are not available.

The normal function and metabolism of βAPP, $sA\beta$, and many amyloid-associated proteins are not understood fully. The effects of age, diet, medication, and presence of inflammatory and noninflammatory diseases on their blood or CSF levels are not well understood. Handling of the samples may vary in different studies and influence the results. For example, the addition of protease inhibitors into plasma influences cytokine levels detected in ELISA (Whiteside, 1994).

The origins of many amyloid and amyloid-associated proteins in CSF, and the relationship between their levels in the brain and CSF, are not known. If the substance is present in blood and can cross the blood-brain barrier (BBB), an increase of their blood levels may lead to a false-positive increase in CSF. Therefore, concentrations in CSF should be normalized in terms of albumin or total protein. Changes in the CSF production rate with age and dilation of the brain ventricles as a result of brain atrophy also may influence the concentration of a given substance in CSF.

The type of assay is another reason for the different results in the studies. Data obtained using quantitative ELISA are easier to interpret and compare than those of qualitative or semiquantitative Western blotting assays. However, the specificity and affinity of the antibodies are of great importance for the sensitivity of an assay. The latter differs from one laboratory to another. One of the main limitations for the widespread use of these assays is the availability of specific antibodies. For example, there are commercial antibodies available against $sA\beta$, but they may not be suitable for ELISA.

Finally, the specificity and sensitivity of a putative marker is intimately related to the role of a given substance in the etiology and pathogenesis of the disease. AD is a complex, genetically and etiologically heterogeneous disorder with a pattern of neuropathological changes rather than a single abnormality in the brain. The biochemical processes that contribute to the pathogenesis of AD are still poorly understood, and may be different in patients with familial and sporadic AD or in those with early-onset and late-onset disease. Hence, it is possible that no single diagnostic marker will be suitable for all forms of AD. For example, the measurement of Aβ in CSF or a fibroblast culture medium may help to identify affected individuals with familial AD associated with APP-mutations, but its usefulness in other forms of AD is unknown.

BIOCHEMICAL MARKER FOR AD—FACT OR FICTION?

As yet, there is no laboratory test to support the clinical diagnosis AD. Thus, is a diagnostic marker for AD a fiction? Due to the heterogeneity and complex nature of AD, it is unlikely that a single marker, with 100% specificity for AD, will be found. There may be, however, different markers that may help to discriminate different subgroups of AD with distinct genetic backgrounds.

One of the main limitations of ELISA for detecting markers specific to AD is the possibility of obtaining false positive and false negative results. A result may be false positive because of the increased presence of cross-reactive antigens in the CSF. In addition, false positive results in nondemented cases could be obtained for individuals with greater than normal levels of amyloid and neurofibrillary changes in their brains. It is possible that such patients are at a preclinical stage of AD. False negative results may be obtained in individuals with borderline AD pathology or who have been clinically misdiagnosed (Bancher et al., 1990).

On the other hand, there may be some assays that will prove useful to confirm the diagnosis of AD or to monitor the progression of the disease. More studies are, however, needed to examine whether measurement of CSF tau discriminates against patients with AD from controls who have no other neurological diseases, and those with other forms of dementia. At present, measurement of CSF Aβ is not useful as a confirmatory test of probable AD, but it may help to identify individuals at risk in familial AD groups associated with βAPP mutations, and may be useful to monitor Aβ accumulation in the brain. The latter will be important when treatment targeted to amyloid formation is available.

REFERENCES

Appleyard, M. E., & McDonald, B. (1992). Acetylcholinesterase and butyrylcholinesterase activities in cerebrospinal fluid from different levels of the neuraxis of patients with dementia of the Alzheimer type. *Journal of Neurology, Neurosurgery, and Psychiatry, 55,* 1074–1078.

Bancher, C., Wisniewski, H. M., Mehta, P. D., Kim, K. S., Grundke-Iqbal, I., & Iqbal, K. (1990). Biochemical markers for Alzheimer disease as reflection of the neuropathology in cerebrospinal fluid. In R. E. Becker & E. Giacobini (Eds.), *Alzheimer's disease, current research in early diagnosis* (pp. 195–216). New York: Taylor and Francis.

Brugge, K., Katzman, R., Hill, L. R., Hansen, L. A., & Saitoh, T. (1992). Serological ∝1-antichymotrypsin in Down's syndrome and Alzheimer's disease. *Annals of Neurology, 32,* 193–197.

Bush, A. I, Whyte, S., Thomas, L. D., Williamson, T. G., Van Tiggelen, C. J., Currie, J., Small, D. H., Moir, R. D., Li, Q. X., Rumble, B., Mönning, Beyreuther, K., & Masters, C. L. (1992). An abnormality of plasma amyloid protein precursor in Alzheimer's disease. *Annals of Neurology, 32,* 57–65.

Cacabelos, R., Barquero, M., Garcia, P., Alvarez, X. A., & Varela-Deseijas, E. (1991). Cerebrospinal fluid interleukin-1 beta (IL-1 beta) in Alzheimer's disease and neurological disorders. *Methods in Experimental Clinical Pharmacology, 13,* 455–458.

Carroll, R. T., Lust, M. R., Kim, K. S., Doyle, P. D., & Emmerling, M. R. (1995). An age-related correlation between levels of β-amyloid precursor protein and β-amyloid in human cerebrospinal fluid. *Biochemical and Biophysical Research Communications, 210,* 345–349.

Chong, J. K., Miller, B. E., & Ghanbari, H. A. (1990). Detection of amyloid beta protein precursor immunoreactivity in normal and Alzheimer's disease cerebrospinal fluid. *Life Science, 47,* 1163–1171.

Delamarche, C., Berger, F., Gallard, L., & Pouplard-Barthelaix, __. (1991). Aging and Alzheimer's disease: Protease inhibitors in cerebrospinal fluid. *Neurobiology of Aging, 12,* 71–74.

Galasko, D., Hansen, L. A., Katzman, R., Wiederholt, W., Masliah, E., Terry, R., Hill, R., Lessin, P., & Thal, L. J. (1994). Clinical-neuropathological correlations in Alzheimer's disease and related dementias. *Archives of Neurology, 51,* 888–895.

Henriksson, T., Barbour, R. M., Braa, S., Ward, P., Fritz, L. C., Johnson-Wood, K., Chung, H. D., Burke, W., Reinikainen, K. J., Riekkinen, P., & Schenk, D. B. (1991). Analysis and quantitation of the β-amyloid precursor protein in the cerebrospinal fluid of Alzheimer's disease patients with a monoclonal antibody-based immunoassay. *Journal of Neurochemistry, 56,* 1037–1042.

Kalaria, R. N. (1993). The immunopathology of Alzheimer's disease and some related disorders. *Brain Pathology, 3,* 333–347.

Katzman, R., & Jackson, J. E. (1991). Alzheimer disease: Basic and clinical advances. *Journal of the American Geriatric Society, 39,* 516–525.

Kitaguchi, N., Tokushima, Y., Oishi, K., Takahashi, Y., Shiojiri, S., Nakamura, S., Tanaka, S., Kodaira, R., & Ito, H. (1990). Determination of amyloid β protein precursors harboring active form of proteinase inhibitor domains in cerebrospinal fluid of Alzheimer's disease patients by trypsin-antibody sandwich ELISA. *Biochemical and Biophysical Research Communications, 166,* 1453–1459.

Kumar, V., Giacobini, E., & Markwell, S. (1989). CSF choline and acetylcholinesterase in early-onset vs. late-onset Alzheimer's disease patients. *Acta Neurologica Scandinavica, 80,* 461–466.

Licastro, F., Morini, M. C., Polazzi, E., & Davis, L. J. (1995). Increased serum $\propto$1-antichymotrypsin in patients with probable Alzheimer's disease: An acute phase reactant without the peripheral acute phase response. *Journal of Neuroimmunology, 57,* 71–75.

Malm, J., Kristensen, B., Ekstedt, J., Adolfsson, R., & Wester, P. (1991). CSF monoamine metabolites, cholinesterases and lactate in the adult hydrocephalus syndrome (normal pressure hydrocephalus) related to CSF hydrodynamic parameters. *Journal of Neurology, Neurosurgery, and Psychiatry, 54,* 252–259.

Matsubara, E., Nirai, S., Amari, M., Shoji, M., Yamaguchi, M., Okamoto, K., Ishiguro, K., Narigaya, Y., & Wakabayashi, K. (1990). $\propto$1-antichymotrypsin as a possible marker for Alzheimer-type dementia. *Annals of Neurology, 28,* 561–567.

McKhann, G., Drachman, D., Folstein, M., Katzman, R., Price, D., & Stadlan, E. M. (1984). Clinical diagnosis of Alzheimer's disease: Report of the NINCDS-ADRDA Work Group under the auspices of the Department of Health and Human Services Task Force on Alzheimer's Disease. *Neurology, 34,* 939–944.

Mehta, P. D., Kim, K. S., & Wisniewski, H. M. (1991). ELISA as a laboratory test to aid the diagnosis of Alzheimer's disease. *Techniques in Diagnostic Pathology, 2,* 99–112.

Mehta, P. D., Pirttilä, T., Mehta, S. P., Dalton, A. J., & Wisniewski, H. M. (1995). Serum levels of interleukin-6 (IL-6) and acute phase proteins in Down's syndrome and Alzheimer's disease (AD). *Neurology, 45*(Suppl. 4), A472.

Mehta, P. D., Thal, L., Wisniewski, H. M., Grundke-Iqbal, I., & Iqbal, K. (1985). Paired helical filaments antigen in CSF. *Lancet, 2,* 35.

Munroe, W. A., Southwick, P. C., Chang, L., Scharre, D. W., Echols, C. L., Jr., Fu, P. C., Whaley, J. M., & Wolfert, R. L. (1995). Tau protein in cerebrospinal

fluid as an aid in the diagnosis of Alzheimer's disease. *Annals of Clinical Laboratory Science, 25,* 207–217.
Nakamura, T., Shoji, M., Harigaya, Y., Watanabe, M., Hosoda, K., Cheung, T. T., Shaffer, L. M., Golde, T. E., Younkin, L. H., Younkin, S. G., & Hirai, S. (1994). Amyloid β protein levels in cerebrospinal fluid are elevated in early-onset Alzheimer's disease. *Annals of Neurology, 1994, 36,* 903–911.
Navaratnam, D. S., Priddle, J. D., McDonald, B., Esiri, M. M., Robinson, J. R., & Smith, A. D. (1991). Anomalous molecular form of acetylcholinesterase in cerebrospinal fluid in histologically diagnosed Alzheimer's disease. *Lancet, 337,* 447–450.
Nitsch, R. M., Rebeck, G. W., Deng, M., Richardson, U. I., Tennis, M., Schenk, D. B., Vigo-Pelfrey, C., Lieberburg, I., Wurtman, R. J., Hyman, B. T., & Growdon, J. H. (1995). Cerebrospinal fluid levels of amyloid β-protein in Alzheimer's disease: Inverse correlation with severity of dementia and effect of apolipoprotein E genotype. *Annals of Neurology, 37,* 512–518.
Palmert, M. R., Usiak, M., Mayeux, R., Raskind, M., Tourtellotte, W. W., & Younkin, S. G. (1990). Soluble derivatives of the β amyloid protein precursor in cerebrospinal fluid: Alterations in normal aging and in Alzheimer's disease. *Neurology, 40,* 1028–1034.
Pirttilä, T., Kim, K. S., Mehta, P. D., Frey, H., & Wisniewski, H. M. (1994b). Soluble amyloid β-protein in the cerebrospinal fluid from patients with Alzheimer's disease, vascular dementia and controls. *Journal of Neurological Science, 127,* 90–95.
Pirttilä, T., Mehta, P. D., Frey, H., & Wisniewski, H. M. (1994a). ∝1-antichymotrypsin and IL-1β are not increased in CSF or serum in Alzheimer's disease. *Neurobiology of Aging, 15,* 313–317.
Pirttilä, T., Mehta, P. D., Lehtimäki, T., Kim, K. S., Sersen, E. A., Frey, H., Nikkari, T., & Wisniewski, H. M. (1994c). Relationship between apolipoprotein E4 allele and CSF amyloid β-protein in Alzheimer's disease and controls. *Neuroscience and Research Communication, 15,* 201–207.
Pirttilä, T., Mehta, P. D., Soininen, H., Kim, K. S., Heinonen, O., Paljärvi, L., Kosunen, O., Riekkinen, P., & Wisniewski, H. M. (1996). Cerebrospinal fluid concentrations of soluble amyloid β-protein and apolipoprotein E in patients with Alzheimer's disease. *Archives of Neurology, 53,* 189–193.
Saunders, A. M., Strittmatter, W. J., Schmechel, D., St. George-Hyslop, P. H., Pericak-Vance, M. A., Joo, S. H., Rosi, B. L., Gusella, J. F., Crapper-MacLachlan, D. R., Alberts, M. J., Hulette, C., Crain, B., Goldgaber, D., & Roses, A. D. (1993). Association of apolipoprotein E allele E4 with late-onset familial and sporadic Alzheimer's disease. *Neurology, 43,* 1467–1472.
Segal, M. B. (1993). Extracellular and cerebrospinal fluids. *Journal of Inherited Metabolic Disorders, 16,* 617–638.
Selkoe, D. (1994). Normal and abnormal biology of the β-amyloid precursor protein. *Annual Review of Neuroscience, 17,* 489–517.

Seubert, P., Vigo-Pelfrey, C., Esch, F., Lee, M., Dovey, H., Davis, D., Shinha, S., Schlossmacher, M., Whaley, J., Swindlehurst, C., McCormack, R., Wolfert, R., Selkoe, D., Lieberburg, I., & Schenk, D. (1992). Isolation and quantitation of soluble Alzheimer's β-peptide from biological fluids. *Nature, 359,* 325–327.

Soininen, H. S., Jolkkonen, J. T., Reinikainen, K. J., Halonen, T. O., & Riekkinen, P. J. (1984). Reduced cholinesterase activity and somatostatin-like immunoreactivity in the cerebrospinal fluid of patients with dementia of the Alzheimer type. *Journal of Neurological Science, 63,* 167–172.

Tabaton, M., Nunzi, M. G., Xue, R., Usiak, M., Autilio-Gambetti, L., & Gambetti, P. (1994). Soluble amyloid β-protein is a marker of Alzheimer amyloid in brain but in cerebrospinal fluid. *Biochemical and Biophysical Research Communication, 200,* 1598–1603.

Tagliavini, F., Giaccone, G., Frangione, B., & Bugiani, O. (1988). Pre-amyloid deposits in the cerebral cortex of patients with Alzheimer's disease and nondemented individuals. *Neuroscience Letter, 93,* 191–196.

Vandermeeren, M., Mercken, M., Vanmechelen, E., Six, J., Van de Voorde, A., Martin, J. J., & Cras, P. (1993). Detection of tau proteins in normal and Alzheimer's disease cerebrospinal fluid with a sensitive sandwich enzymelinked immunosorbent assay. *Journal of Neurochemistry, 61,* 1828–1834.

Van Duijn, C. M., Hofman, A., & Nagelkerken, L. (1990). Serum levels of interleukin-6 are not elevated in patients with Alzheimer's disease. *Neuroscience Letter, 108,* 350–354.

Van Gool, W. A., Kuiper, M. A., Walstra, G. J. M., Wolters, E. C., & Bolhuis, P. A. (1995). Concentrations of amyloid β protein in cerebrospinal fluid of patients with Alzheimer's disease. *Annals of Neurology, 37,* 277–279.

Van Gool, W. A., Schenk, D. B., & Bolhuis, P. A. (1994). Concentrations of amyloid-β protein in cerebrospinal fluid increase with age in patients free from neurodegenerative disease. *Neuroscience Letter, 172,* 122–124.

Van Nostrand, W. E., Wagner, S. L., Shankle, W. R., Farrow, J. S., Dick, M., Rozemuller, J. M., Kuiper, M. A., Wolters, E. C., Zimmerman, J., Cotman, C. W., & Cunningham, D. D. (1992). Decreased levels of soluble amyloid β-protein precursor in cerebrospinal fluid of live Alzheimer disease patients. *Proceedings of the National Academy of Science, USA, 89,* 2551–2555.

Vigo-Pelfrey, C., Seubert, P., Barbour, R., Blomquist, C., Lee, M., Lee, D., Coria, F., Chang, L., Miller, B., Lieberburg, I., & Schenk, D. (1995). Elevation of microtubule-associated protein tau in the cerebrospinal fluid of patients with Alzheimer's disease. *Neurology, 45,* 788–793.

Whiteside, T. L. (1994). Cytokine measurements and interpretation of cytokine assays in human disease. *Journal of Clinical Immunology, 14,* 327–339.

Wisniewski, H. M., Wegiel, J., & Popovitch, E. R. (1994). Age-associaetd development of diffuse and thioflavin-S-positive plaques in Down syndrome. *Development Brain Dysfunction, 7,* 330–339.

Wisniewski, H. M., & Wegiel, J. (1995). The neuropathology of Alzheimer's disease. *Neuroimaging Clinics of North America, 5*, 45–57.

Wolozin, B., & Davies, P. (1987). Alzheimer-related neuronal protein A68: Specificity and distribution. *Annals of Neurology, 22*, 521–526.

PART THREE

Treatment Updates

CHAPTER **9**

Diagnosis and Treatment of Alzheimer's Disease and Comorbid Depression

Barnett S. Meyers
Fughik Tirumalasetti

Psychiatric complications from Alzheimer's disease (AD) are present in up to 50% of the cases. During the last 2 decades, increasing attention has been given to the diagnosis, prevalence, treatment, and outcomes of depressive syndromes occurring in AD patients. In this chapter, the authors will:

1. discuss conceptual and methodological issues bearing on the relationships between AD and depression; and
2. review studies addressing the treatment of AD patients suffering from this combination of disorders. Emphasis will be given to treatment studies of patients meeting diagnostic criteria for both AD and major depression.

The overlap of signs and symptoms of depression with those of dementia can confound diagnosis and management. Literature about the relationships between depression and dementia has conceptualized syndromes in which diagnostic confusion or syndromal overlap commonly occur (Emery & Oxman, 1992; Teri & Wagner, 1992). Described categories include (a) pseudodementia (depression "appearing like" or imitating dementia); (b) depressive dementia (a true reversible dementia secondary to depression); (c) "pseudodepression" (dementia in which signs and symptoms "appear like" and can be mistaken for depression and the coexisting dementia and major depression. The latter category refers to instances of true comorbidity. Definitions generally require that the onset of depression follow a period of cognitive deterioration. The diagnosis of dementia with comorbid depression does not address causation; the major depression could be secondary to or independent of the dementing disorder. We will focus on the diagnosis and treatment of patients suffering from these affective and cognitive disorders concurrently. Consideration of the important questions of mechanisms and pathogenesis, including whether AD may predispose a patient to development of major depression, is beyond the scope of this chapter. Although depression has been found to exist in association with types of degenerative dementing disorders other than AD, including multi-infarct dementia (Cummings, Miller, Hill, & Neshkes, 1987; Sultzer, Levin, Mahler, High, & Cummings, 1993), Parkinson's disease (Cummings, 1985), Huntington's disease (Folstein, Abbott, Chase, Jensen, & Folstein, 1983), and Pick's disease (Liston, 1977), our focus will be on the treatment of depression occurring specifically in association with AD.

The effective treatment of major depression associated with AD merits special consideration because of findings that patients with these comorbid disorders suffer excess disability (Pearson, Teri, Reifler, & Raskind, 1989; Rovner et al., 1989). Depression in association with AD predicts poorer functioning on measures of instrumental functioning in patients with mild cognitive impairment and lower functioning on more basic measures in patients with severe impairment (Fitz & Teri, 1994). Furthermore, AD victims with comorbid depression have significantly increased mortality rates over the 1st year of follow-up (Rovner et al., 1991).

EPIDEMIOLOGY

Prevalence and Risk Factors

A wide range of prevalence rates for depression in AD has been reported with estimates from 0% (Burns, Jacoby, & Levy, 1990) to 86% (Merriam,

Aronson, Gaston, Wey, & Katz, 1988). Differences in diagnostic methodology, setting, and source of clinical information contribute to discrepancies in the literature. Higher prevalence rates have been found in studies using caregiver reports (Merriam et al., 1988; Mackenzie, Robiner, & Knopman, 1989), a finding related to the higher endorsement of depressive symptoms in collateral informants than in AD patients themselves (Burke, Rubin, Morris, & Berg, 1988). Although setting presumably influences prevalence rates, differences in diagnostic criteria also confound interpretation of reported findings. Thus prevalences between 11% (Greenwald et al., 1989) and 20% have been reported in mental health settings (Ballinger, Reid, & Heather, 1982), and a range of 17%–31% among outpatients attending geriatric medical or Alzheimer's disease clinics (Reding, Haycox, & Blass, 1985; Reifler, Larson, Teri, & Paulsen, 1986; Rovner et al., 1990). Among systematically diagnosed AD admissions to nursing homes, 10% have been found to meet criteria for concurrent major depression (Rovner, Kafonek, Filipp, Lucas, & Folstein, 1986).

Earlier age of onset (Lawlor, 1994), a positive family history of depression (Pearlson et al., 1990), and female gender (Reifler et al., 1986; Lazarus, Newton, Cohler, Lesser, & Schwoen, 1987; Migliorelli, Tesona Sabe, Petracchi, Leiguarda, & Starkstein, 1995) have been reported to increase the association between AD and depression. Controversy persists about the relationship between severity of cognitive dysfunction and prevalence of comorbid major depression, with higher rates reported in association with better function in some (Reifler et al., 1982) but not all (Gottlieb, Gur, & Gur, 1988; Migliorelli et al., 1995; Rovner, Broadhead, & Spenser, 1989) studies.

Incidence

Recent studies have assessed the incidence of major depression in prospectively studied AD patients with rates approximating 1% reported over follow-up periods of 2 to 3 years (Burke et al., 1988; Weiner, Edland, Luszczynkska, 1994). These data contrast with the finding that 22% of 32 prospectively studied AD patients developed major depression over the 6 years until all cases reached postmortem confirmations of AD (Rosen & Zubenko, 1991). Because 40%–50% of AD plus depression patients have a history of major depression before the onset of AD (Migliorelli et al., 1995; Reifler et al., 1986), the exclusion of patients with prior depression from the largest prospectively studied sample (Weiner et al., 1994) may have decreased the reported incidence rate.

A relationship between previous depression and subsequent dementia is suggested strongly by the follow-up of nondemented depressed patients referred for assessment to a memory disorders clinic (Reding et al., 1985). In this study, 70% of referrals without dementia met DSM-III (American Psychiatric Association, 1980) criteria for major depression or dysthymia, and 57% of these individuals developed dementia during approximately 3 years of follow-up. The selection bias inherent in studying nondemented depressives referred for memory assessment presumably contributed to the high incidence in this study.

Comparison of reported differences for rates of major depression in patients with AD must consider diagnostic criteria applied by investigators. Use of DSM-III-R (American Psychiatric Association, 1987) and DSM-IV (American Psychiatric Association, 1994) criteria results in lower prevalence rates than DSM-III (American Psychiatric Association, 1980) because recent DSMs do not include irritability as a symptom of mood disturbance or impaired cognition that could be secondary to another existing condition as criteria (Mackenzie et al., 1989). Nevertheless, a recent study using a structured clinical interview to reach a DSM III-R diagnosis demonstrated that 23% of AD seen in an outpatient neurology clinic met criteria for major depression, with another 28% diagnosed with dysthymia (Migliorelli et al., 1995).

DIAGNOSTIC CONSIDERATIONS

Conceptual Issues: Pseudodementia, Depression with Reversible Dementia, and Comorbid Depression

Reports that prior depression is a risk factor for the occurrence of depression in association with AD bear on the problem of pseudodementia. As described by Kiloh (1961), pseudodementia refers to a syndrome that combines an exaggeration of cognitive symptoms with another psychiatric disorder. The prefix *pseudo* indicates that the cognitive disturbance is apparent rather than real. Wells (1979) elaborated on this syndrome, pointing out that patients with pseudodementia are typically older depressives whose clinical pictures are marked by: (a) exaggerated memory complaints and (b) the absence of behavioral evidence of true cognitive dysfunction that is proportional to the severity of complaints. We previously used the alternative term "cognitive hypochondriasis" to refer to this symptomatic picture (Meyers, 1987).

M. F. Folstein, Folstein, and McHugh (1978) used the term "dementia syndrome of depression" to describe a subset of depressives with true reversible cognitive dysfunction in association with an affective episode. This syndrome has been described as pseudodementia by some investigators (Caine, 1981) and as depression with reversible dementia by others (Rabins, Merchant, & Nedstadt, 1984). Data demonstrating that individuals suffering major depression with reversible cognitive impairment have biological abnormalities comparable to those with irreversible dementia and (Alexopoulos, Young, Lieberman, & Shamoian, 1987) that reversible dementia predicts the development of an irreversible cognitive decline in some (Kral & Emery, 1989; Alexopoulos, Meyers, Young, Mattis, & Kakuma, 1993) highlight the prognostic importance of a dementia syndrome occurring in association with major depression, even when recovery of the cognitive function occurs in association with remission of the depressive episode. Studies addressing the treatment response of patients with major depression associated with reversible cognitive impairment will be considered next.

Problems of Measurement: Symptomatic Overlap

As noted previously, because cognitive deficits that develop in association with a major depression may reverse with recovery from the mood disorder, the diagnosis of AD with comorbid depression is generally reserved for patients in whom clear evidence of dementia preceded the onset of affective symptoms. Nevertheless, assessment of mood symptoms in patients with AD is confounded by the overlap of signs and symptoms of dementia with those of depressive disorders. Thus patients with dementia are known to score higher than age-matched controls on depression rating scales (Knesevich, Martin, Berg, & Danziger, 1983; Lazarus et al., 1987). Note also that item analysis of depression scores has revealed AD patients to score higher for diminished work and activity, psychomotor retardation, and ideational symptoms of depression but not on measures of neurovegetative disturbance (Lazarus et al.).

A study of the endorsement of Feigner symptoms of major depression (Feighner et al., 1972) in patients without prior depressive episodes demonstrates increased endorsement of diagnostic criteria for depression as well (Burke et al., 1988). Although AD patients and age-matched controls did not differ for the overall number of Feighner symptoms reported at index or 15-month follow-up, AD patients were significantly more likely to endorse change in psychomotor activity or symptoms of disturbed thinking or concentration at one of these time points. Collateral informants of the AD patients reported a significantly higher number of depressive symptoms than those of controls at all time points, with psychomotor disturbance, diminished energy, loss of interest, and difficulty thinking and concentrating all reported at a greater frequency by collaterals of the AD patients. Finally, AD patients' ability to report depressive symptoms is influenced by the severity of cognitive impairment (Teri & Wagner, 1992); thus the sensitivity of the self-report Geriatric Depression Scale (Yesavage et al., 1983) is decreased in patients with severe dementia (Parmalee, Katz, & Lawton, 1989). Studies demonstrating that cognitive dysfunction contributes to scores on objective measures of depression and that severity of cognitive dysfunction influences the reporting of symptoms highlight the need for sensitive and specific measures of depression in controlled trials of AD patients who meet criteria-based diagnoses for concurrent major depression.

Dimensional Scales for Depression in AD

The complexity of assessing the severity of depression in AD has led to the development of dimensional measures to improve the sensitivity and specificity of depression assessment in this population. The Cornell Scale for Depression in Dementia (CSDD) (Alexopoulos, Abrams, Young, & Shamoian, 1988) is a 19-item measure derived, in part, from the 17-item Hamilton Scale for Depression (Ham-D) (Hamilton, 1960). The CSDD is rated by clinicians using information obtained from caregivers and has demonstrated greater sensitivity to major depression than the Ham-D (Alexopoulos et al., 1988; Logsdon & Teri, 1995). Additional scales have been developed for use in patients with dementia. The Alzheimer's Disease Assessment Scale (Mohs, Rosen, Greenwald, & Davis, 1983), applied primarily to assess the severity and course of cognitive dysfunction, includes a limited number of items for depression. The Dementia Mood Assessment Scale (Sunderland et al., 1988), a 24-item scale that uses a semistructured interview and direct observation over time, was designed for possible use in treatment trials. Future studies are needed to assess and compare the sensitivity of these measures to changes in subjects with dementia and coexisting depression treated in randomized protocols.

TREATMENT

Depressive Symptoms

AD patients who do not meet diagnostic criteria for clinical depression have higher depression scores than age-matched controls. It is, therefore, interesting that a number of pharmacologic interventions have been associated with decreased depression scores in nondepressed samples of AD patients. Dihydroergotoxin (Hydergine) has had Food and Drug Administration approval for the treatment of organic brain disease for more than 30 years. The mild improvement in functioning on multidimensional dementia measures reported with Hydergine treatment may be mediated by improvement in mood, perhaps through the drug's weak effect on central dopamine and serotonin receptors (Hollister & Yesavage, 1984). This interpretation of Hydergine's efficacy parallels the studies reviewed by Teri and Wagner (1992) demonstrating that a variety of centrally acting medications can improve depression scores in nondepressed AD patients. The reported benefits of psychostimulants for withdrawal and apathy in elderly patients with dementia (Chiarello & Cole, 1987) should be interpreted similarly: improvement in depression rating scale items does not demonstrate effectiveness for the treatment of major depression.

Clinical Depression

There are remarkably few systematic studies of treatment response in patients with AD and comorbid major depression; controlled studies are rarer still. A chart review study of outpatients with AD found that 85% of patients treated for major depression demonstrated clear evidence of improved mood (Reifler et al., 1986). Prospective studies have shown an association between inpatient psychiatric treatment and significant improvement in Ham-D scores. Effectiveness of treatment has been demonstrated across phenomenologic subgroups of AD, with the greatest improvement occurring in patients meeting criteria for comorbid major depression (Greenwald et al., 1989; Zubenko et al., 1992). An open study of treatment response to intensive treatment with nortriptyline or electroconvulsive therapy in elderly major depressives with comorbid cognitive impairment demonstrated that 81.3% achieved predischarge Ham-D scores of ≤ 10 (Reynolds et al., 1987). Overall, decreased Ham-D scores were significantly correlated with improvements in dementia ratings. The patients with impairment arising in the context of a major depression demonstrated greater improvement in Ham-D and cognitive functioning scores than did patients in whom dementia preceded the onset of the depressive episode.

In the single placebo-controlled study of somatic therapy for patients meeting criteria for both AD and major depression, moderately intense imipramine treatment, with average doses and plasma concentrations of 83 mg a day and 119 ng/ml, respectively, was associated with significant improvements in depression scores during the 8-week study period (Reifler et al., 1989). Imipramine treatment of depressed AD patients was associated with significant improvements in mini-mental state examination scores, and none of these subjects developed an anticholinergic delirium; however, imipramine was associated with significant deterioration on the more sensitive Dementia Rating Scale (Mattis, 1978). Results of this study cannot be interpreted as demonstrating efficacy for imipramine, because placebo-treated patients had comparable levels of improvement. Furthermore, the fact that imipramine plasma levels were below the generally accepted therapeutic concentrations may have decreased drug-placebo differences.

Our knowledge of dose and response relationships in patients with AD and comorbid depression is limited. Note that a preliminary study demonstrated that the customary concentration and response relationship for nortriptyline does not hold for patients suffering from depression associated with cognitive impairment (Young et al., 1991).

Case reports indicate that other classes of antidepressants, including monamine oxidase inhibitors and serotonin reuptake inhibitors (SSRIs) (Burke, Folks, Roccaforte, & Wengel, 1994), may be effective for patients with AD and comorbid depression. In a placebo-controlled study of AD patients with mixed mood and behavioral symptoms, treatment with citalopram, an SSRI not currently available in the United States, was associated with significant reductions in affective symptoms, including depressed mood (Gottfries, Karlsson, & Nyth, 1992). Although a subgroup of patients with AD and comorbid depression demonstrated improved cognitive functioning in association with citalopram treatment, data on the antidepressant efficacy of citalopram in this subsample were not provided.

The nonpharmacologic approach of behavioral therapy for patients and caregivers has been studied in the treatment of depression associated with AD. Although data from controlled studies are needed, investigators report that preliminary findings indicate that caregivers are able to apply behavioral therapy principles and reduce depressive symptoms in AD patients (Teri & Wagner, 1992).

Note that controlled treatment studies of patients with major depression and reversible dementia are also lacking. Although observational studies have reported that the great majority of these patients improve in association with intensive somatic therapy (Rabins et al., 1984; Reynolds et al., 1987), nothing is known about the degree and frequency of responses in these patients compared to cognitively intact elderly depressives and patients with AD and comorbid depression.

Course

Longitudinal studies of patients with depression and cognitive impairment have focused particularly on the course of cognitive functioning. Patients with major depression associated with dementia demonstrated improved mood and cognition after acute treatment and a 2-year follow-up (Rabins et al., 1984). Similarly, only one of nine subjects diagnosed initially as suffering major depression associated with cognitive impairment demonstrated cognitive decline at a 2-year follow-up, in contrast to the deterioration in the subsample diagnosed initially as having AD and comorbid depression (Reynolds et al., 1986). In contrast, a larger 3-year longitudinal study comparing elderly depressives with reversible dementia to an age-matched sample of cognitively intact depressives demonstrated a higher risk for dementia in subjects with depression-related impairment (Alexopoulos et al., 1993). These data suggest that reversible dementia is prodromal for dementia in a subset of elderly major depressives. None of these investigations assessed the course of depression in AD patients with comorbid depression or compared the course of depression in these subjects with that in cognitively intact elderly depressives or depressives with reversible dementia.

FUTURE DIRECTIONS

Controlled studies are required to clarify the efficacy and safety of various antidepressants in the treatment of AD associated with comorbid major depression. Comparison groups should include patients with cognitive impairment occurring contemporaneously with the depressive episode and age-matched depressives without cognitive impairment.

Little is known about the dose or concentration and response relationships in patients with AD and comorbid depression or in reversible dementia secondary to depression. Although this issue is somewhat mitigated by treatment with SSRIs, the question remains relevant when these subgroups are treated with standard secondary amine TCAs and newer agents with broad dosage ranges such as buproprion, venlafaxine, and nefazadone.

Finally, essentially nothing is known about the course of depression in patients with depression and comorbid dementia. Placebo-controlled continuation and maintenance studies are needed to determine the appropriateness of long-term therapy. The use of sensitive measures of both depressive symptoms and cognitive functioning is crucial. Overlap of signs and symptoms limits the sensitivity to change of scales customarily used in treatment studies. Sensitive measures of cognition are needed to assess the possible untoward effect of long-term pharmacologic treatment with anticholinergic agents in a population known to suffer degeneration of cholinergic neurons. Given the prevalence and the excessive rate of morbidity and mortality of depression occurring in the context of AD, it is surprising how little is known about the optimal acute and longer term management of this population.

REFERENCES

Alexopoulos, G. S., Abrams, R. C., Young, R. C., & Shamoian, C. A. (1988). Cornell Scale for depression in dementia. *Biological Psychiatry, 23,* 271–284.

Alexopoulos, G. S., Meyers, B. S., Young, R. C., Mattis, S., & Kakuma, T. (1993). The course of geriatric depression with "reversible dementia": A controlled study. *American Journal of Psychiatry, 150,* 1693–1699.

Alexopoulos, G. S., Young, R. C., Lieberman, K. W., & Shamoian, C. A. (1987). Platelet MAO activity in geriatric patients with depression and dementia. *American Journal of Psychiatry, 144,* 1480–1483.

American Psychiatric Association. (1980). *Diagnostic and statistical manual of mental disorders* (3rd ed.). Washington, DC: American Psychiatric Association.

American Psychiatric Association. (1987). *Diagnostic and statistical manual of mental disorders* (3rd ed. rev.). Washington, DC: American Psychiatric Association.

American Psychiatric Association. (1994). *Diagnostic and statistical manual of mental disorders* (4th ed.). Washington, DC: American Psychiatric Association.

Ballinger, B. R., Reid, A. H., & Heather, B. B. (1982). Cluster analysis of symptoms in elderly demented patients. *British Journal of Psychiatry, 140*, 257–262.

Burke, W. J., Folks, D. J., Roccaforte, W. H., & Wengel, S. V. (1994). Serotonin-reuptake inhibitors for the treatment of coexisting depression and psychosis in dementia of the Alzheimer's type. *American Journal of Geriatric Psychiatry, 2*, 352–354.

Burke, W. J., Rubin, E. H., Morris, J. C., & Berg, I. (1988). Symptoms of depression in dementia of the Alzheimer's type. *Alzheimer Disease and Associated Disorders, 2*, 356–362.

Burns, A., Jacoby, R., & Levy, R. (1990). Psychiatric phenomena in Alzheimer's disease. Pt. 3. Disorders of mood. *British Journal of Psychiatry, 157*, 81–86.

Caine, E. (1981). Pseudodementia: Current concepts and future directions. *Archives of General Psychiatry, 38*, 1359–1364.

Chiarello, R. J., & Cole, J. O. (1987). The use of psychostimulants in general psychiatry. *Archives of General Psychiatry, 24*, 286–295.

Cummings, J. L. (1985). Psychosomatic aspects of movement disorders. In M. R. Trimble (Ed.), *Interface between neurology and psychiatry* (pp. 111–132). New York: S. Karger.

Cummings, J. L., Miller, B., Hill, M. A., & Neshkes, R. (1987). Neuropsychiatric aspects of multi-infarct dementia and dementia of the Alzheimer type. *Archives of Neurology, 44*, 389–393.

Emery, V. O., & Oxman, T. E. (1992). Update on the dementia spectrum of depression. *American Journal of Psychiatry, 149*, 305–317.

Feighner, J. P., Robins, E., Guze, S. B., Woodruff, Jr., R. A., Winokur, G., & Munoz, R. (1972). Diagnostic criteria for use in psychiatric research. *Archives of General Psychiatry, 26*, 57–63.

Fitz, A. G., & Teri, L. (1994). Depression, cognition and functional ability in patients with Alzheimer's disease. *Journal of the American Geriatrics Society, 42*, 186–191.

Folstein, S. E., Abbott, M. H., Chase, G. A., Jensen, B. A., & Folstein, M. F. (1983). The association of affective disorder with Huntington's disease in a case series and in families. *Psychology and Medicine, 13*, 537–542.

Folstein, M. F., Folstein, S. E., & McHugh, P. R. (1975). "Mini-mental state": A practical method for grading the cognitive state of patients for the clinician. *Journal of Psychiatric Research, 12*, 189–198.

Folstein, M. F., Folstein, S. E., & McHugh, P. R. (1978). Dementia syndrome of depression. In R. Katzman, R. D. Terry, & K. L. Bick (Eds.), *Alzheimer's disease: Senile dementia and related disorders*. New York: Raven Press.

Gottfries, C. G., Karlsson, I., & Nyth, A. L. (1992). Treatment of depression in elderly patients with and without dementing disorders. *International Clinical Psychopharmacology*, 6(Suppl. 5), 55–64.

Gottlieb, G. L., Gur, R. E., & Gur, R. C. (1988). Reliability of psychiatric scales in patients with dementia of the Alzheimer's type. *American Journal of Psychiatry*, 145, 857–860.

Greenwald, B. S., Kramer-Ginsberg, E., Marin, D. B., Laitman, L. B., Hermann, C. K., Moths, R. C., & Davis, K. L. (1989). Dementia with coexistent major depression. *American Journal of Psychiatry*, 146, 1472–1478.

Hamilton, M. (1960). A rating scale for depression. *Journal of Neurology, Neurosurgery, and Psychiatry*, 23, 56–62.

Hollister, L. E., & Yesavage, J. (1984). Ergolyoid mesylates for senile dementias: Unanswered questions. *Annals of Internal Medicine*, 100, 894–898.

Jenike, M. A. (1985). Monamine oxidase inhibitors as treatment for depressed patients with primary degenerative dementia (Alzheimer's disease). *American Journal of Psychiatry*, 21, 65–71.

Kiloh, L. G. (1961). Pseudo-dementia. *Acta Psychiatrica Scandinavica*, 37, 336–351.

Knesevich, J. W., Martin, R. L., Berg, L., & Danziger, W. (1983). Preliminary report on affective symptoms in the early stages of senile dementia of the Alzheimer's type. *American Journal of Psychiatry*, 140, 233–236.

Kral, V., & Emory, O. (1989). Long term follow-up of depressive pseudodementia. *Canadian Journal of Psychiatry*, 34, 445–447.

Lawlor, B. A., Ryan, T. M., Schmeidler, J., Mohs, R. C., & Davis, K. L. (1994). Clinical symptoms associated with age at onset in Alzheimer's disease. *American Journal of Psychiatry*, 11, 1646–1649.

Lazarus, L. W., Newton, N., Cohler, B., Lesser, J., & Schweon, C. (1987). Frequency and presentation of depressive symptoms in patients with primary degenerative dementia. *American Journal of Psychiatry*, 144, 41–45.

Liston, E. H., Jr. (1977). Occult presenile dementia. *Journal of Nervous Mental Disorders*, 164, 263–267.

Logsdon, R. G., & Teri, L. (1995). Depression in Alzheimer's disease patients: Caregivers as surrogate reporters. *Journal of the American Geriatrics Society*, 43, 150–155.

Mackenzie, T. B., Robiner, W. N., & Knopman, D. S. (1989). Differences between patient and family assessments of depression in Alzheimer's disease. *American Journal of Psychiatry*, 146, 1174–1178.

Mattis, S. (1978). Dementia Rating Scale. Odessa, FL: Psychological Resources.

Merriam, A. E., Aronson, M. K., Gaston, P., Wey, S. L., & Katz, I. (1988). The psychiatric symptoms of Alzheimer's disease. *Journal of the American Geriatric Society*, 35, 7–12.

Meyers, B. S. (1987). Adverse cognitive effects of tricyclic antidepressants in the treatment of geriatric depression: Fact or fiction? In C. A. Shamoian

(Ed.), *Psychopharmacological treatment complications in the elderly* (pp. 1–16). Washington, DC: American Psychiatric Press.
Migliorelli, R., Tesona Sabe, L., Petracchi, M., Leiguarda, R., & Starkstein, S. E. (1995). Prevalence and correlates of dysthymia and major depression among patients with Alzheimer's disease. *American Journal of Psychiatry, 152,* 37–44.
Mohs, R. C., Rosen, W. G., Greenwald, B. S., & Davis, K. L. (1983). Neuropathologically validated scales for Alzheimer's disease. In T. Crook, S. Ferris, & R. Artus (Eds.), *Assessment in geriatric psychopharmacology* (pp. 37–41). New Canaan, CT: Mark Powley Associates.
Parmalee, P. A., Katz, I. R., & Lawton, M. P. (1989). Depression among the institutionalized aged: Assessment and prevalence estimation. *Journal of Gerontology and Medical Science, 44,* M22–M29.
Pearlson, G. D., Ross, C. A., Lohr, W. D., Rovner, B. W. Chase, G. A., & Folstein, M. F. (1990). Association between family history of affective disorder and the depressive syndrome of Alzheimer's disease. *American Journal of Psychiatry, 147,* 452–456.
Pearson, J. L., Teri, L., Reifler, B. V., & Raskind, M. A. (1989). Functional status and cognitive impairment in Alzheimer's patients with and without depression. *Journal of the American Geriatric Society, 37,* 1117–1121.
Rabins, P. V., Merchant, A., & Nedstadt, G. (1984). Criteria for diagnosing reversible dementia caused by depression: Validation by a two-year follow-up. *British Journal of Psychiatry, 144,* 488–492.
Reding, M., Haycox, J., & Blass, J. (1985). Depression in patients referred to a dementia clinic. *Archives of Neurology, 42,* 894–896.
Reifler, B. V., Larson, E., & Hanley, R. (1982). Coexistence of cognitive impairment and depression in geriatric outpatients. *American Journal of Psychiatry, 139,* 623–626.
Reifler, B. V., Larson, E., Teri, L., & Poulsen, M. (1986). Dementia of the Alzheimer's type and depression. *Journal of the American Geriatric Society, 34,* 855–859.
Reifler, B. V., Teri, L., Raskind, M., Veith, R., Barnes, R., White, E., & McLean, P. (1989). Double-blind trial of imipramine in Alzheimer's disease patients with and without depression. *American Journal of Psychiatry, 146,* 45–49.
Reynolds, C. R., Kupfer, D. J., Hoch, C. C., Stack, J. A., Houck, P. R., & Sewitch, D. E. (1986). Two-year follow-up of elderly patients with mixed depression and dementia. *Journal of the American Geriatric Society, 34,* 793–799.
Reynolds, C. R., Perel, J. M., Kupfer, D. J., Zimmer, B., Stach, J. A., & Hoch, C. (1987). Open-trial response to antidepressant treatment in elderly patients with mixed depression and cognitive impairment. *Journal of Psychiatric Research, 21,* 111–122.
Rosen, J., & Zubenko, G. S. (1991). Emergence of psychosis and depression in the longitudinal evaluation of Alzheimer's disease. *Biology and Psychiatry, 29,* 224–232.

Rovner, B. W., Broadhead, J., Spenser, M., & Carlson, K., & Folstein, M. F. (1989). Depression and Alzheimer's disease. *American Journal of Psychiatry, 146,* 350–353.

Rovner, B. W., German, P. S., Brant, L. J., Clark, R., Burton, L., & Folstein, M. F. (1991). Depression and mortality in nursing homes. *Journal of the American Medical Association, 265,* 993–996.

Rovner, B. W., German, P. S., Broadhead, J., Morris, R. K., Brant, L. J., Blausetine, J., & Folstein, M. F. (1990). The prevalence and management of dementia and other psychiatric disorders in nursing homes. *International Psychogeriatrics, 2,* 13–24.

Rovner, B. W., Kafonek, S., Filipp, L., Lucas, M., & Folstein, M. F. (1986). Prevalence of mental illness in a community nursing home. *American Journal of Psychiatry, 143,* 144–149.

Sultzer, D. L., Levin, H. S., Mahler, M. E., High, W. M., & Cummings, J. L. (1993). A comparison of psychiatric symptoms in vascular dementia and Alzheimer's disease. *American Journal of Psychiatry, 150,* 1806–1812.

Sunderland, T., Alterman, I. S., Young, D., Hill, J. L., Tariot, P. N., Newhouse, P. A., Mueller, E. A., Mellow, A. M., & Cohen, R. M. (1988). A new scale for the assessment of depressed mood in demented patients. *American Journal of Psychiatry, 145,* 955–959.

Teri, L., & Wagner, A. (1992). Alzheimer's disease and depression. *Journal of Consulting and Clinical Psychology, 60,* 379–391.

Weiner, M. F., Edland, S. D., & Luszczynkska, H. (1994). Prevalence and incidence of major depression in Alzheimer's disease. *American Journal of Psychiatry, 151,* 1006–1009.

Wells, C. E. (1979). Pseudodementia. *American Journal of Psychiatry, 136,* 895–900.

Yesavage, J. A., Brink, T. L., Rose, T. L., Lum, O., Huang, V., Adey, M. B., & Leiser, V. O. (1983). Development and validation of a geriatric depression screening scale: A preliminary report. *Journal of Psychiatric Research, 17,* 37–49.

Young, R. C., Mattis, S., Alexopoulos, G. S., Meyers, B. S., Schindeldecker, R. D., & Dhar, A. K. (1991). Verbal memory and plasma drug concentrations in elderly depressives treated with nortriptyline. *Psychopharmacology Bulletin, 27,* 291–294.

Zubenko, G. S., Rosen, J., Sweet, R. A., Mulsant, B. H., & Hind Rifai, A. (1992). Impact of psychiatric hospitalization on behavioral complications of Alzheimer's disease. *American Journal of Psychiatry, 149,* 1484–1491.

CHAPTER 10

Diagnosis and Management of Paranoia, Delusion, Agitation, and Other Behavioral Problems in Alzheimer's Disease Patients

J. Thad Lake
George T. Grossberg

Because advances in medicine have led to longer lives for much of the world's population, the dementing illnesses are being pushed to the forefront of the research and clinical arenas of medicine. Progressive cognitive decline along with psychiatric and behavioral disturbances characterize the most common of the dementing illnesses, Alzheimer's disease. Until recently, most of the research conducted on dementia of the Alzheimer's type (DAT) has focused on altering the natural history of the disease by decreasing or halting the cognitive decline that is characteristic of this illness. The results have not been promising. Thus the attention has begun to shift toward diagnosis and management of troublesome behaviors that complicate the long-term care of the DAT patients. Some of the more common behavioral symptoms that accompany DAT include agitation, sundowning, wandering, social inappropriateness, sexual impulsiveness, and repetitive purposeless activity. Common psychiatric disturbances include depression and psychosis. In this chapter, the authors will focus on the recent advances in the diagnosis and management of psychosis, agitation, and other behavioral problems in Alzheimer's disease patients.

CLINICAL IMPORTANCE

In order for the behavioral and psychiatric disturbances to be worthy of research efforts, they should be highly prevalent, burdensome, and treatable. First of all, these symptoms must be present in a significant percentage of DAT patients to warrant investigation of management options. In addition to the high prevalence, these symptoms must cause a significant burden on the patient or caregiver. Once prevalence and burden are established, treatability must be addressed. Treatment involves appropriate diagnosis and application of tested management options, ranging from environmental modification to pharmacologic treatment. In the older DAT patient, it is essential always to include an assessment of whether or not the benefits outweigh the risks or side effects.

PREVALENCE

Alois Alzheimer included psychiatric and behavioral symptoms in his initial description of the disease (Alzheimer, 1977). The prevalence of psychopathology and troublesome behaviors in DAT has been investigated in modern times to establish further the importance of these problems. The prevalence of behavioral symptoms ranged from 66% to 100% in several studies (Cohen et al., 1993; Merriam, Aronson, Gatson, Wey, & Katz, 1988; Swearer, Drachman, O'Donnell, & Mitchell, 1988; Teri, Larson, & Reifler, 1988). The most frequent symptoms cited were agitation, angry outbursts, wandering, sleep and dietary disturbances, paranoia, delusions, and hallucinations. Two of these studies also have correlated increased dementia severity with increased prevalence of behavioral disturbances (Swearer et al.; Teri et al.). They showed that as cognitive impairment worsened, a higher number of problems occurred in each patient. Teri et al. demonstrated three or more behaviors present in only

8% of the mildly impaired as opposed to 41% and 88% in the moderate and severe groups, respectively.

Because psychosis is a psychiatric phenomenon rather than a behavioral problem, it has been considered separately in a few studies. The occurrence of delusions in DAT patients ranged from 15.7% (Burns, Jacoby, & Levy, 1990) to 43.5% (Deutsch, Bylsma, Rovner, Steele, & Folstein, 1991), whereas misidentifications (30%) and hallucinations (23%) were reported equally in both studies. Another study of 230 DAT patients identified a high prevalence of perceptual disturbances (40.1%) that included a higher rate of hallucinations (29.1%) (Gilley, Whalen, Wilson, & Bennett, 1991). Visual hallucinations superseded auditory hallucinations in all three studies. This prevalence of both behavioral and psychotic symptoms firmly establishes their clinical importance in the long-term care of DAT patients. As the population continues to age, an increasingly large portion will be at risk for DAT. Because behavioral and psychiatric symptoms are present in the majority of these patients, these problems deserve further investigation.

BURDEN

Establishment of the negative effect that these behaviors have on the DAT patient also is vital to demonstrating their clinical importance. Behavioral symptoms are not infrequently the result of an underlying need that the DAT patient is unable to express. Thus, addressing the problematic behavior also may satisfy the patient's needs and improve his or her quality of life. In addition to the reduction in the patient's own quality of life, the presence of problematic behaviors can overwhelm caregivers. Rabins, Mace, and Lucas (1982) assessed caregiver burden by interviewing the families of 55 demented patients. Of the caregivers interviewed, 87% complained of fatigue, anger, and depression directly linked to caring for the demented family member. Among the most distressing behaviors cited were physical agitation, accusatory behavior, and suspiciousness. Because symptoms such as these have been associated with increased institutionalization, control of these problems likely would decrease the need and result in improved quality of life for the patient as well as decreased health care costs (Steele, Rovner, Chase, & Folstein, 1990). Thus appropriate diagnosis and management of these symptoms can improve quality of life, avoid the large burden that the demented patient places on his or her caregivers, and prevent institutionalization.

DIAGNOSIS

The prevalence studies described previously differed in their method of assessment or diagnosis of psychiatric and behavioral symptoms. Some groups used direct observation of the patient, while others used primary caregiver questionnaires or interviews. Both methods have strengths and weaknesses. Direct observation provides objective collection of data that can be standardized and repeated. However, the patient is observed only for a specified time period that may miss the occurrence of troublesome behavior. In addition, caregiver opinion is not included. The caregiver interview or questionnaire reveals the behaviors that are the most troublesome in the management of the patient in his or her home environment. Because the caregivers' opinions commonly guide clinical management, the importance of their assessment is intuitive. In other words, treatment success often is directly proportional to the happiness of the caregiver. Thus, although the objective collection of data obtained through observational methods may provide more accurate data for research purposes, the caregiver ratings remain highly applicable to clinical management.

To achieve a high level of clinical applicability when investigating behavioral problems, the method of standardized assessment must be based on caregiver ratings. One such research tool is the Cohen-Mansfield Agitation Inventory (CMAI) (Cohen-Mansfield, 1995). Cohen-Mansfield has established a standardized method of assessing agitation or behavioral disruptions that not only is based on caregiver rating but also is applicable to the spectrum of DAT patients. This inventory is useful in assessing both the nursing home patients and the patients that remain at home in the community. The term "agitation" is used interchangeably with disruptive behaviors in the CMAI and is defined as "inappropriate verbal, vocal, or motor activity that is not judged by an outside observer to result from the needs or confusion of the agitated patient" (Cohen-Mansfield). In contrast to the prior generalized use of agitation, the definition using the CMAI improves the investigative consistency and clinical applicability of this term.

As already mentioned, Cohen-Mansfield divides agitated behavior into three main categories: physically aggressive, physically nonaggressive, and verbally agitated. These main categories are represented in the CMAI by 29 specific target behaviors. This tool for standardized assessment contains 29 behaviors that the caregiver rates according to a 7-point scale of frequency, with 7 being the highest frequency of occurrence. Because the identification of target symptoms is at the foundation of the management of psychiatric disorders, well-defined agitated behaviors are important in guiding clinical decision making. To assess critically the literature and apply successful treatment options to individual patients, target symptoms responsive to intervention must be identified. A standardized approach to rating behavioral problems, such as the CMAI, will ensure clinical applicability only if individual target symptoms are mentioned in addition to the overall rating scale. Because improvement in specific target symptoms is more clinically relevant than improvement in a standardized rating, identification of modifiable target symptoms can assist the clinician in initiating management of these behaviors accordingly. Likewise, psychotic symptoms such as delusions, hallucinations, and misidentification must be assessed individually to ensure accurate and applicable study of the diagnosis and treatment of these problems.

NONPHARMACOLOGIC MANAGEMENT

The etiology of behavioral problems often is difficult to discern because of the level of cognitive impairment and resulting lack of communication skills. In demented patients, common causes can be related directly to the inability to impart their needs. Thus it is important to identify any underlying triggers before proceeding to pharmacologic treatment of problem behavior. A good history and physical exam are invaluable in the initial approach to these behaviors. Possible etiologies include hunger, pain, boredom, overstimulation, loneliness, fear, acute confusion or disorientation, and conflicts with other residents or staff. Manipulation or treatment of any of these triggers should be attempted as the first step in the management of behavioral disturbances. Psychotic symptoms should likewise receive a thorough work-up before initiating medical management. Any prior history of a psychiatric disorder should be determined. Toxicity from either prescribed or illicit drugs should be assessed. Benzodiazepine withdrawal and alcohol withdrawal or intoxication also are possible causes of psychosis in these patients. Initial lab and radiographic screening may be a warranted step in evaluating the psychotic DAT patient. Underlying medical causes of delirium that should be ruled out include infection, urinary or fecal retention, dehydration, hypoxia, thyroid disease, B_{12} and thiamine deficiency, hyperadrenalism, hypo- or hyperglycemia, hypercalcemia, sodium and potassium imbalance, stroke, or intracranial pathology. Once these problems have been considered and appropriately ruled out, modification of behavioral symptoms can be pursued.

In a recent review of behavioral approaches to management, Gugel (1994) stressed the basic needs of the individual as causing all behavior. This article outlined human needs as originally developed by Maslow. The physiologic needs of ''hunger, thirst, stimulation, relaxation, elimination, sex, sleep, and bodily integrity'' (Gugel) are at the most primitive level. These basic needs are followed in order by safety needs, the need for love, and finally the need for self-esteem. Therefore, an initial behavioral approach to these problematic DAT patients will assess whether or not these needs are being sufficiently met.

Behavioral modification in DAT patients has been defined as ''any intervention that attempts to change the frequency, intensity, duration, or location of a specific behavior or set of behaviors by systematically varying antecedent stimuli or consequential events'' (McGovern & Koss, 1994). The behavioral treatment outlined by Gugel, operant conditioning, attempts to exchange problematic behaviors for more acceptable behaviors. This method identifies and alters reinforcers of problematic behaviors to reinforce positive behaviors. Gugel points out that the demented elderly patients usually are responsive to positive reinforcers such as praise rather than scolding or negative reinforcement.

Discerning the behaviors that may respond only to behavioral modification from those that usually respond to pharmacologic treatment is important when managing DAT patients. This issue has been addressed in a previous review (Maletta, 1994). Maletta lists the following ''behaviors'' as generally responsive to medication: (a) delusions, (b) hallucinations, (c) verbal and physical agitation, and (d) regressed behavior. He further described behaviors generally not responsive to medication management. These problems include wandering, socially inappropriate activities, purposeless repetitive activities, difficult personalities, hoarding, and stealing. Although categorization of behaviors may be helpful, the initial work-up for modifiable causes should not be abandoned in the pharmacologically amenable group.

Wandering is a commonly cited behavioral problem in DAT patients and traditionally is not responsive to medication and may simply be best remedied by providing an enclosed area for the patient to walk. The repetitive purposeless behaviors can be lessened by providing daily activities for the DAT patients. This strategy may work with any of the problem behaviors that are caused by an underlying boredom or lack of stimulation. Sundowning, another common disruptive behavior, is characterized by increased agitation in the evening and may be improved by increasing daytime activity, preventing daytime napping, and enforcing a regular sleep schedule. On the other hand, overstimulation or sudden changes in daily routine also may precipitate behavioral symptoms. Thus any changes in the activity or environment should be made gradually to allow the patient or patients time to adjust. When problem behaviors are related directly to cognitive loss, a reassuring, empathic caregiver is the key to managing the medication-resistant behaviors. To allow efficacious use of environmental, social, and behavioral modification, nonpharmacologic treatments need to be tested further through randomized, controlled clinical trials. After the aforementioned modifications are exhausted, the clinician usually must proceed to pharmacologic treatment options.

PHARMACOLOGIC MANAGEMENT

As previously mentioned, the first step in initiating pharmacologic treatment is the identification of target symptoms. With target symptoms in mind, medication should be used based on current knowledge of efficacy and adverse effects. In keeping with a medical model, the underlying pathophysiology of specific disturbances should guide not only research trials but also the clinical prescription of medication. This approach obviously is not possible with some of the ill-defined problematic behaviors. However, one of the most troublesome behaviors, aggression, has some fairly well defined neurochemical correlates (Eichelman, 1987).

Eichelman reviewed the role of certain neurotransmitters, including acetylcholine, dopamine, GABA, norepinephrine, and serotonin. While both acetylcholine and dopamine increase aggressive behavior in animal studies, GABA and serotonin have been shown to inhibit animal aggression. Serotonin has had the strongest correlation with human aggression research, whereas the effect of norepinephrine has been equivocal in animal and human studies. Therefore, serotonergic, GABAergic, and dopamine-blocking medications appear to be intuitive choices corresponding to these mechanisms. Because a deficiency in acetylcholine has been implicated in the pathogenesis of DAT, anticholinergic treatment is not an acceptable option. Because tryptophan is a serotonin precursor, Eichelman points out that the use of lithium takes advantage of the neurochemistry by increasing the tryptophan uptake into the brain. Eichelman's paper also mentioned a possible role of limbic kindling in episodic aggressive behavior. The anticonvulsant carbamezapine has a speculated limbic anti-kindling effect, which possibly explains its efficacy in treating aggressive behavior. The use of neuroleptics in the agitated DAT patient generally has been for the sedative properties of this class of drugs. However, with dopamine implicated in the neurochemistry of aggression, these drugs may act more directly on pathophysiology.

The selection of a specific medication always must be made by weighing its benefits against its inherent risks. The elderly patients that comprise the DAT population are more sensitive to the immediate adverse effects of medication and to the accumulative long-term effects. This must be kept in mind when determining which medication and which dose to use. The clinician always should individualize titration of psychotropic medications to an effective minimal dose.

NEUROLEPTICS

The neuroleptic medications conventionally have been used to treat the troublesome behaviors of the DAT patient. In contrast to the patient exhibiting behavioral agitation, the patient who experiences unrelenting psychotic symptoms will remain the best candidate for neuroleptic treatment. Although neuroleptics are the most efficacious drugs for managing psychosis in these patients, their long-term adverse effects outweigh their efficacy in treating behavioral problems. The meta-analysis done by Schneider, Pollack, and Lyness (1990) revealed that only 18 of every 100 patients in the analyzed studies benefited from treatment with a neuroleptic. This previously belabored, modest efficacy pales in comparison to the risk of anticholinergic, autonomic, and cardiac side effects associated with the low potency neuroleptics and the risk of extrapyramidal symptoms and tardive dyskinesia that are associated with long-term use of the high potency neuroleptics (Grossberg, 1990; Grossberg & Manepalli, 1995). Because the high potency neuroleptics have less of the anticholinergic and cardiac side effects, short-term use of these medications when necessary may be acceptable. The high potency medications such as haloperidol can be effective when initiated at low doses such as 0.5 mg and then titrated upward until symptomatic improvement occurs (Grossberg & Manepalli, 1995). The new antipsychotic, risperidone, may be particularly useful in this patient population, having the benefits of the high potency neuroleptics but with lower extrapyramidal side effects. The clinician always should consider trials of decreased dose or discontinuation of the medication when target symptoms are under control. The clinician also should keep in mind that environmental, social, and behavioral modifications are often helpful in the DAT patients with psychotic symptoms. Although large randomized, controlled trials are lacking in support of alternative medications, initial case studies and small trials appear promising.

TRAZADONE

The serotonergic agent trazadone seems to be an efficacious alternative in the treatment of the agitated DAT patient. The proposed mechanism is that of serotonergic inhibition of aggressive behavior. However, the presence of comorbid depression expressed as a behavioral symptom also may play a role in the success of this agent and other medications with antidepressant efficacy. A retrospective study of 16 patients meeting NINCDS criteria for probable Alzheimer's disease revealed that trazadone treatment resulted in at least mild benefits in 13 of these patients (Aisen, Johannessen, & Marin, 1993). However, 5 of the 16 patients had to discontinue use secondary to possible adverse effects. The listed adverse effects were hypotension, ileus, increased agitation, and worsened confusion. Pedal edema was noted in all patients receiving trazadone but was not sufficient to warrant discontinuation. Because all of the patients studied had comorbid medical illnesses and multiple medication regimens, the adverse effects could not be attributed solely to trazadone. Although four patients were identified as much improved, the target symptoms that improved were not noted in this report. In this study, the dose ranged from 100 to 300 mg per day, with a mean dose of 180 +/− 70 mg per day. In another report of six demented patients treated with trazadone and adjunctive tryptophan, four showed improvements (Wilcock, Stevens, & Perkins, 1987). The three improved patients showed a reduction in aggression, noisy behavior, and temper tantrums. Trazadone was started at 50 mg twice daily and tryptophan at 500 mg twice daily. Both medications were titrated upward until target symptom improvement or side effects occurred. In addition, several case reports of trazadone use in demented patients with behavioral disruptions also have demonstrated favorable reductions in problematic behavior with minimal adverse effects (Greenwald, Marin, & Silverman, 1986; O'Neil, Page, & Adkins, 1986; Simpson & Foster, 1986). Obviously, the literature on trazadone treatment of behavioral problems is in its early stage. Because this medication is generally well tolerated in the elderly population, it merits further investigation. Large, long-term, controlled trials are needed to confirm the efficacy of this option in pharmacologic treatment of agitated behavior.

BUSPIRONE

Buspirone is another medication with proposed serotonergic activity that has been used in DAT patients with problematic behaviors. Several case reports have demonstrated significant reductions in behavioral agitation using buspirone at doses ranging from 15 to 45 mg per day in divided doses (Colenda, 1988; Lebert, Pasquier, Goudemand, & Petit, 1993; Tiller, Dakis, & Shaw, 1988). These successful case study reports led Sakauye, Camp, and Ford to perform an open-label study involving 10 patients who met NINCDS-ADRDA criteria for Alzheimer's disease (Sakauye et al.). They used CMAI to assess behavioral response to treatment with buspirone. A 22% reduction in the baseline CMAI was achieved with an initial dose of 5 mg three times per day increased at 5 mg per day to a maximum of 60 mg per day. Through clinical judgment, they observed maximal benefit from a dose of 30 to 40 mg per day at weeks 5 through 7. The only side effect mentioned in the study was nausea and resulted in one patient's dropping out. Similar to trazadone, buspirone is usually well tolerated; however, good, long-term trials also are lacking for this medication.

BENZODIAZEPINES

Like the neuroleptics, this class of drugs also has been employed for its sedative effects. Although the sedative properties are useful in the extremely agitated patients, relief of underlying anxiety may prove efficacious in treating some disruptive patients. When compared to the long half-life benzodiazepines such as diazepam and chlordiazepoxide, the short half-life benzodiazepines such as oxazepam, lorazepam, and temazepam have been better tolerated in elderly patients (Salzman, Shader, Greenblatt, & Harmatz, 1983). The longer half-life medications are associated with more sedation and higher prevalence of paradoxical agitation and worsening confusion. This is due to the accumulation of the long half-life drugs and their metabolites complicated by the reduced oxidative biotransformation seen in elderly people.

Previously reviewed literature revealed no studies that tested the use of benzodiazepines solely in DAT patients (Stern, Drachman, O'Donnell, & Mitchell, 1991). The studies reviewed supported the use of short half-life agents with the specific target symptom of agitation due to an underlying anxiety showing the best results. The most efficacious of the short-acting benzodiazepines has been oxazepam, with effective doses ranging from 15 to 80 mg per day. Because it is well absorbed intramuscularly, orazepam generally has been useful for short-term management of severely agitated patients. However, this use may not be applicable to the DAT patient because of the decrease in cognitive function and the increase in confusion that the benzodiazepines are occasionally known to cause. This effect can lead to a vicious cycle when the agitated DAT patient receives repeated as-needed doses causing increased confusion and increased agitation. The long-term risks of dependence and withdrawal also limit the use of this medication. Clinical trials specifically dealing with DAT patients are needed to justify the use of these medications for uses other than anxiety.

BETA ADRENERGIC BLOCKERS

Beta-blocking medications such as propranolol have reported efficacy in younger organically impaired patients (Elliot, 1977). Again, large randomized, controlled trials are lacking involving the DAT patient population. The largest double-blind, placebo-controlled study to date assessed the effects of pindolol on 11 organically impaired patients with behavioral abnormalities (Greendyke & Kanter, 1986). In comparison to placebo, pindolol significantly reduced assaultiveness, hostility, uncommunicativeness, uncooperativeness, and repetitive behaviors. These results were observed within 2 weeks of beginning treatment and at an optimal dose of 40 to 60 mg per day. Furthermore, the patients improved without the occurrence of significant bradycardia or hypotension, which are two of the important side effects of the beta-blocking agents. This likely was due to the inherent sympathomimetic effect of pindolol, which results in better sympathetic tone than other beta-blockers. Comorbid medical problems such as heart failure, obstructive lung disease, or diabetes must be considered when employing these agents. In addition, rapid withdrawal of these medications can result in rebound hypertension. Because initial reports have demonstrated significant efficacy along with minimal side effects in a selected population, these medications may be beneficial in carefully selected patients.

ANTICONVULSANTS

The aforementioned limbic kindling that is believed to play a role in the pathophysiology of aggression may explain the initial success of this class of medications. Carbamezapine has been employed recently in the treatment of agitated behavior. Gleason and Schneider (1990) used carbamezapine in treating nine patients who met the NINCDS-ADRDA criteria for probable Alzheimer's disease. According to changes in the Brief Psychiatric Rating Scale (BPRS), substantial improvement occurred in five of the patients. They further cited specific improvements in tension, hostility, uncooperativeness, and agitation. Doses ranged from 200 to 1000 mg per day, with a corresponding range in serum drug levels from 2.3 to 9.6 ug per ml. Ataxia was the most common side effect and was present in three of the patients studied. One of the affected patients had to discontinue the medication. In a more recent placebo-controlled trial, carbamazepine reduced BPRS scores significantly more than placebo (Tariot, Erb, Leibovici, Podgorski, Cox, & Asnisetal, 1994). Clinical global impression improved on 16 of the 25 agitated, demented nursing home patients without a decrease in the Mini-Mental State Exam (MMSE). The preservation of cognitive function is an important asset to any medication treating the behavioral problems in DAT patients. The doses in this study ranged from 100 to 800 mg per day, with an average dose near 300 mg per day. Despite the heterogeneous demented sample, this study is a good start toward establishing carbamezapine as a proven pharmacologic treatment option for DAT patients with agitation.

Another anticonvulsant, sodium valproate, has been efficacious in initial case reports (Mellow, Solano-Lopez, & Davis, 1993). The reports demonstrated significant improvement in two of four agitated, demented patients. The two responsive patients met diagnostic criteria for DAT and benefited from a dose ranging from 1000 to 2500 mg per day. The medication was well tolerated by all four participants. This initial report warrants further investigation of sodium valproate as a treatment option in agitated DAT patients.

When using either of these anticonvulsant medications, the clinician periodically should check liver enzymes because both drugs can sometimes cause hepatotoxicity. Carbamazepine also sometimes causes leukopenia or can precipitate aplastic anemia. Thus the clinician is justified in periodic assessment of complete blood counts. Despite these infrequent adverse effects, these two medications have very minimal side effect profiles when compared with neuroleptics, benzodiazepines, and beta-blockers.

OTHER TREATMENTS

Lithium also has been used in the treatment of behavioral problems in the DAT patient. Although some initial case studies have shown significant benefits, more recent small trials have been equivocal (Havens & Cole, 1982; Holton & George, 1985). Lithium carries the potential for exacerbating cognitive defects, causing neurotoxicity, nephrotoxicity, and drug interactions. As with the alternatives, mentioned previously, large randomized, controlled trials are needed to establish efficacy of lithium use in DAT patients.

Bright-light treatment has been targeted specifically at the behavior of sundowning. In a study of 10 patients meeting NINCDS-ADRDA criteria for Alzheimer's disease, daily exposure to 2 hours of bright light reduced the clinical rating of sundowning behavior in 8 of the 10 patients (Satlin, Volicer, Ross, Herz, & Campbell, 1992). A light box containing three U-shaped fluorescent bulbs provided 1500–2000 lux of light treatment in each 2-hour period. This appears to be a very simple and benign treatment for the often troublesome behavior of sundowning. A subsequent trial of 14 demented inpatients also showed improvements in behavioral symptoms with the use of bright-light therapy (Mishima, Okawa, Hishikawa, Hozumi, Hori, & Takahashi, 1994). It is hoped that further clinical trials will build on these promising initial results.

In a case report of two elderly demented men, estrogen significantly reduced physically aggressive behavior without occurrence of any adverse effects (Kyomen, Nobel, & Wei, 1991). Because testosterone has been shown to increase aggression, the use of estrogen seems intuitive in treating aggressively agitated DAT patients. Clinical trials involving estrogen will need to be done to support initially positive case reports.

In addition to the medication options listed previously, short-term psychiatric hospitalization has been beneficial to the agitated DAT patient (Zubenko et al., 1992). In a prospective study of 120 Alzheimer's disease patients, short-term inpatient stays were effective in returning patients to their homes and preventing institutionalization. These brief visits were used to reevaluate pharmacologic regimens and initiate comprehensive treatment plans. Both the patient and the burdened caregiver may benefit from brief separation and reorientation of management. The clinician should keep this option in mind when dealing with stressed caregivers and their agitated patients or family members afflicted with Alzheimer's disease.

SUMMARY

Although it has been established that a majority of patients with Alzheimer's disease will develop burdensome behavior problems during the course of this chronic debilitating disease, the only common theme established in the treatment of these symptoms is the lack of large, well controlled clinical trials. Therefore, as research efforts fill this void, diagnosis or identification of specific target symptoms will allow the critically thinking clinician to apply up-to-date research to his or her patients. Once the modifiable, environmental, and social factors have been identified, manipulation of these triggers should be attempted in the first step of treatment. Because aggressive agitation and psychotic symptoms are the most pharmacologically responsive behavioral disturbances, medication trials are warranted when these target symptoms are present. Whether employing behavioral modification or medication, preservation of cognitive functioning should be a primary goal in this group of sensitive patients. Although clinicians historically have taken advantage of the sedative properties of neuroleptics in the agitated patient, options with less severe side effects and more specific actions on proposed pathophysiologic mechanisms are available and under further investigation.

REFERENCES

Aisen, P., Johannessen, D., & Marin, D. (1993). Trazadone for behavioral disturbance in Alzheimer's disease. *American Journal of Geriatric Psychiatry, 4*(1), 349–350.
Alzheimer, A. (1977). A unique illness involving the cerebral cortex. In D. Rottenberg & F. Rottenberg (Eds.), *Neurological Classics in Modern Translation.* New York: Hafner.
Burns, A., Jacoby, R., & Levy, R. (1990). Psychiatric phenomena in Alzheimer's disease. *British Journal of Psychiatry, 157,* 72–93.
Cohen, D., Eisdorfer, C., Gorelick, P., Luchins, D., Freels, S., Ashford, J., Semla, T., Levy, P., & Hirschman, R. (1993). Psychopathology associated with Alzheimer's disease and related disorders. *Journal of Gerontology, 48*(6), M255–M260.
Cohen-Mansfield, J. (1995). Assessment of disruptive behavior/agitation in the elderly: Function, methods, and difficulties. *Journal of Geriatric Psychiatry and Neurology, 8,* 52–60.
Colenda, C. (1988). Buspirone in treatment of agitated demented patient[s]. *Lancet, 1,* 1169.
Deutsch, L., Bylsma, F., Rovner, B., Steele, C., & Folstein, M. (1991). Psychosis and physical aggression in probable Alzheimer's disease. *American Journal of Psychiatry, 148,* 1159–1163.
Eichelman, B. (1987). Neurochemical bases of aggressive behavior. *Psychiatric Annals, 17*(6), 371–374.
Elliot, F. (1977). Propranolol for the control of belligerent behavior following acute brain damage. *Annals of Neurology, 1,* 489–491.
Gilley, D., Whalen, M., Wilson, R., & Bennett, D. (1991). Hallucinations and associated factors in Alzheimer's disease. *Journal of Neuropsychiatry, 3,* 371–376.
Gleason, R., & Schneider, L. (1990). Carbamezapine treatment of agitation in Alzheimer's outpatients refractory to neuroleptics. *Journal of Clinical Psychiatry, 51*(3), 115–118.
Greendyke, R., & Kanter, D. (1986). Therapeutic effects of pindolol on behavioral disturbances associated with organic brain disease: A double-blind study. *Journal of Clinical Psychiatry, 478,* 423–426.
Greenwald, B., Marin, D., & Silverman, S. (1986). Serotonergic treatment of screaming and banging in dementia. *Lancet, 2,* 1464–1465.
Grossberg, G. (1990). The pitfalls of meta-analysis. *Journal of the American Geriatric Society, 38,* 607.
Grossberg, G., & Maneppuli, J. (1995). The older patient with psychotic symptoms. *Psychiatric Services, 46,* 55–59.

Gugel, R. N. (1994). Behavioral approaches for managing patients with Alzheimer's disease and related disorders. *Medical Clinics of North America, 78,* 861–867.
Havens, W., & Cole, J. (1982). Successful treatment of dementia with lithium. *Journal of Clinical Psychopharmacology, 2,* 71–72.
Holton, A., & George, K. (1985). The use of lithium carbonate in severely demented patients with behavioral disturbance. *British Journal of Psychiatry, 146,* 99–100.
Kyomen, H., Nobel, K., & Wei, J. (1991). The use of estrogen to decrease aggressive physical behavior in elderly men with dementia. *Journal of the American Geriatric Society, 39,* 1110–1112.
Lebert, F., Pasquier, F., Goudemand, M., & Petit, H. (1993). Euphoria with buspirone after fluoxetine treatment. *American Journal of Psychiatry, 150*(1), 167.
Maletta, G. (1994). Pharmacologic treatment and management of the aggressive demented patient. *Psychiatric Annals, 20*(8), 446–455.
McGovern, R., & Koss, E. (1994). The use of behavior modification with Alzheimer patients: Values and limitations. *Alzheimer Disease and Associated Disorders, 8*(3), 82–91.
Mellow, A., Solano-Lopez, C., & Davis, S. (1993). Sodium valproate in the treatment of behavioral disturbance in dementia. *Journal of Geriatric Psychiatry and Neurology, 6,* 205–209.
Merriam, A., Aronson, M., Gatson, P., Wey, S., & Katz, I. (1988). The psychiatric symptoms of Alzheimer's disease. *Journal of the American Geriatric Society, 36,* 7–12.
Mishimi, K., Okawa, M., Hishikawa, Y., Hozumi, S., Hori, H., & Takahashi, K. (1994). Morning bright light therapy for sleep and behavior disorders in elderly patients with dementia. *Acta Psychiatrica Scandinavica, 89,* 1–7.
O'Neil, M., Page, N., & Adkins, W. (1986). Tryptophan-trazadone treatment of aggressive behavior. *Lancet, 2,* 859–860.
Rabins, P., Mace, N., & Lucas, M. J. (1982). The impact of dementia on the family. *Journal of the American Medical Association, 248*(3), 333–335.
Sakauye, K., Camp, C., & Ford, P. (1993). Effects of buspirone on agitation associated with dementia. *American Journal of Geriatric Psychiatry, 1*(1), 82–84.
Salzman, C., Shader, R., Greenblatt, D., & Harmatz, J. (1983). Long vs. short half-life benzodiazepines in the elderly. *Archives of General Psychiatry, 40,* 293–297.
Satlin, A., Volicer, L., Ross, V., Herz, L., & Campbell, S. (1992). Bright light treatment of behavioral and sleep disturbances in patients with Alzheimer's disease. *American Journal of Psychiatry, 149*(8), 1028–1032.
Schneider, L., Pollock, V., & Lyness, S. (1990). A meta-analysis of controlled trials of neuroleptic treatment in dementia. *Journal of the American Geriatric Society, 38,* 553–563.

Simpson, D., & Foster, D. (1986). Improvement in organically disturbed behavior with trazadone treatment. *Journal of Clinical Psychiatry, 47*(4), 191–193.
Steele, C., Rovner, B., Chase, G., & Folstein, M. (1990). Psychiatric symptoms and nursing home placement of patients with Alzheimer's disease. *American Journal of Psychiatry, 147,* 1049–1051.
Stern, R., Duffelmeyer, M., Zemishlani, Z., & Davidson, M. (1991). The use of benzodiazepines in the management of behavioral symptoms in demented patients. *Psychiatric Clinics of North America, 14*(2), 375–384.
Swearer, J., Drachman, D., O'Donnell, B., & Mitchell, A. (1988). Troublesome and disruptive behaviors in dementia. *Journal of the American Geriatric Society, 36,* 784–790.
Tariot, P., Erb, R., Leibovici, A., Podgorski, C., Cox, C., Asnis, D., Kolassa, J., & Irvine, C. (1994). Carbamazepine treatment of agitation in nursing home patients with dementia: A Preliminary Study. *Journal of the American Geriatric Society, 42,* 1160–1166.
Teri, L., Larson, E., & Reifler, B. (1988). Behavioral disturbance in dementia of the Alzheimer's type. *Journal of the American Geriatric Society, 36,* 1–6.
Tiller, J., Dakis, J., & Shaw, J. (1988). Short-term buspirone treatment in disinhibition with dementia. *Lancet, 2,* 510.
Wilcock, G., Stevens, J., & Perkins, A. (1987, April). Trazadone/tryptophan for aggressive behavior. *Lancet,* 929–930.
Zubenko, G., Rosen, J., Sweet, R., Mulsant, B., & Rifai, A. (1992). Impact of psychiatric hospitalization on behavioral complications of Alzheimer's disease. *American Journal of Psychiatry, 149*(11), 1484–1491.

CHAPTER 11

Noncholinergic Drugs in the Treatment of Memory Problems in Alzheimer's Disease Patients

Maurice W. Dysken
Kathleen M. Hoover

A variety of noncholinergic agents have been tested in clinical trials to determine if they offer any benefit in improving cognition or slowing cognitive decline in patients with Alzheimer's dementia. These agents all have compelling rationales, either theoretical or empirical or both, that have provided the impetus for testing in human subjects. In this chapter, we will review 20 clinical trials involving 14 noncholinergic agents that were published between 1984 and 1995. The theoretical justification, preclinical empirical data, and methodology are presented for each

---

This work was supported in part by research funds from the Department of Veterans Affairs. The authors gratefully acknowledge the able assistance of Susan B. Love, Susan Anton-Johnson, and Nancy J. Reimers.

study. Table 11.1 summarizes these points as well as the results of each study. For the purposes of this review, a noncholinergic agent is defined as a pharmacologic agent whose mechanism of action does not involve direct stimulation of muscarinic receptors or inhibition of acetylcholinesterase.

ACETYL-L-CARNITINE

Acetyl-L-carnitine (ALC) is an endogenous substance that is found in mitochondria and is involved in the uptake into mitochondria of activated long-chain fatty acids (Fritz, 1963; Morris & Carey, 1983). ALC has been shown to increase acetyl-CoA and choline acetyltransferase activities, choline uptake, and acetylcholine release (Imperato, Ramacci, & Angelucci, 1989), and for these reasons is believed to enhance cholinomimetic activity (Onofrj, Bodis-Wollmer, Pola, & Calvani, 1988). In aged rats, chronic ALC treatment decreases histologic and behavioral deterioration (Angelucci, Ramacci, Amenta, Lorentz, & Maccari, 1988), improves discrimination learning and tasks of spatial learning (Caprioli, Ghirardi, Ramacci, & Angelucci, 1990), increases longevity, and improves long-term memory performance without affecting sensory-motor performance (Barnes et al., 1990; Markowska et al., 1990).

Spagnoli et al. (1991) reported a 10-center, double-blind, placebo-controlled, parallel group study of ALC in patients with Alzheimer's disease. The 130 Alzheimer patients (F = 92; M = 38) met DSM-III (American Psychiatric Association, 1980) criteria for primary degenerative dementia (PDD) and had an illness duration of at least 6 months. Patients were excluded who had severe disability as manifested by a Katz index (Katz, Ford, Moskowitz, Jackson, & Jaffe, 1963) of 12 or more or a Blessed Dementia Scale score of more than 20. Either ALC (1,000 mg bid) or a matching placebo was taken orally for 1 year. Fourteen efficacy measures were used: two measures assessed behavior and disability through interviews with caregivers, nurses or clinical observation, and the remaining efficacy measures provided direct evaluations of patients' cognitive performances. All outcome measures were carried out at baseline and after 1 year of treatment. Some of the measures also were repeated at 3 and 6 months.

After 1 year of double-blind treatment, the group on ALC ($N = 63$) showed a significantly lower rate of deterioration compared with the

TABLE 11.1 (*continued*)

Drug/Study/Yr.	Dx	N	Route	Dosages	Duration	Result
Acetyl-L-carnitine						
Spagnoli et al., 1991	PDD	130	P.O.	2,000 mg/d	1 yr.	+
Alaproclate						
Dehlin et al., 1985	PDD/MID	40	P.O.	0, 400 mg/d	2 wk. P, 4 wk. DB, 2 wk. P	−
Buflomedil						
Levinson et al., 1985	DAT/MID	46	P.O.	0, 600 mg/d	24 wk.	+
Ceranapril						
Sudilovsky et al., 1993	PDD	30	P.O.	0, 10, 80 mg/d	4 wk. × 4 wk. × 4 wk. 1st wk. of each period = P	−
Cycloserine						
Mohr et al., 1995	AD*	40	P.O.	0, 10, 30, 100 mg/d	1 wk. P, 6 mo.	−
Desferrioxamine						
Crapper-McLachlan et al., 1991	AD	48	IM	0, 250 mg	24 mo. × 5 d/wk.	±

Monosialoganglioside					
Ala et al., 1990	AD	42	IM	0, 100 mg/d	12 wk	−
Flicker et al., 1994	DAT	12	IM	0, 100 mg/d	6 wk. × 6 wk. 3 wk. P between	−
Indomethacin					
Rogers et al., 1993	AD	44	P.O.	0, 100, 125 or 150 mg/d	6 mo.	+
Milacemide					
Dysken et al., 1992	DAT	228	P.O.	0, 1,200 mg/d	1 wk. P, 4 wk. DB, 4 wk. P	−
Cutler et al., 1993	AD	148	P.O.	0, 400, 800, 1,200 mg/d	4 wk. DB, 4 wk. P	−
Nerve Growth Factor					
Olson et al., 1992	AD*	1	IVt	6.6 mg (total)	3 mo.	±

(continued)

TABLE 11.1 (continued)

Drug/Study/Yr.	Dx	N	Route	Dosages	Duration	Result
Nimodipine						
Ban et al., 1990	PDD/MID	178	P.O.	0, 90 mg/d	12 wk.	+
Tollefson, 1990	PDD	195	P.O.	0, 90, 180 mg/d	2 wk. P, 12 wk. DB	+
Phosphatidylserine						
Delwaide et al., 1986	DAT	35	P.O.	0, 300 mg/d	6 wk.	±
Amaducci et al., 1988	AD	142	P.O.	0, 200 mg/d	3 mo. DB, 3 mo. F/U	±
Thiamine						
Blass et al., 1988	AD	11	P.O.	0, 3 g/d	3 mo. × 3 mo.	+
Nolen et al., 1991	AD	12	P.O.	0, 3 g/d	1 yr.	–
Meador et al., 1993	AD*	18	P.O.	0, 3 g/d	1 mo. × 1 mo.	±
	AD*	17	P.O.	0, best dose (up to 6 g/d)	1 mo. × 1 mo.	+
Zimeldine						
Cutler et al., 1985	PDD	4	P.O.	low dose: 125 ± 50 mg/d high dose: 225 ± 50 mg/d	2 wk. P 4 wk. 6 wk. P 4 wk.	–

Note. References are cited fully in the Reference List.
*Also met criteria for PDD.

Dx = diagnosis; N = number of subjects; PDD = primary degenerative dementia; MID = multi-infarct dementia; DAT = dementia of the Alzheimer type; AD = probable Alzheimer's dementia; P.O. = by mouth; IM = intramuscular; IVt = intraventricular; wk = week; mo = month; DB = double-blind; F/U = follow-up.

placebo group ($N = 67$) on 13 of the 14 variables. The differences were statistically significant for the Blessed Dementia Scale, logical intelligence, ideomotor and buccofacial apraxia (De Renzi, Motti, & Nichelli, 1980), and selective attention. Seventeen percent ($N = 22$) of the patients dropped out of the study: half dropped out because of death (six on active drug and five on placebo), and four were dropped because of agitation (three on active drug and one on placebo).

ALAPROCLATE

Postmortem studies in patients with senile dementia have shown reduced levels of 5-HT in the hippocampus. Alaproclate is a potent 5-HT reuptake inhibitor with regional selectivity in the hippocampus and hypothalamus. It also has been shown to potentiate cholinergic mediated activity in the brain (Ögren, Norström, Danielsson, Peterson, & Bartfoi, 1985). An open trial of alaproclate in patients with senile dementia demonstrated an improvement in emotional functions in five of the nine patients (Bergman et al., 1983).

Dehlin, Hedenrud, Jansson, and Nörgärd (1985) conducted a randomized, double-blind, parallel-group, placebo-controlled study of alaproclate in 40 inpatients ages 65 or older who met DSM-III criteria for primary degenerative dementia (PDD) or multi-infarct dementia (MID). Those with severe psychiatric, cardiac, renal, or liver diseases as well as malabsorption syndromes or markedly abnormal laboratory values were excluded from the study. Initially, 43 subjects (F = 24, M = 19) were randomized to either active medication ($n = 20$) or placebo ($n = 23$). Their age range was 65–93 years with a mean ($\pm$ SD) age of 82 ($\pm$ 6) years. They were given either oral doses of alaproclate (200 mg bid) or placebo for 4 weeks, preceded and followed by 2-week placebo washout periods. Forty subjects, 20 in each group, were used for efficacy evaluations. Dementia severity was assessed at baseline, at weeks 2 and 4 during active treatment, and after the terminal placebo washout phase. Three rating scales were used as efficacy measures: one was the dementia rating scale by Gottfries, Bråne, and Steen (GBS) (1982), which assessed intellectual, emotional, and motor functions; one was a clinical global evaluation performed by a nurse and ward physician; and the last were selected items (7, 18, 19) from the Comprehensive Psychological Rating Scale (CPRS) (Åsberg, Montgomery, Perris, Schalling, & Sedvall, 1978) to assess suicidal thoughts, reduced appetite, and reduced sleep.

No differences in efficacy were seen in this mixed group of patients suffering from PDD & MID between active drug and placebo except on the intellectual factor of the GBS scale. This difference, indicating a statistically significant lower score of intellectual functioning in the alaproclate group, was deemed by the authors to have no clinical relevance. It was concluded that 4 weeks of treatment with alaproclate showed no clinically significant effects on dementia symptoms. Although no serious adverse experiences were reported, eight patients (five in the drug group) had their dosages reduced due to adverse events.

BUFLOMEDIL

Buflomedil is a vasodilator that increases cerebral blood flow in patients with cerebrovascular disease (Touya, 1981). Its mode of action, however, is still unknown. Several studies in patients with symptoms of senility showed that buflomedil produced definite improvements in performance on psychometric tests (Kugler, Krauskopf, & Dersch, 1981; Seus, 1980).

Levinson, Wright, and Barklem (1985) conducted a 6-month, randomized, double-blind, placebo-controlled, parallel group study of buflomedil on patients with either primary dementia of the Alzheimer's type (DAT) or MID. Patients were required to be 60 years of age or older, currently residing in a geriatric nursing home, and having mild to moderate dementia symptoms. Patients were excluded if they scored ≥ 20 on the HAM-D or ≥ 40 on the HAM-A. During a single-blind, 1-month placebo lead-in phase, patients who showed improvement in over 50% of the screening and efficacy items were excluded as placebo responders. Those patients remaining were randomly assigned to either 600 mg a day of buflomedil (300 mg before breakfast, 150 mg before lunch, 150 mg before supper) or matching placebo. Symptom severity was assessed at baseline and then at weeks 8, 12, 16, and 24. Efficacy measures included the 19 variables of the Sandoz Clinical Assessment-Geriatric Scale (SCAG), the six variables of the supplemental clinical assessment scale for nurse's observation (SCASNO), and the total raw score of the Luna-Nebraska Memory Test.

A total of 65 patients were recruited into the study, but 10 were excluded as placebo responders. The data from the remaining 55 patients were evaluated for safety parameters, but for various reasons, the data from 9 of these patients were not usable for efficacy measures. Of the remaining 46 patients, 33 were considered to have AD. Sixteen of them received buflomedil and 17 received placebo. The other 13 patients were presumed to be suffering from multi-infarct dementia. Eight received the active medication and 5 were treated with placebo. The total SCAG & SCASNO scores favored the buflomedil group over the placebo group ($p < 0.05$). The buflomedil-treated patients showed significantly greater ($p < 0.05$) improvement on 10 of the 18 SCAG items, including symptoms in each of the three functional areas of interest: cognitive function, psychosomatic function, and interpersonal relations. Four of the six SCASNO Scale items showed greater improvement in the group treated with the active medication. No significant within-group or between-group differences were found on the Luna-Nebraska Memory Test. The results of the efficacy measures were that a statistically significant improvement was found in those patients taking buflomedil in such characteristics as alertness, anxiety, emotional lability, hostility, indifference, and mood. Based on the SCASNO Scale, indifference to surroundings, hostility, and uncooperativeness showed statistically and clinically significant improvements in the group treated with the active medication. Self-care showed borderline improvements of buflomedil over placebo. The authors concluded that buflomedil is effective in both dementia types, but that it is more effective in primary dementia of the Alzheimer type than in multi-infarct dementia. Although a few adverse events were noted, most were transient and none of them were considered to be drug related.

CERANAPRIL

Increased activity of angiotensin-converting enzyme (ACE) has been found in postmortem brains from Alzheimer's patients compared to controls (Arregui, Perry, Rossor, & Tomlinson, 1982). Animal studies have demonstrated impairment in learning and memory with angiotensin II administration as well as improved cognition with ACE inhibitors. Pretreatment with ACE inhibitors block the amnestic effects of scopolamine. A clinical trial in humans using the ACE inhibitor captopril indicated a similar effect in humans (Croog, Sudilovsky, Levine, & Testa, 1987).

Sudilovsky et al. (1993) conducted a pilot clinical trial of the ACE inhibitor ceranapril in Alzheimer's disease. This 15-week, double-blind, placebo-controlled, three-way crossover study evaluated the cognitive effects of ceranapril in 30 patients with DSM-III-(American Psychiatric Association, 1980) defined primary degenerative dementia. The age range for the 30 patients (F = 14, M = 16) was 54 to 75 years, with a mean (± SD) age of 67.5 (± 5.6). Inclusion criteria included a Mini-Mental State Examination score from 12 to 26, a Global Dementia Score (GDS) (Reisberg, Ferris, de Leon, & Crook, 1982) from 3 to 5, and a vocabulary score of 8 or higher on the Wechsler Adult Intelligence Scale (WAIS). Patients were excluded if they had a Ham-D score of ≥ 17 or a modified Ischemia Scale Score (ISS) of ≥ 4. Each patient received medication doses of 5 mg bid, 40 mg bid, and placebo bid, divided into periods of 5 weeks each, with the 1st week of each block designated as a placebo week. The Computerized Neuropsychological Test Battery (Veroff et al., 1991) as well as noncomputerized cognitive test batteries were used as outcome measures at weeks 1, 5, 6, 10, 11, and 15. The noncomputerized tests of psychological performance consisted of the Benton Work Fluency Test, Parts A and B of the Trail Making Test, and the Digit Symbol Substitution Test from the WAIS.

No significant results were obtained, although it was concluded that a study of longer duration or higher dosages may be warranted. There were no clinically significant adverse events.

CYCLOSERINE

N-Methyl-D-Asparate (NMDA) receptor activation is believed to result in long-term potentiation, which has been hypothesized as a mechanism for memory formation. Cycloserine activates NMDA receptors by modulating NMDA receptor-associated glycine recognition sites. Cycloserine has been shown to have positive cognitive effects in elderly patients (Mohr et al., 1995) and to ameliorate some of the scopolamine-induced deficits in young, healthy volunteers (Jones, Wesnes, & Kirby, 1991).

Mohr and coworkers (Mohr et al., 1995) took part in a multicenter trial to study cycloserine in patients with probable Alzheimer's disease as defined by NINCDS-ADRDA criteria and DSM-III-R criteria. Patients were required to be at least 50 years of age, score 12–24 on the MMSE, ≤ 4 on the Hachinski Ischemic Scale, and ≤ 12 on the Hamilton Depression Scale. Patients were randomly assigned to 5, 15, or 50 mg doses of cycloserine bid or placebo following a 7-day single-blind, placebo lead-in period. The Computerized Drug Research (CDR) Cognitive Assessment System of Wesnes and the Mattis Dementia Rating Scale (MDRS) (Mattis, 1989) were used as measures of cognitive status. The CDR provides measures of cognitive processing speed and accuracy, and the MDRS assesses attention, memory, structural ability, and executive function. Two self-rating scales, the Behavioral Pathology in AD worksheet and the Brief Cognitive Rating Scale (BCRS) (Reisberg, 1983), were completed. Global impressions were measured by the Clinical Global Improvement scale (CGI), completed by the investigator, the Patient Global Improvement Rating (PGIR), completed by the caregiver, and the Clinical Interview Based Impression of Change (CIBIC) (Leber, 1991), completed by a clinician blind to the study conditions. Quantified electroencephalography (QEEG) also was used to assess CNS activity at baseline and at 2, 14, and 26 weeks after treatment.

A total of 29 subjects (F = 15, M = 14) were studied with a mean (± SD) age of 71.5 (± 9.1). No significant improvement was found in either the cognitive or global rating scales. No changes in CNS activity were detected by the QEEG. No serious adverse events were reported.

DESFERRIOXAMINE

Increased aluminum concentrations have been found in several brain regions of patients dying with Alzheimer's dementia (Edwardson & Candy, 1989). Epidemiological studies reported an association between aluminum concentrations in drinking water and the occurrence of Alzheimer's dementia (Neri & Hewitt, 1991). Although there is no convincing proof that aluminum toxicity causes disease progression, decreasing brain exposure to circulating aluminum by use of a chelating agent has been proposed as potentially beneficial.

Crapper-McLachlan et al. (1991) described 48 outpatients (F = 25; M = 23) who were selected with probable AD as defined by NINCDS-ADRDA (McKhann et al., 1984), Hachinski Ischemic Scores (HIS) of < 4, and an age of 73 or less. They were randomly assigned to receive desferrioxamine (a trivalent ion chelator of aluminum and also iron), lecithin, or no treatment in a single-blind study. The desferrioxamine group (F = 13, M = 12, mean age (± SD) of 63.2 (± 6.4)) received a treatment dose of 125 mg intramuscularly twice a day, 5 days per week, for 24 months. Within the no treatment group (F = 12, M = 11, mean age (± SD) of 63.0 (± 6.2)), those patients receiving lecithin were given 500 mg bid orally on a daily basis for 24 months. Video recordings of activities of daily living were completed at weeks 6, 12, 18, and 24, and were considered the primary efficacy measures. Cognitive measures were not included in the outcome assessment. The tapes were scored by trained raters who were blind to treatment assignment.

The mean rate of decline assessed by daily living skills was twice as rapid in the no treatment groups compared to the group treated with desferrioxamine. There were no reported serious adverse events. Abdominal pain, anorexia, lethargy, and nausea, however, were reported in 30% of the patients taking desferrioxamine. Five patients on desferrioxamine and one patient in the no treatment group died during the trial. In 1993, Crapper-McLachlan, Smith, and Kruck reported a trace metal analysis of the autopsied brains of the six patients who died during the trial. Neocortical brain aluminum concentrations were reduced to nearly control levels in those patients on extended desferrioxamine treatment in the weeks immediately before death.

MONOSIALOGANGLIOSIDE (GM-1)

Monosialoganglioside (GM-1) is a neuronal glycolipid that potentiates nerve growth factor effects by increasing neuronal survival and neurite outgrowth in vitro. GM-1 has shown potential usefulness in treating cognitive impairment associated with stroke, motor dysfunction following spinal cord injury, and sensory dysfunction associated with diabetic neuropathy. One study reported a positive effect in the treatment of dementia (Miceli, Caltagirone, & Gianotti, 1977).

Ala, Romero, Knight, Feldt, and Frey (1990) conducted a double-blind, placebo-controlled study to evaluate the efficacy and safety of GM-1 in patients suffering from mild-to-moderate AD as defined by NINCDS-ADRDA. Of the original 46 participants (F = 28, M = 18; 21 drug, 25 placebo; age range 51–84 years), 42 completed the study. Patients were randomly assigned to receive either 12 weeks of 100 mg a day of the active drug IM or the saline placebo IM. Study selection criteria included symptom duration of ≥ 2 years, an eighth grade education, a MMSE score of 13–23, an Hachinski Ischemic Score (HIS) of ≤ 4, a Blessed Dementia Scale (BDS) score ranging from 6 to 19, and a Ham-D of ≤ 15. Outcome measures included 10 cognitive and 17 psychosocial scales.

No significant differences were found between the GM-1 and placebo groups at 12 and 24 weeks. Patients in both the active drug and placebo groups remained cognitively stable over the duration of the study. The psychosocial scales, however, suggested that patients worsened over this same 24-week period. Two of the four dropout patients withdrew from the study because they developed an allergic rash.

In 1994, Flicker, Ferris, Kalkstein, and Serby conducted a double-blind, placebo-controlled, crossover study of 100 mg a day monosialoganglioside (GM-1) versus placebo in 12 patients with dementia of the Alzheimer type (11 female, 1 male). The subjects, all outpatients, had a mean age of 68.1 (range 56–81) and had a rating of 4 or 5 on the Global Deterioration Scale (GDS). The duration of the trial was 15 weeks and consisted of two 6-week, double-blind treatment periods with an intervening 3-week washout period. Placebo and drug treatments were administered in a counterbalanced order. During the first week of each treatment, patients were hospitalized. Monosialoganglioside sodium (100 mg) and placebo were administered IM each day. During each of the 6-week treatment periods, the subjects were evaluated at baseline and after 2 and 6 weeks of treatment. Efficacy evaluations included tests of immediate memory (digit-span), telephone number recall, verbal recall (shopping list task), visuospatial recall (delayed spatial recall), visual recognition memory (visual recognition span), facial recognition, language (object naming), concept formation (object sorting), visuospatial praxis (digit symbol), block construction, visuoperceptual function (judgment of line orientation), psychomotor speed (finger tapping speed), and perseveration (intrusions on the shopping list task).

Of the 20 outcome measures, only the object function recognition test elicited a significant change; in this case, an improvement from baseline in the placebo group and a decline from baseline in the GM-1 group. The authors concluded that overall GM-1 was not effective in improving cognitive functions in patients with AD.

INDOMETHACIN

Although inflammation is not characteristically found in the brains of patients dying with Alzheimer's disease, many immune-related markers have been identified in association with β-amyloid deposits (McGeer & Rogers, 1992). Two retrospective studies have suggested that rheumatoid arthritis patients who typically take anti-inflammatory medication have a lower than expected frequency of Alzheimer's disease (McGeer, McGeer, Rogers, & Sibley, 1991; Jenkinson, Bliss, Brain, & Scott, 1989). Indomethacin, a nonsteroidal anti-inflammatory drug that crosses the blood-brain barrier, was therefore considered as a possible treatment for AD based on the hypothesis that anti-inflammatory agents may be beneficial in this disease.

Rogers et al. (1993) studied 44 patients who had a diagnosis of probable Alzheimer's disease and scored ≥ 16 on MMSE. Patients were treated with either weight adjusted doses of indomethacin (100, 125, or 150 mg a day) or placebo administered three times daily for a period of 6 months. The cognitive test battery was made up of the MMSE, the Alzheimer Disease Assessment Scale (ADAS), the Boston Naming Test (BNT), and the Token Test (TK). The efficacy measures were expressed as change scores that were calculated as percent change from baseline to 6 months.

Of the original 44 volunteers, 28 completed the study, divided equally between the drug and placebo groups. Averaged across the battery of mental status tests, the patients on active medication improved 1.3% ± 1.8% (M ± SD), whereas the placebo group declined by 8.4% ± 2.3% (M ± SD). The most consistent differences in efficacy between the groups were found in the MMSE and the ADAS, although these differences were significant by one-tailed but not two-tailed tests. More than 20% of the patients on active drug developed adverse events, primarily gastrointestinal, that were severe enough to result in removal from the study.

MILACEMIDE

Milacemide (2-n-pentylaminoacetamide hydrochloride), a monoamine oxidase-β inhibitor, is a pro-drug for glycine and is believed to play a stimulatory role through glycine receptors on NMDA receptors (Bowery, 1987). Animal models have indicated that milacemide may have beneficial effects on cognition. In rats, for example, milacemide reversed memory impairment induced by electroshock, memory loss induced by scopalamine and diazepam (Quartermain, Nuygen, Sheu, & Herting, 1991), and facilitated memory consolidation and retrieval during passive-avoidance learning (Handelman, Mueller, & Cordi, 1988).

Dysken et al. (1992) and Cutler et al. (1993) tested this medication in multicenter, double-blind, placebo-controlled clinical trials in Alzheimer's disease. Dysken et al. (1992) reported data collected at 16 study sites. A total of 228 outpatients (F = 112; M = 116) received either milacemide treatment of 1,200 mg a day (n = 113) or placebo (n = 115) for a period of 1 month following a 1-week lead-in placebo period and followed by a 4-week placebo washout period. Patients who met study criteria were ≥ 50 years of age with dementia of the Alzheimer type and between the ages of 40 and 80 for the onset of Alzheimer's. MMSE scores ranged from 14 to 24, GDS scores ranged from 3 to 5, Hamilton Depression Rating Scale scores were < 18, Wechsler Adult Intelligence Scale (WAIS-R) vocabulary scores were less that 1.5 standard deviation below the mean adjusted for GDS stage, and Modified Hachinski Ischemic Scale (MHIS) scores were < 4. The primary efficacy measures were the Alzheimer's Disease Assessment Scale and the MMSE. Other measures of efficacy included the Clinical Global Impression Scale (CGI), Patients' Global Improvement Rating (PGIR), Wechsler Memory Scale, WAIS-R vocabulary score, Verbal Fluency Score (VFS), and a modified Instrumental Activities of Daily Living Scale (IADLS) (Lawton & Brody, 1969). The Behavioral Pathology in Alzheimer's Disease Rating Scale (Reisberg, Borenstein, & Franssen, 1987) was completed at the end of the placebo lead-in, the double-blind, and placebo washout phases. The GDS was completed at the end of the treatment and washout phases. Efficacy measures were obtained at screening, after the placebo washout phase, and after the double-blind treatment phase and at the end of the trial.

The efficacy measures did not demonstrate significant improvement in the milacemide treated group compared to the control group. Six members of the drug-treated group were removed from the study because of adverse events. Of these six, the four milacemide patients were dropped because of elevated liver enzymes. Two participants taking placebo were removed from the study because of an episode of myocardial ischemia and a spontaneous bone fracture.

In Cutler et al. (1993), 148 AD patients (73 women, 75 men) with a mean age of 71.5 years (range 52–91) were enrolled for participation, and 129 patients completed the study. Patients were required to meet NINCDS criteria for AD, be ≥ 50 years of age, score between 10 and 27 on the MMSE and 3 to 5 on the GDS. The scores on the HIS and the Dementia Rating Scale (DRS) were required to be less than 4 and 20, respectively. Patients received single oral doses of 400 mg a day (n = 40), 800 mg a day (n = 38), or 1,200 mg a day (n = 33) of milacemide or placebo (n = 37) for 1 month followed by 1 month of single-blind placebo treatment. Efficacy measures included the ADAS, the CGI, the

PGIR, the Physical Self-Maintenance Scale, and the IADLS. The HAM-D was obtained at baseline and at the end of the double-blind treatment phase. Efficacy measures were obtained at the screening visit and biweeky thereafter.

No statistically significant differences were found between the drug and placebo groups. Nineteen patients did not complete the study: ten of these patients were dropped because of adverse events. Clinically significant liver enzyme levels were found in five of the patients receiving the active medication.

NERVE GROWTH FACTOR

Nerve growth factor (NGF) has been shown to rescue neurons, stimulate axonal growth, and improve cholinergic function in animals with lesioned cholinergic projections (Hefti, 1986; Williams et al., 1986). NGF treatment also has been found to counteract memory deficits in aged rats (Fischer et al., 1987). Data from aged rodent brains suggest that NGF mRNA and protein levels are decreased (Lärkvors et al., 1987) and that decreased levels of NGF in the hippocampus correlate with spatial learning deficits.

Olson et al. (1992) carried out a study of NGF in a 69-year-old female patient who had signs of AD for 8 years. This participant met DSM-III-R for PDD and NINCDS-ADRDA criteria for probable AD. Her baseline MMSE was 16 and she also had marked cholinergic deficiencies on PET scanning using ^{11}C-nicotine as a marker for nicotinic receptors. Mouse NGF was infused directly into the brain by means of an implantable remote-controlled infusion system. Over a 3-month period, a total of 6.6 mg was delivered intraventricularly. A cognitive test battery was given twice prior to treatment, 1 month after the start of the infusion, and 2.5 months after termination of NGF treatment. A test session was planned at the time of NGF termination but could not be carried out. The cognitive battery consisted of the MMSE as a general measure of cognitive functioning as well as face and word recognition (Bäckman, 1991), spatial memory, selective reminding, digit-span memory, and verbal fluency (Lezak, 1983). EEG measurements, PET measures of blood flow using 11C-butanol, and PET measures of cholinergic binding using 11C-nicotine were also done.

Verbal episodic memory (delayed word recognition, selective reminding task parameters) was improved after 1 month of treatment. Two and a half months later, this improvement was no longer seen. No other cognitive improvements were noted throughout the trial, and in fact cognitive decline was seen in a number of areas. For example, general cognitive functioning (MMSE), delayed face recognition, semantic memory (verbal fluency), and short-term memory (digit-span) deteriorated during the study. The treatment resulted in a marked but transient increase in uptake and binding of ^{11}C-nicotine in the frontal and temporal cortex, a persistent increase in cortical blood flow, and progressive decreases of slow wave EEG activity. There were no serious adverse events ascribed to this treatment.

NIMODIPINE

Nimodipine is a calcium antagonist that can reduce the age-related increases of total calcium content in the hippocampus and other neurons. Nimodipine has been shown to improve memory in brain-damaged and old rats, restore sensory-motor function and abnormal walking patterns in old rats, and accelerate acquisition of associative learning in aging rabbits by reversing age-related changes in calcium-dependent processes (Deyo, Straube, & Disterhoft, 1989). In fibroblasts from AD patients, the increase in the total (bound) cell calcium content is greater than in normal aging (Peterson & Goldman, 1985). These findings suggest that nimodipine may have a therapeutic effect on the cognitive decline of elderly patients with dementia.

Ban et al. (1990) reported on a multicenter, placebo-controlled, double-blind clinical trial of oral nimodipine in 178 elderly patients with cognitive decline. Patients were diagnosed with either PDD or MID (DSM-III) and had mild to moderately severe cognitive decline on the GDS (Reisberg et al., 1982). Patients with significant concurrent medical conditions were excluded. The participants ranged in age from 55 to 95 with a mean (± SD) of 75.4 (± 9.6). Fifty-nine percent ($n = 105$) of the patients were women and 41% ($n = 73$) were men. Most of the participants were inpatients and were diagnosed as PDD or MID based on a HIS (Hachinski et al., 1975) score of ≤ 4 or ≥ 7, respectively. Those with ischemic scores of 6 or 7 were classified as mixed dementia (MD). Based on these criteria, 86 participants were classified as PDD, 52 as MID, and 40 with MD. Each participant took 30 mg of nimodipine t.i.d. or a matching placebo for 12 weeks following a 2-week washout period. Assessments were completed prior to randomization at the 30th, 60th, and 90th day of double-blind treatment. Outcome measurements included the WMS, the MMSE, GDS, Sandoz Clinical Assessment Geriatric Scale, the Plutchik Geriatric Rating Scale, the Severity of Illness and Global Improvement Scales of Clinical Global Impression, and the Hamilton Psychiatric Rating Scale for Depression.

Nimodipine treatment for the combined PDD and MID sample was significantly better than placebo on the following scales: CGI-Severity of Illness, CGI-Global Improvement, Ham-D, MMSE, GDS, Sandoz Clinical Assessment Geriatric, one of the seven scales of the Plutchik Geriatric Rating Scale, and the WMS. Thus the superiority of active drug over placebo was seen in all of the efficacy ratings as well as in psychopathology, performance, social behavior, and overall impression. Ten types of adverse events were reported by 19 subjects (10 nimodipine treated, 9 placebo treated). Only one of these events, specifically, a report of "transient cerebral ischemic attack" in a nimodipine patient, was sufficiently severe to have resulted in discontinuation of treatment. In general, adverse events in patients assigned to nimodipine were few and mild.

Tollefson (1990) reported on a 12-week multicenter, double-blind, placebo-controlled, randomized clinical trial of nimodipine in patients with DSM-III-R PDD. Of the 234 patients screened into the study, 227 began the study and 195 (M = 72, F = 123) were included in the final efficacy analysis. Patients needed to be at least 45 years of age, score < 4 on the HIS, score from 4 and 23 on the MMSE, have a score of 4 to 6 on the GDS, and score < 16 on the 21-item HAM-D at both screening and after a 2-week placebo lead-in period. Patients with clinically significant concomitant illnesses were excluded. The mean age at baseline was 69.5 years with an average symptom duration of 3.8 years. Patients were assigned to one of three treatment groups: placebo, nimodipine 30 mg tid, or nimodipine 60 mg t.i.d. Efficacy measures included the Buschke Selective Reminding Task, the Word Fluency Subtest, the Standardized Road Map Test, First and Last Names Test, Symbol Digit Modality Test, and Tapping Speed. A tester who was blind to the drug condition completed the CGI, and relatives completed the Relatives' Assessment of Global Symptomatology (RAGS) and Activities of Daily Living (ADL). Patients were seen weekly for 3 weeks and then at 2-week intervals.

As a group, those receiving active medication at a dose of 30 mg t.i.d. showed prophylactic benefit in eight measures over 3 months of treatment compared to controls. This benefit was not demonstrated in the group receiving active medication at a dose of 60 mg t.i.d. Fifty-four of the original 234 participants (23%) reported adverse events. Seven of the adverse events were considered serious and included urinary frequency, fecal impactions, rash, suspicion, agitation, flatulence, and nausea. Of the three patients who discontinued the study because of adverse events, two were on placebo.

PHOSPHATIDYLSERINE

Phosphatidylserine is a natural phospholipid obtained from the brain cortex that appears to play a role in cerebral metabolism during the aging process. Protection against age-dependent biochemical and behavioral changes was observed in old rats after its administration. Phosphatidylserine also has shown facilitative effects in aged rats in a variety of learning and memory tasks that included both active and passive avoidance tests (Corwin, Dean, Bartus, Rotrosen, & Watkins, 1985).

To determine whether phosphatidylserine would have similar effects in humans, Delwaide, Gyselynck-Mambourg, Hurlet, and Ylieff (1986) conducted a double-blind, randomized, placebo-controlled study in 42 hospitalized patients who suffered from senile dementia of the Alzheimer's type. All patients had a HIS (Hachinski et al., 1975) of 1 to 6. The efficacy measures used were the Crichton Scale (Robinson, 1961), the Peri Scale, which was designed on site (see Appendix A of the original article), and a circle crossing test. Compared to the Crichton Scale, the Peri Scale was more descriptive and has a larger number of items. An initial washout period was followed by a 6-week period of 100 mg t.i.d. of phosphatidylserine or placebo. Seventeen patients received the drug and 18 received placebo. The patients were tested at baseline, and at the end of 1 and 6 weeks of treatment, as well as 3 weeks after treatment. Thirty-five of the 42 patients completed the double-blind portion of the study. The seven patients who dropped out (four placebo, three drug) did so because of intercurrent disease or trauma. None of the premature terminations were believed to have resulted from the medication.

Although the Crichton Rating Scale showed a trend toward improvement in the drug-treated group, it was not statistically significant. No difference was found in the two groups on the circle crossing test. The Peri Scale, however, showed a significant improvement ($p < 0.05$) for the drug group compared to the placebo group. The treated group returned to its pretreatment level after discontinuation of the drug.

Amaducci and the SMID group (1988) (Studio Multicenterico Italiano sulla Demenze-Italia [Multicenter Study of Dementia]) studied 142 patients from seven neurology departments in a 3-month double-blind randomized placebo-controlled trial of phosphatidylserine. Patients were between the ages of 40 and 80, generally met NINCDS-ADRDA diagnostic criteria, and scored less than 6 on the first three items of the Ham-D. Participants were randomly assigned to active medication or placebo based on sex, age, and severity of illness (above and below a score of 14 on Part 1 of the Blessed Dementia Scale). After the 3-month treatment study, patients were followed off medication/placebo for 21 months. Patients were evaluated at baseline, at the end of treatment, 3 months after treatment, and at 6-month intervals after that. At the time of publication, data were available for 6 months. Nine efficacy measures were used: the Blessed Dementia Scale, the Randt Memory Test, the Babcock Story Recall Test, a digit-span test, the Block-Tapping Task, the Token Test, the Set Test (Isaacs & Kennie, 1973), the Clifton Assessment Scale for the Elderly (Pattie, 1981), and a test requiring subjects to copy drawings from memory. Either bovine brain phosphatidylserine or matching placebo in 100 mg capsules bid was administered.

Data from 133 (66 on active drug and 64 on placebo) patients were analyzed after 3 months of treatment, and data from 115 (60 on active drug and 55 on placebo) were analyzed at 3 months posttreatment. Three of the outcome measures (Set Test, Blessed Dementia Scale-Nonpersonal Memory, and Block-Tapping Task) reached trend significance at the 0.1 level or beyond in a subgroup of patients with severe impairment who were on the active medication. Because of the number of efficacy variables, these results are not striking. Three months after the termination of the drug, however, the improvement favoring the drug group was maintained and in some cases was enhanced. The authors speculated that these relatively long-term results may reflect the action of phosphatidylserine in producing structural neuronal changes rather than transient metabolic changes.

THIAMINE

Thiamine, or vitamin B-1, is necessary for the metabolism of acetylcholine as well as for its release from the presynaptic neuron. Biochemical, clinical, and pathological data suggest that thiamine-dependent enzymes are reduced in AD patients (Gibson et al., 1988). Slight abnormalities in the thiamine-dependent enzyme transketolase were found in red blood cells and cultured skin fibroblasts taken from AD patients. A double-blind crossover study (Haycox, 1984) in eight healthy young adults demonstrated that a single 5 gram dose of oral thiamine partially reversed the cognitive deficits induced by the anticholinergic agent scopalamine.

Blass, Gleason, Brush, DiPonte, and Thaler (1988) tested this putative relationship in a short-term, double-blind, placebo-controlled crossover study in 16 patients with probable Alzheimer's disease (NINCDS-ADRDA criteria) who were not thiamine deficient clinically. Of the 16 patients, 5 withdrew from the study prematurely. Three of these people required antidepressant medication and two were hospitalized. The mean (± SD) baseline MMSE of the 11 outpatients who completed the study was 14.2 (± 1.4), and the mean age was 72. The double-blind medication was given tid and consisted of 1 g capsule of either thiamine hydrochloride or 250 mg capsules of niacinamide placebo, which was weight adjusted to match the active medication. The patients were randomized to one of the two treatments for 3 months, with a subsequent 3-month crossover period. Six patients received the active medication first, and five received the placebo first. Patients were seen at monthly intervals and were rated on the MMSE, the Blessed Dementia Rating Scale, and the caregiver scored Haycox (1984) Behavioral Scale.

Slightly higher, but statistically significant MMSE total scores were found with thiamine treatment compared to placebo. The mean (± SEM) difference score for the MMSE for the two groups was only 0.72 (± .14) ($p < 0.001$). The behavioral ratings did not demonstrate significant differences. Although this short-term thiamine effect was modest, the small difference in the MMSE could become greater if it were maintained over a long period of time.

As a follow-up to the Blass, Gleason, Brush, DiPonte, and Thaler (1988) short-term study, Nolan, Black, Sheu, Langberg, and Blass (1991) conducted a 12-month double-blind parallel-group study of 3 g a day of thiamine versus placebo. Of the 15 subjects enrolled, 10 completed the study and 2 participated through 9 months of the study. Each patient had a diagnosis of possible ($n = 2$) or probable ($n = 13$) Alzheimer's disease. Of the 15 patients, 10 were female and 5 were male, and they ranged in age from 59 to 87, with a mean age of 76.3. At study entry, their MMSE scores ranged from 8 to 23, with a mean score of 16.4. The double-blind medication consisted of either 1 g of thiamine or placebo taken tid. The study participants were seen at 3-month intervals. The Consortium to Establish a Registry for Alzheimer's Disease (CERAD) neuropsychological battery was administered at each visit. The CERAD Battery includes verbal fluency measures, the Boston Naming Test (15-item), MMSE, and constructional praxis. Because behavioral ratings did not appear to be affected by thiamine in the Blass study, this study used only measures of cognitive function. A 10-item, word-learning list coupled with recall and recognition testing also was included.

No significant differences were found on any of the efficacy measures. Thus the results of this study suggest that oral thiamine ingested over a 12-month period neither improves cognition nor slows the progression of cognitive deterioration in Alzheimer's patients.

As a further follow-up to the previous two studies, Meador et al. (1993) examined the effects of 3 to 8 mg of oral thiamine daily in patients with Alzheimer's disease. Two experiments were incorporated in the Meador study. Eighteen patients (F = 13; M = 5) with probable Alzheimer's disease and an HIS score ≤ 4 participated in the first experiment. In this study, participants were given thiamine hydrochloride tablets three to four times a day to equal a daily dose of 3 g. Subjects received thiamine or placebo, in randomized order, for 1 month each in a crossover design without an intervening washout period. The ADAS was chosen as the major dependent variable. The MMSE was also chosen as a comparative measure to the study conducted by Blass. The CGI physician rating was used as well. In 13 of 17 patients, the ADAS scores were better in the thiamine treated group compared to the placebo treated group. The authors concluded that there was a mild beneficial effect of thiamine, but that this effect was small.

The second experiment was conducted with the participation of 17 subjects, 6 of whom participated in the first experiment. For these six subjects, the mean time between studies was 6 months with a minimum elapsed time of 3.5 months. The 17 study participants (F = 8; M = 9) had a mean age of 69 (range 54–93) and a mean education level of 14 (range 7–20). The second experiment had three phases. The first phase, which was 3 months in duration, was an open label best-dose titration phase with a maximum of 6 g a day of oral thiamine. This was followed by a single-blind best-dose versus placebo crossover phase in which participants took the single blind medication for 1 month in each of the crossover stages. The third phase was conducted with the last seven subjects. In this phase, thiamine was incrementally increased by 0.5 g a day each month up to a maximum of 8 g a day. Efficacy testing, using the same scales as in the first experiment, was conducted each month through the 9 months and every 8 weeks thereafter.

The results of the study showed that high-dose thiamine significantly improved the ADAS scores at months 1, 6, and 7 compared to baseline. The MMSE scores, however, showed no significant improvement throughout the study. The CGI scores improved in most patients at dosages > 4 g a day. Three patients dropped out during the study, two because of concurrent illnesses and one because of refusal to continue. The authors concluded that the results from their 3 g a day study of oral thiamine were consistent with the Blass study and that their preliminary studies of dosages up to 8 g a day suggested mild benefits of higher dose thiamine in AD.

ZIMELDINE

Catecholaminergic, dopaminergic, and serotonergic systems in AD have been studied in Alzheimer's disease. Serotonin has been measured biochemically in autopsied Alzheimer's brain tissue (Gottfries et al., 1983), and this has been shown to be reduced in the hippocampus, cortex, caudate, and hypothalamus compared to controls (Bowen, 1983). Postsynaptic serotonin receptors in postmortem AD brains also have been found to be significantly decreased compared to controls. Zimeldine, a bicyclic compound that is a specific serotonin reuptake inhibitor, recently has been demonstrated to reverse the adverse effects of alcohol on memory function in normal volunteers. Cutler et al. (1985) hypothesized that zimeldine may have a beneficial effect on Alzheimer symptoms through activation of the serotonergic system.

Cutler et al. (1985) designed a double-blind, placebo-controlled crossover study of 23 weeks duration in Alzheimer's patients to evaluate the effects of zimeldine on memory. A total of two 4-week drug phases were each preceded by a placebo period. Following double-blind treatment, there was a 4-week recovery phase during which no medications were administered. Concentrations of 5-hydroxyindoleacetic acid (5-HIAA), homovanillic acid (HVA), 3-methoxy-4-hydroxyphenylglycol (MHPG), and platelet serotonin uptake were measured in the peripheral and cerebrospinal fluid. All patients were required to meet DSM-III criteria for PDD, be free of depressive illness as determined by DSM-III, be free of any clinically significant medical conditions, and have a HIS score of < 4. In addition, all patients were required to have an MDS score of > 110 and a MMSE score of > 20. Of the five men enrolled in the study, four completed the protocol. The fifth patient had to be dropped because of a zimeldine hypersensitivity reaction that consisted of fever and hematuria without alterations in liver function and hematologic profile. No further study participants were enrolled because the study was withdrawn from further worldwide investigative trials by the manufacturer.

The mean age of the four patients was 63 years, with a mean duration of illness of 3.8 years and a mean (± SD) educational level of 15.75 (± 2.63). At baseline, the mean (± SD) MMSE score was 23.5 (± 3.42), the mean Blessed Memory Information Concentration Test score was 26 (± 3.74), the mean (± SD) Blessed Dementia Scale score was 6.25 (± 3.07), the mean (± SD) MDS score was 124.75 (± 5.44), the mean (± SD) full score for the Wechsler Adult Intelligence Scale was 109.75 (± 15.65), and the mean (± SD) HIS was 1.50 (± .58). All patients initially received a single 100 mg dose of the active medication to determine pharmacokinetic parameters. Seventy-two hours later, all patients began taking three tablets of placebo at 8:00 a.m. and 8:00 p.m. for a 2-week washout period (weeks 4 and 5). At the beginning of weeks 6 and 16, patients were randomly assigned to receive active medication in doses sufficient to maintain desired plasma concentrations (low: 50–75 ng/mL or high: 100–150 ng/mL). All patients received placebo from week 10 to week 15. The patients had blood drawn weekly for measurements of plasma zimeldine concentrations. Neuropsychological tests included a continuous performance test, paired associate learning (verbal and visual-verbal tasks), paired associate delayed memory (recognition and recall), and object memory.

The authors concluded that there were no significant effects of zimeldine on memory or reaction time as compared to placebo. Zimeldine reduced 5-HIAA concentration in the cerebral spinal fluid by 3%. There was a 90% reduction in platelet serotonin reuptake. These changes were unaccompanied by measurable changes in reaction time in AD patients. Two patients had severe side effects. One of the patients was described earlier and was not included in the study. The second patients developed bilateral paresthesias that resolved on discontinuation of zimeldine.

Comments

Of the 14 noncholinergic agents reviewed, only four showed unequivocal improvement: acetyl-L-carnitine, buflomedil, indomethacin, and nimodipine. The other agents were either insignificant in demonstrating cognitive improvement (alaproclate, ceranapril, cycloserine, GM-1, milacemide, and zimeldine) or showed mixed results (desferrioxamine, NGF, phosphatidylserine, and thiamine). Three agents demonstrating efficacy each had different mechanisms of action that included indirect cholinomimetic stimulation (acetyl-L-carnitine), anti-inflammation (indomethacin), and Ca antagonism (nimodipine). The mechanism of action of the vasodilator, buflomedil, is unknown. Additional studies are needed to replicate these positive findings and also to test the efficacy and safety of additional NSAIDs and Ca antagonists.

Six of the noncholinergic agents were clearly ineffective in enhancing cognition. Two agents are 5-HT reuptake inhibitors (alaproclate, zimeldine), two are NMDA receptor agonists (cycloserine, milacemide), one is an ACE inhibitor (ceranapril), and one is a NGF potentiator (GM-1). These limited data suggest that 5-HT reuptake inhibitors and NMDA receptor agonists will prove to be ineffective cognition enhancers, but additional work needs to be done with these classes of pharmacologic agents. It is clearly too early to assess the efficacy of ACE inhibitors and gangliosides because so little data are available from clinical trials.

The remaining four noncholinergic agents were equivocal in demonstrating efficacy. Desferrioximine showed improvement in activities of daily living, but failed to demonstrate improved cognition because cognitive measures were not utilized in assessing outcomes. Intraventricular administration of NGF in one patient showed unsustained improvement in verbal episodic memory. Phosphatidylserine study demonstrated improvement in some neuropsychological tests but not others. The other study showed improvement 3 months after drug discontinuation. Of the three thamine studies, one was positive, one mixed, and one was negative.

REFERENCES AND BIBLIOGRAPHY

Ala, T., Romero, S., Knight, F., Feldt, K., & Frey, W. H. (1990). GM-1 treatment of Alzheimer's disease. A pilot study of safety and efficacy. *Archives of Neurology, 47*, 1126–1130.

Amaducci, L. (1988). Phosphatidylserine in the treatment of Alzheimer's disease: Results of a multicenter study. *Psychopharmacology Bulletin, 24*, 130–134.

American Psychiatric Association. (1980). *Diagnostic and Statistical Manual of Mental Disorders (DSM-III)*. Washington, DC: American Psychiatric Association.

American Psychiatric Association. (1987). *Diagnostic and Statistical Manual of Mental Disorders (DSM-III-R)*. Washington, DC: American Psychiatric Association.
Angelucci, L., Ramacci, M. T., Amenta, F., Lorentz, C. & Maccari, F. (1988). Acetyl-L-carnitine in the rat's hippocampus and aging: Morphological, endocrine and behavioral correlates. In A. Borio, J. R. Perez-Polo, J. de Vellis, & B. Haber (Eds.), *Neural development and regeneration. Cellular and molecular aspects* (pp. 57–66). Berlin: Springer-Verlag.
Arregui, A., Perry, E. K., Rossor, M., & Tomlinson, B. E. (1982). Angiotensin converting enzyme in Alzheimer's disease increased activity in caudate nucleus and cortical areas. *Journal of Neurochemistry, 38*, 1490–1492.
Arrigoni, G., & De Renzi, E. (1964). Constructional apraxia and hemispheric locus of lesion. *Cortex, 1*, 170–197.
Åsberg, M., Montgomery, S. A., Perris, C., Schalling, D., & Sedvall, G. (1978). A comprehensive psychopathological rating scale. *Acta Psychiatrica Scandinavica, 271*, 5–27.
Babcock, H., & Levy, L. (1930). An experiment in the measurement of mental deterioration. *Archives of Psychology, 117*, 105–107.
Ban, T. A., Morey, L., Aguglia, E., Azzarelli, O., Balsano, F., Marigliano, V., Caglieris, N., Sterlicchio, M., Capurso, A., Tomasi, N. A., Crepaldi, G., Volpe, D., Palmieri, G., Ambrosi, G., Polli, E., Cortellaro, M., Zanussi, C., & Froldi, M. (1990). Nimodipine in the treatment of old age dementias. *Progress in Neuro-Psychopharmacology and Biological Psychiatry, 14*, 525–551.
Barnes, C. A., Markowska, A. L., Ingram, D. K., Kametani, H., Spangler, E. L., Lemken, V. J., & Olton, D. S. (1990). Acetyl-L-carnitine 2: Effects on learning and memory performance of aged rats in simple and complex mazes. *Neurobiology of Aging, 11*, 499–506.
Bassi, S., Albizzati, M. G., Sbacchi, M., Frattola, L., & Massarotti, M. (1984). Double-blind evaluation of monosialoganglioside (GM-1) therapy in stroke. *Journal of Neuroscience Research, 12*, 493–498.
Bäckman, L. (1986). Adult age differences in cross-modal recoding and mental tempo, and older adults' utilization of compensatory task conditions. *Experimental Aging Research, 12*, 135–140.
Bäckman, L. (1991). Recognition memory across the adult life span: The role of prior knowledge. *Memory and Cognition, 19*, 63–71.
Benton, A., & Hamsher, K. D. S. (1976). *Multilingual Aphasia Examination*. Iowa City: University of Iowa.
Benton, A. L., Hamsher, K., Varney, N. R., & Spreen, O. (1983). *Contributions to Neuropsychological Assessment: A Clinical Manual*. New York: Oxford University Press.
Bergman, I., Bråne, G., Gottfries, C. G., Jostell, C., Karlsson, I., & Svennerholm, L. (1983). Alaproclate: A pharmacokinetic and biochemical study in patients with dementia of Alzheimer type. *Psychopharmacology, 80*, 279–283.

Blass, J. P., Gleason, P., Brush, D., DiPonte, P., & Thaler, H. (1988). Thiamine and Alzheimer's disease. A pilot study. *Archives of Neurology, 45,* 833–835.

Blessed, G., Tomlinson, B. E., & Roth, M. (1968). The association between quantitative measures of dementia and of senile change in the cerebral grey matter of elderly subjects. *British Journal of Psychiatry, 114,* 797–811.

Bowen, D. M. (1983). Biochemical assessment of neurotransmitter and metabolic dysfunction and cerebral atrophy in Alzheimer's disease. In R. Katzman (Ed.), *Biological aspects of Alzheimer's disease, Banbury Report 15* (pp. 219–231). Cold Spring Harbor, New York: Cold Spring Harbor Laboratory.

Bowery, N. (1987). Glycine-binding sites and NMDA receptors in brain. *Nature, 326,* 338.

Bristow, D., Bowery, N., & Woodruff, G. (1986). Light microscopic autoradiographic localization of [3H]glycine and [3H]strychnine binding sites in rat brain. *European Journal of Pharmacology, 126,* 303–307.

Buschke, H. (1973). Selective reminding for analysis of memory and learning. *Journal of Verbal Learning and Verbal Behavior, 12,* 543–550.

Calderini, G., Aporti, F., Bellini, F., Bonettim, A. C., Teolato, S., Zanotti, A., & Toffano, G. (1985). Pharmacological effect of phosphatidylserine on age-dependent memory dysfunction. *Annals of the New York Academy of Science, 444,* 504–506.

Caprioli, A., Ghirardi, O., Ramacci, M. T., & Angelucci, L. (1990). Age-dependent deficits in radial maze performance in the rat: Effect of chronic treatment with acetyl-L-carnitine. *Progress in Neuropsychopharmacology and Biological Psychiatry, 14,* 359–369.

Carlsson, A., Adolfsson, R., Aquiloniou, S. M., Gottfries, C., Oreland, L., Svennerholm, L., & Winblad, B. (1980). Biogenic amines in human brain in normal aging, senile dementia and chronic alcoholism. In M. Goldstein, D. B. Calne, & A. Lieberman (Eds.), *Ergot compounds and brain function: Neuroendocrine and neuropsychiatric aspects* (pp. 295–314). New York: Raven Press.

Corwin, J., Dean, R. L., Bartus, R. T., Rotrosen, J., & Watkins, D. L. (1985). Behavioral effects of phosphatidylserine in the aged Fisher 344 rat: Amelioration of passive avoidance deficits without changes in psychomotor task performance. *Neurobiology of Aging, 6,* 11–15.

Costall, B., Horovitz, Z. P., Kelly, M. E., Naylor, R. J., & Tomkins, D. M. (1988). Captopril improves basic performance and antagonizes scopolamine impairment in a mouse habituation test. *British Journal of Pharmacology, 95,* 882.

Crapper, D. R., Quittkat, S., Krishnan, S. S., Dalton, A. J., & DeBoni, U. (1980). Intranuclear aluminum content in Alzheimer's disease, dialysis, encephalopathy, and experimental aluminum encephalopathy. *Acta Neuropathologica, 50,* 19–24.

Crapper-McLachlan, D. R., Dalton, A. J., Kruck, T. P., Bell, M. Y., Smith, W. L., Kalow, W., & Andrews, D. F. (1991). Intramuscular desferrioxamine in patients with Alzheimer's disease. *Lancet, 337,* 1304–1308.

Crapper-McLachlan, D. R., Smith, W. L., & Kruck, T. P. (1993). Desferrioxamine and Alzheimer's disease: Video home behavior assessment of clinical course and measures of brain aluminum. *Therapeutic Drug Monitoring, 15,* 602–607.

Croog, S. H., Levine, S., Testa, M., Brown, B., Bulpitt, C. J., Jenkins, C. D., Klerman, G. L., & Williams, G. H. (1986). The effects of antihypertensive therapy on the quality of life. *New England Journal of Medicine, 314,* 1657–1664.

Croog, S. H., Sudilovsky, A., Levine, S., & Testa, M. (1987). Work performance, absenteeism, and antihypertensive medications. *Journal of Hypertension, 5,* 547–554.

Crook, T., Ferris, S. H., McCarthy, M., & Rae, D. (1980). The utility of digit recall tasks for assessing memory in the aged. *Journal of Consulting and Clinical Psychology, 48,* 228–233.

Cutler, N. R., Fakouhi, D., Smith, W. T., Hendrie, H. C., Matsuo, F., Sramek, J. J., & Herting, R. L. (1993). Evaluation of multiple doses of milacemide in the treatment of senile dementia of the Alzheimer's type. *Journal of Geriatric Psychiatry and Neurology, 6,* 115–119.

Cutler, N. R., Haxby, J., Kay, A. D., Narang, P. K., Lesko, L. J., Costa, J. L., Ninos, M., Linnoila, M., Potter, W. Z., Renfrew, J. W., & Moore, A. M. (1985). Evaluation of zimeldine in Alzheimer's disease. Cognitive and biochemical measures. *Archives of Neurology, 42,* 744–748.

Dehlin, O., Hedenrud, B., Jansson, P., & Nörgärd, J. (1985). A double-blind comparison of alaproclate and placebo in the treatment of patients with senile dementia. *Acta Psychiatrica Scandinavica, 71,* 190–196.

Delwaide, P. J., Gyselynck-Mambourg, A. M., Hurlet, A., & Ylieff, M. (1986). Double-blind randomized controlled study of phosphatidylserine in senile demented patients. *Acta Neurologica Scandinavica, 73,* 136–140.

De Renzi, E., & Vignolo, L. A. (1962). The Token Test: A sensitive test to detect disturbances in aphasics. *Brain, 85,* 665–678.

De Renzi, E., Motti, F., & Nichelli, P. (1980). Imitating gestures: A quantitative approach to ideomotor apraxia. *Archives of Neurology, 37,* 6–10.

De Renzi, E., Pieczuro, A., & Vignoli, L. A. (1966). Oral apraxia and aphasia. *Cortex, 2,* 50–73.

Deyo, R. A., Straube, K. T., & Disterhoft, J. F. (1989). Nimodipine facilitates associative learning in aging rabbits. *Science, 248,* 809–811.

Drago, F., Canonico, P. L., & Scapagnini, U. (1981). Behavioral effects of phosphatidylserine in aged rats. *Neurobiology of Aging, 2,* 209–213.

Dysken, M. W., Mendels, J., LeWitt, P., Reisberg, B., Pomara, N., Wood, J., Skare, S., Fakouhi, J. D., & Herting, R. L. (1992). Milacemide: A placebo-controlled study in senile dementia of the Alzheimer type. *Journal of the American Geriatric Society, 40*, 503–506.

Edwardson, J. A., & Candy, J. M. (1989). Aluminum and the pathogenesis of senile plaques in Alzheimer's disease, Down's syndrome and chronic renal dialysis. *Annals of Medicine, 21*, 95–97.

Ferris, S. H., Crook, T., Sathanatha, G., & Gershan, S. (1976). Reaction time as a diagnostic measure of cognitive impairment in senility. *Journal of American Geriatrics, 24*, 529–533.

Fischer, W., Wictorin, K., Börklund, A., Williams, L. R., Varon, S., & Gage, F. H. (1987). Amelioration of cholinergic neuron atrophy and spatial memory impairment in aged rats by nerve growth factor. *Nature, 329*, 65–68.

Flaten, T. P. (1990). Geographical associations between aluminum in drinking water and registered death rates with dementia (including Alzheimer's disease, Parkinson's disease and amytrophic lateral sclerosis) in Norway. *Environmental Geochemistry and Health, 12*, 152–167.

Flicker, C., Bartus, R. T., Crook, T. H., & Ferris, S. H. (1984). Effects of aging and dementia upon recent visuospatial memory. *Neurobiology of Aging, 5*, 275–283.

Flicker, C., Ferris, S. H., Crook, T., & Bartus, R. T. (1986). The effects of aging and dementia on concept formation as measured on an object-sorting task. *Developmental Neuropsychology, 2*, 65–72.

Flicker, C., Ferris, S. H., Crook, T., & Bartus, R. T. (1987a). Implications of memory and language dysfunction in the naming deficit of senile dementia. *Brain and Language, 31*, 187–200.

Flicker, C., Ferris, S. H., Crook, T., & Bartus, R. T. (1987b). A visual recognition memory test for the assessment of cognitive function in aging and dementia. *Experimental Aging Research, 13*, 127–132.

Flicker, C., Ferris, S. H., Crook, T., & Bartus, R. T. (1990). Impaired facial recognition memory in aging and dementia. *Alzheimer Disease and Associated Disorders, 4*, 43–54.

Flicker, C., Ferris, S. H., Kalkstein, D., & Serby, M. (1994). A double-blind, placebo-controlled crossover study of ganglioside GM-1 treatment for Alzheimer's disease. *American Journal of Psychiatry, 151*, 126–129.

Folstein, M., Folstein, S., & McHugh, R. (1975). Mini-Mental State: A practical method for grading the cognitive state of patients for the clinician. *Journal of Psychiatric Research, 12*, 189–198.

Fritz, I. B. (1963). Carnitine and its role in fatty acid metabolism. *Advances in Lipid Research, 1*, 285–334.

Geisler, F. H., Dorsey, F. C., & Coleman, W. P. (1991). Recovery of motor function after spinal-cord injury—A randomized, placebo-controlled trial with GM-1 ganglioside. *New England Journal of Medicine, 324*, 1829–1838.

Ghirardi, O., Milano, S., Ramacci, M. T., & Angelucci, L. (1988). Effect of acetyl-L-carnitine chronic treatment on discrimination models in aged rats. *Physiological Behavior, 44*, 769–773.

Ghirardi, O., Milano, S., Ramacci, M. T., & Angelucci, L. (1989). Long-term acetyl-L-carnitine preserves spatial learning in the senescent rat. *Progress in Neuropsychopharmacology and Biological Psychiatry, 13,* 237–245.

Gibson, G. E., Sheu, K. F. R., Blass, J. P., Baker, A., Carlson, K. C., Harding, B., & Perrino, P. (1988). Reduced activities of thiamine-dependent enzymes in the brains and peripheral tissues of patients with Alzheimer's disease. *Archives of Neurology, 45,* 841–845.

Gottfries, C. G., Adolfsson, R., Aquiloniou, S. M., Carlsson, A., Eckernas, S. A., Nordberg, A., Oreland, L., Svennerholm, L., Wiberg, A., & Winblad, B. (1983). Biochemical changes in dementia disorders of Alzheimer's type (AD/SDAT). *Neurobiology of Aging, 4,* 261–271.

Gottfries, C. G., Bråne, G., & Steen, G. (1982). A new rating scale for dementia syndromes. *Gerontology, 28,* 20–31.

Guy, W., & Bonato, R. R. (1970). *Manual for the ECDEU Assessment Battery.* Washington, DC: U.S. Department of Health, Education, & Welfare.

Hachinski, V. C., Iliff, L. D., Zilkha, E., Boulay, G. H., McAllister, V. L., Marshall, J., Russell, R. W., & Symon, L. (1975). Cerebral blood flow in dementia. *Archives of Neurology, 32,* 632–637.

Hachinski, V., Lassen, N., & Marshall, J. (1974). Multi-infarct dementia—A cause of mental deterioration in the elderly. *Lancet, 2,* 207–209.

Hamilton, M. (1960). A rating scale for depression. *Journal of Neurology, Neurosurgery and Psychiatry, 23,* 56–62.

Handelman, G. E., Mueller, L. L., & Cordi, A. A. (1988). Glycinergic compounds facilitate memory formation and retrieval in rats. *Society for Neuroscience Abstracts, 14,* 249.

Haycox, J. A. (1984). A simple, reliable clinical behavioral scale for assessing demented patients. *Journal of Clinical Psychiatry, 45,* 23–24.

Hefti, F. (1986). Nerve growth factor promotes survival of septal cholinergic neurons after fimbrial transections. *Journal of Neuroscience, 6,* 2155–2162.

Horowitz, S. H. (1986). Ganglioside therapy in diabetic neuropathy. *Muscle Nerve, 9,* 531–536.

Imperato, A., Ramacci, M. T., & Angelucci, L. (1989). Acetyl-L-Carnitine enhances acetylcholine release in the striatum and hippocampus of awake freely moving rats. *Neuroscience Letters, 107,* 251–255.

Isaacs, B., & Kennie, A. T. (1973). The Set Test as an aid to the detection of dementia in old people. *British Journal of Psychiatry, 123,* 467–470.

Jenkinson, M. L., Bliss, M. R., Brain, A. T., & Scott, D. L. (1989). Rheumatoid arthritis and senile dementia of the Alzhemer's type. *British Journal of Rheumatology, 26,* 86–88.

Jones, R. W., Wesnes, K. A., & Kirby, J. (1991). Effects of NMDA modulation in scopolamine dementia. *Annals of the New York Academy of Sciences, 640,* 241–244.

Katz, S., Ford, A. B., Moskowitz, R. W., Jackson, B. A., & Jaffe, M. W. (1963). Studies of illness in the aged: The Index of ADL, a standardized measure of biological and psychological function. *Journal of the American Medical Association, 185,* 914–919.

Kugler, J., Krauskopf, R., & Dersch, J. E. (1981, October). *Comparison of the effects of buflomedil and placebo on the EEG in psychometric test performance of patients with cerebrovascular insufficiency.* Proceedings of the Conference on Microcirculation and Ischemic Vascular Diseases, Rio de Janeiro, New York.

Landfield, P. W., Pitler, T. A., & Applegate, M. D. (1986). The aged hippocampus: A model system for studies on mechanisms of behavioral plasticity and brain aging. In R. I. Isaacson & K. H. Pribram (Eds.), *The hippocampus.* New York: Plenum Press.

Lärkvors, L., Ebendal, T., Whittemore, S. R., Perrson, J., Hoffer, B., & Olson, L. (1987). Decreased level of nerve growth factor (NGF) and its messenger RNA in the aged rat brain. *Molecular Brain Research, 3,* 55–60.

Lawton, B., & Brody, E. (1969). Assessment of older people: Self-maintaining and instrumental activities of daily living. *Gerontologist, 9,* 179–186.

Lehman, H. E., & Ban, T. A. (1970). Psychometric tests in evaluation of brain pathology responsive to drugs. *Geriatrics, 25,* 142–147.

Leon, A., Benvegnu, D., Dal Toso, R., Presti, D., Facci, L., Giorgi, O., & Toffano, G. (1984). Dorsal root ganglia and nerve growth factor: A model for understanding the mechanism of GM-1 effects on neuronal repair. *Journal of Neuroscience Research, 12,* 277–287.

Levinson, B., Wright, P., & Barklem, S. (1985). Effect of buflomedil on behaviour, memory, and intellectual capacity in patients with dementia. A placebo-controlled study. *South African Medical Journal, 68,* 302–307.

Lezak, M. D. (1983). *Neuropsychological Assessment.* New York: Oxford University Press.

Markowska, A. L., Ingram, D. K., Barnes, C. A., Spangler, E. L., Lemken, V. J., Kametani, H., Yee, W., & Olton, D. S. (1990). Acetyl-L-carnitine 1 effects on mortality pathology and sensory-motor performance in aging rats. *Neurobiology of Aging, 11,* 491–498.

Martyn, C. N., Osmond, C., Edwardson, J. A., & Lacey, R. F. (1989). Geographical relation between Alzheimer's disease and aluminum in drinking water. *Lancet, 338,* 390.

Mattis, S. (1976). Mental status examination for organic mental syndrome in the elderly patient. In L. Bellak & T. Katasu (Eds.), *Geriatric psychiatry: A handbook for psychiatrists and primary care physicians* (pp. 71–122). New York: Grune Stratton.

Mattis, S. (1989). *Dementia Rating Scale.* Odessa, FL: Psychological Assessment Resources.

McGeer, P. L., McGeer, E., Rogers, J., & Sibley, J. (1991). Anti-inflammatory drugs and Alzheimer disease. *Lancet, 335*, 1037.

McGeer, P. L., & Rogers, J. (1992). Anti-inflammatory agents as therapeutic approach to Alzheimer's disease. *Neurology, 42*, 447–449.

McKhann, G., Drachman, D., Folstein, M., Katzman, R., Price, D., & Stadlan, E. N. (1984). Clinical diagnosis of Alzheimer's disease: Report of the NINCDS-ADRDA Work Group under the auspices of the Department of Health and Human Services Task Force on Alzheimer's Disease. *Neurology, 34*, 939–944.

Meador, K., Loring, D., Nichols, M., Zamrini, E., Rivner, M., Posas, H., Thompson, E., & Moore, E. (1993). Preliminary findings of high-dose thiamine in dementia of Alzheimer's type. *Journal of Geriatric Psychiatry and Neurology, 6*, 222–229.

Melo, J. C., & Graeff, F. G. (1975). Effect of intracerebroventricular bradykinin and related peptides on rabbit operant behavior. *Journal of Pharmacology and Experimental Therapy, 193*, 1–10.

Miceli, G., Caltagirone, C., & Gainotti, G. (1977). Gangliosides in the treatment of mental deterioration: A double-blind comparison with placebo. *Acta Psychiatrica Scandinavica, 55*, 102–110.

Milner, B. (1971). Interhemispheric differences in the localization of psychological processes in man. *British Medical Bulletin, 27*, 272–277.

Mohr, E., Knott, V., Sampson, M., Wesnes, K., Herting, R., & Mendis, T. (1995). Cognitive and quantified electroencephalographic correlates of cycloserine treatment in Alzheimer's disease. *Clinical Neuropharmacology, 18*, 28–38.

Mohs, R., Rosen, W., & Davis, K. (1983). The Alzheimer's Disease Assessment Scale: An instrument for assessing treatment efficacy. *Psychopharmacology Bulletin, 19*, 448–450.

Monaghan, D., & Cotman, C. (1985). Distribution of N-methyl-D-aspartate-sensitive L-[3H]glutamate-binding sites in rat brain. *Journal of Neuroscience, 5*, 2909–2919.

Money, J., Alexander, D., & Walker, H. T. (1965). *Manual for a standardized road-map test of direction sense.* Baltimore: Johns Hopkins University Press.

Morgan, J. M., & Routtenberg, A. (1977). Angiotensin injected into the neostriatum after learning disrupts retention performance. *Science, 196*, 87–89.

Morris, A. J., & Carey, E. M. (1983). Postnatal changes in the concentration of carnitine and acetylcarnitines in rat brain. *Brain Research, 284*, 381–384.

Morris, J. C., Heyman, A., Mohs, R. C., Huhes, J. P., VanBelle, G., Fillenbaum, G., Mellits, E. D., & Clark, C. (1989). The consortium to establish a registry for Alzheimer's disease (CERAD) I: Clinical and neuropsychological assessment of Alzheimer's disease. *Neurology, 39*, 1159–1165.

Neri, L. C., & Hewitt, D. (1991). Aluminum, Alzheimer's disease and drinking water. *Lancet, 338*, 1594–95.

Nolan, K. A., Black, R. S., Sheu, K. F., Langberg, J., & Blass, J. P. (1991). A trial of thiamine in Alzheimer's disease. *Archives of Neurology*, *48*, 81–83.
Olson, L., Nordberg, A., von Holst, H., Böckman, L., Ebendal, T., Alafuzoll, I., Amberla, K., Hartvig, P., Herlitz, A., Lilja, A., Lundqvist, H., Ångström, B., Meyerson, B., Persson, A., Viitanen, M., Winblad, B., & Seiger, Å. (1992). Nerve growth factor affects 11C-nicotine binding, blood flow, EEG, and verbal episodic memory in an Alzheimer patient (Case Report). *Journal of Neural Transmission*, *4*, 79–95.
Ögren, S. O., Holm, A. C., Hall, H., & Lindberg, U. H. (1984). Alaproclate, a new selective 5-HT uptake inhibitor with therapeutic potential in depression and senile dementia. *Journal of Neural Transmission*, *59*, 265–288.
Ögren, S. O., Norström, Danielsson, E., Peterson, L. L., & Bartfoi, T. (1985). In vivo and in vitro studies on the potentiation of muscarinic receptor stimulation by alaproclate, a selective 5-HT uptake blocker. *Journal of Neural Transmission*.
Onofrj, M., Bodis-Wollmer, I., Pola, P., & Calvani, M. (1988). Central cholinergic effects of levo-acetylcarnitine. *Drugs in Experimental and Clinical Research*, *9*, 161–169.
Pattie, A. H. (1981). A survey version of the Clifton Assessment Procedure for the Elderly (CAPE). *British Journal of Clinical Psychology*, *20*, 173–178.
Peterson, C., & Goldman, J. E. (1985). Alterations in calcium uptake in cultured skin fibroblasts from patients with Alzheimer's disease. *New England Journal of Medicine*, *312*, 1063–1065.
Quartermain, D., Nuygen, T., Sheu, J., & Herting, R. L. (1991). Milacemide enhances memory storage and alleviates spontaneous forgetting in mice. *Pharmacology and Biochemical Behavior*, *39*, 31–35.
Randt, C. T., Brown, E. R., & Osborne, D. P. J. (1980). A memory test for longitudinal measurement of mild to moderate deficits. *Clinical Neuropsychology*, *2*, 184–194.
Reisberg, B. (1983). The Brief Cognitive Rating Scale and Global Deterioration Scale. In I. Crook, S. Ferris, & R. Bartus (Eds.), *Assessment in Geriatric Psychopharmacology*, 19–35. New Canaan, CT: Mark Powell Association.
Reisberg, B., Borenstein, J., & Franssen, E. (1987). Behave-AD: A clinical rating scale for the assessment of pharmacologically remediable behavioral symptomatology in Alzheimer's disease. In H. J. Altman (Ed.), *Alzheimer's disease: Problems, prospects and perspectives*. New York: Plenum.
Reisberg, B., Ferris, S. H., de Leon, M. J., & Crook, T. (1982). The Global Deterioration Scale for assessment of primary degenerative dementia. *American Journal of Psychiatry*, *139*, 1136–1139.
Robinson, R. A. (1961). Problems of drug trials in elderly people. *Gerontology Clinic*, *3*, 247–257.
Rogers, J., Kirby, L. C., Hempelman, S. R., Berry, D. L., McGeer, P. L., Kaszniak, A. W., Zalinski, J., Cofield, M., Mansukhani, L., Willson, P., & Kogan, F.

(1993). Clinical trial of indomethacin in Alzheimer's disease. *Neurology, 43,* 1609–1611.

Rosen, W. G., Terry, R. D., Fuld, P., Katzman, R., & Peck, A. (1980). Pathological verification of ischemic scores in differentiation of dementias. *Annals of Neurology, 7,* 486.

Scraibine, A., Schuurman, T., & Traber, J. (1989). Pharmacological basis for the use of nimodipine in central nervous system disorders. *The FASEB Journal, 3,* 1799–1806.

Seus, R. (1980). Evaluación psicométrico y EEG de los farmacos. In A. Portera Sanchez (Ed.), *Simposio Internacional sobre Isquemia Cerebral, Madrid, 6-7 June,* Amsterdam.

Sharpes, M. J., & Gollin, E. S. (1987). Memory for object locations in young and elderly adults. *Journal of Gerontology, 42,* 336–341.

Sheu, K. F. R., Clark, D. D., Kim, Y. T., Blass, J. P., Harding, B. J., & DeCicco, J. (1988). Studies of transketolase abnormality in Alzheimer's disease. *Archives of Neurology, 45,* 841–845.

Shimizu, M. (1991). Current clinical trials of cognitive enhancers in Japan [Review]. *Alzheimer Disease and Associated Disorders, 5*(Suppl. 1), S13–S24.

Skaper, S. D., Katoh-Semba, R., & Varon, S. (1985). GM-1 ganglioside accelerates neurite outgrowth from primary peripheral and central neurons under selected culture conditions. *Developmental Brain Research, 23,* 19–26.

Spagnoli, A., Lucca, U., Menasce, G., Bandera, L., Cizza, G., Forloni, G., Tettamanti, M., Frattura, L., Tiraboschi, P., Comelli, M., Senin, U., Longo, A., Petrini, A., Brambilla, G., Belloni, A., Negri, C., Cavazzuti, F., Salsi, A., Calogero, P., Parma, E., Stramba-Badiale, M., Vitali, S., Andreoni, Inzoli, M. R., Santus, G., Caregnato, R., Peruzza, M., Favaretto, M., Bozeglav, C., Alberoni, M., De Leo, D., Serraiotto, L., Baiocchi, A., Scoccia, S., Culotta, P., & Ieracitano, D. (1991). Long-term acetyl-L-carnitine treatment in Alzheimer's disease. *Neurology, 41,* 1726–1732.

Spreen, O., & Benton, A. L. (1977). *Manual of instructions for the Neurosensory Center Comprehensive Examination for Aphasia.* Victoria, British Columbia, Canada: University of Victoria.

Stone, B. J., Gray, J. W., Dean, R. S., & Wheeler, T. E. (1988). An examination of the Wechsler Adult Intelligence Scale (WAIS) subsets from a neuropsychological perspective. *Int Journal of Neuroscience, 40,* 31–39.

Sudilovsky, A., Cutler, N. R., Sramek, J. J., Wardle, T., Veroff, A. E., Mickelson, W., Markowitz, J., & Repetti, S. (1993). A pilot clinical trial of the angiotensin-converting enzyme inhibitor ceranapril in Alzheimer disease. *Alzheimer Disease and Associated Disorders, 7,* 105–111.

Suzuki, K. (1987). Gangliosides and neuropathy. In H. Rahmann (Ed.), *Gangliosides and modulation of neuronal functions* (pp. H7–531–545). New York: Springer-Verlag.

Tollefson, G. D. (1990). Short-term effects of the calcium channel blocker nimodipine (Bay-e-9736) in the management of primary degenerative dementia. *Biological Psychiatry, 27,* 1133–1142.
Touya, C. (1981). Cerebral blood flow in diffuse cerebrovascular diseases. *Angiology, 32,* 40.
Towart, R., & Kazda, S. (1979). The cell and mechanism of action of nimodipine. A new calcium antagonist. *British Journal of Pharmacology, 67,* 409–410.
Tuszynski, M. H., U, H. S., Amaral, D. C., & Gage, F. H. (1990). Nerve growth factor infusion in the primate brain reduces lesion-induced cholinergic neuronal degeneration. *Journal of Neuroscience, 10,* 3604–3614.
Veroff, A. E., Cutler, N. R., Stramek, J. J., Prior, P. L., Mickelson, W., & Hartman, J. K. (1991). A new assessment tool for neuropsychopharmacologic research: The Computerized Neuropsychological Test Battery. *Journal of Geriatric Psychiatry and Neurology, 4,* 211–217.
Wechsler, D. (1945). A standardized memory scale for clinical use. *Journal of Psychology, 19,* 87–95.
Wechsler, D. (1955). *Manual for the Wechsler Adult Intelligence Scale.* New York: Psychological Corp.
Wechsler, D. (1981). *WAIS-R Manual.* New York: Psychological Corporation.
Wesnes, K. (1989). A fully automated psychometric test battery for human psychopharmacology. In Anonymous, *Abstracts of the IVth World Congress of Biological Psychiatry, 153.* Philadelphia, PA.
Will, B., & Hefti, F. (1985). Behavioural and neurochemical effects of chronic intraventricular injections of nerve growth factor in adult rats with fimbria lesions. *Behavioral Brain Research, 17,* 17–24.
Williams, L. R., Varon, S., Peterson, G. M., Wictorin, K., Börklund, A., & Gage, F. H. (1986). Continuous infusion of nerve growth factor prevents basal forebrain neuronal death after fimbria fornix transection. *Proceedings of the National Academy of Sciences, USA, 33,* 9231–9235.

CHAPTER **12**

Cholinergic System Therapy for Alzheimer's Disease

John S. Kennedy
Joseph A. Kwentus
Vinod Kumar
Dennis Schmidt

CHOLINERGIC SYSTEM THERAPY FOR ALZHEIMER'S DISEASE

Acetylcholine, the neurotransmitter found in cholinergic system neurons, has been subject to study for a very long time. Examination of acetylcholine's role in normal cellular communication was initiated in 1907 when it was proposed that acetylcholine was a mediator of cellular function and was subsequently highlighted in 1914 when Dale noted that the normal actions of acetylcholine were similar to those of parasympathetic nerve stimulation.

Recently, many advances in the understanding of the normal structure and functioning of the human cholinergic system have occurred. Yet, because this system of nerves defined by the use of acetylcholine as its neurotransmitter is exceedingly complex, it remains only incompletely understood (Fibiger & Vincent, 1987; Mesulam, 1995). Mirroring current incomplete understanding of the normal functioning of the cholinergic system, the role of the abnormally functioning cholinergic system in Alzheimer's Disease (AD) also remains incompletely understood. It is clear that the cholinergic system is one of the brain's more important regulatory neuronal systems (Mesulam, 1995). It also is evident that changes in the functioning of the cholinergic system affect many other neurotransmitter systems (Decker & McGaugh, 1991). The converse is also true. Precise understanding of the effects of specific cholinergic system changes observed with normal aging and in disease states such as AD await further clarification of the normal structure and functions of its components. As a better understanding of the cholinergic system emerges, the value and limitations of animal lesion models commonly employed in drug development, such as lesions of the neuronal tracts coursing through the Basal Forebrain to approximate the effects of AD (Ownman, Fuxe, Jason, & Kahrstrom, 1989), will become clearer.

Neuroanatomical Taxonomy of the Cholinergic System: Normal Architecture and Changes Associated with Alzheimer's Disease

The cholinergic system and its constituent components are among the most phylogenetically ancient and ubiquitous brain structures. As might be expected of neuronal systems that emerged early in evolution, the cholinergic system courses to and through many neuroanatomical structures in the brain. Considerable effort has been expended to clarify the structural taxonomy of the cholinergic system in the brain. This effort anticipates that an accurate map of the relationship of cholinergic neuronal populations to different brain structures would provide a means of elucidating the various structure-function associations attributable to the cholinergic system.

Cholinergic neurons have been proposed to be neuroanatomically classifiable into eight major cell groups that share in common the presence of choline acetyl transferase (ChAT), acetylcholinesterase (AChE), and either muscarinic (m-ACh-r) or nicotinic (n-ACh-r) receptors (Mesulam & Geula, 1988). These eight cholinergic cell groups have been classified as groups Ch_1–Ch_8 (Taylor, 1991). First, this review will focus primarily on the characteristics of groups Ch_1–Ch_4, the cell groups that arise in the Basal Forebrain. Second, it is noted where relevant that the striatal cholinergic neuronal population also is important in some aspects of disorders such as AD. In large measure, the striatal cholinergic innervations in the brain arise from cholinergic interneurons not associated directly with the cell groups Ch_1–Ch_4 (Mesulam, 1995).

In human beings, in addition to containing acetylcholinesterase and ChAT, most if not all of the Ch_1–Ch_4 cells contain Calbindin D-28K (Guela, Schatz, & Mesulam, 1993) and the nerve growth factor receptor (NGF-r) (Mufson, Bothwell, Hersh, & Kordower, 1989). Also, these cells do not express galanin (Kordower & Mufson, 1990). This pattern of: $^+$Acetylcholinesterase; $^+$ChAT; $^+$Calbindin D-28K; $^+$NGF-r; $^-$galanin allows most Ch_{1-4} cells to be traced using modern histological and immunological techniques. The Ch_1 cell group consists of about 10% of the neurons in the medial septal nucleus and, together with cells from Ch_2, is considered to be the major source of cholinergic innervation of the hippocampus (Mesulam, 1995). The Ch_2 cell group is associated with the vertical nucleus of the diagonal band where cholinergic neurons comprise 70% of that structure (Mesulam, 1995). The Ch_3 cell group is associated with the horizontal limb of the diagonal band nucleus where about 1% of cells are of the cholinergic type (Mesulam, 1995). In monkeys, Ch_3 is believed to be the major source of cholinergic innervation to the olfactory bulb (Mesulam, 1995). The Ch_4 is a large cholinergic cell group and is associated with 90% of the neurons in the basalis of the substantia innominata (i.e., Nucleus Basalis of Meynert [NBM]). The presence of noncholinergic neurons accounting for at least 10% of neurons in the NBM, as well as the presence of other features, highlights the fact that Ch_4 and NBM are not equivalent terms. The Ch_4/NBM group is of substantial interest in disorders such as AD. The Ch_4/Basal Forebrain neuronal cell group has been noted to undergo selective cholinergic cell loss in AD (Whitehouse, Price, Clark, Coyle, & Delong, 1981), and the Basal Forebrain has been shown to be the primary source of cortical cholinergic innervation damage in AD (Whitehouse, Price, Struble, Clark, Coyle, & Delong, 1982). The cell loss in the NBM has been significantly correlated with the extent of loss of the cholinergic cell marker ChAT in the cerebral cortex in AD (Etienne, Robitaille, Wood, Gauthier, Nair, & Quirion, 1986). Across species, the Ch_4 cell group demonstrates increasing differential complexity as evolution progresses (Mesulam, 1995). In the monkey, Ch_4 appears as the chief source of cholinergic innervation to the entire cerebral cortex and the amygdala (Mesulam, 1995). In the monkey, the Ch_4 system can be classified further by regions innervated into four subgroups: Ch_{4am}; Ch_{4AL}; $Ch_{4id\text{-}iv}$; Ch_{4p} (Mesulam, 1995). The Ch_{4am} subgroup innervates the medial cortical areas including the ungulate gyrus; Ch_{4AL} innervates the parietal and opercular regions as well as the ungulate gyrus; $Ch_{4id\text{-}iv}$ innervates the laterodorsal frontoparietal, peristriate and midtemporal regions; and Ch_{4p} supplies the temporal and temporopolar areas (Mesulam, Mufson, Levey, & Wainer, 1983).

In human beings, the highest density of cholinergic axons is seen in the limbic system structures, including the Ch_1 and Ch_2 derived hippocampus and the Ch_4 derived amygdala cholinergic neurons (Mesulam, 1995). This schemata delineating the normal pattern of projection of cholinergic neurons may be of particular relevance to understanding the variability in presentation of some subtypes of AD-afflicted patients, as well the variable response of patients to cholinomimetic therapies. A few cases of AD have been described that show differential involvement of the Ch_4 subsystems (Mesulam et al., 1988). Such differential Ch_4 subsystem degeneration may be more likely to be evident earlier in the course of the illness than later. It also has been noted that while research has focused on the role of the NBM in AD, it should not be overlooked that the entire rostral Cholinergic Basal Forebrain is involved in AD and eventually degenerates (Fibiger & Vincent, 1987). Although explanations as to why the Basal Forebrain Cholinergic system is specifically vulnerable in AD have been proposed (Kennedy & Whitehouse, 1993), no concise explanation has been accepted broadly by the research community.

PHARMACOLOGIC TREATMENT STRATEGIES INTENDED TO ENHANCE ACETYLCHOLINE SYNTHESIS INSIDE AND RELEASE FROM THE NEURON

The inability of AD-affected neurons to release adequate amounts of acetylcholine is thought to be responsible for many of the cognitive and psychobiological symptoms of the disorder. The failure of the neurons to release acetylcholine also is thought to possibly contribute to the disorder's progression. The possible role of deficient release of acetylcholine in AD is described next.

Current attempts to modulate the functioning of cholinergic cells involve several different pharmacologic approaches. The historical principal foci of treatment trials in AD have been based on attempts to reverse acutely cognitive symptoms of the disorder by increasing acetylcholine synthesis or release, prolonging acetylcholine intrasynaptic availability or pharmacologically mimicking the actions of acetylcholine on muscarinic and nicotinic receptors. Secondary foci have involved attempts to modify noncognitive symptoms that are often the most prominent changes, and more recently interest has begun to focus on whether cholinomimetic treatments are neuroprotective and thereby slow the relentless progression of neurodegeneration seen in AD.

Overview of the Synthesis of Acetylcholine

While it is summarily accurate to state that the synthesis of acetylcholine requires two intermediate precursors: choline and acetyl coenzyme A and that the reaction-forming acetylcholine is catalyzed by the cytoplasmic enzyme, choline acetyl transferase [ChAT], this does not imply that the process that results in the presence of acetylcholine in the synapse is simple. In fact, as discussed below, acetylcholine is synthesized inside cholinergic neurons via a complex series of steps, each of which has been considered as a potential focus of treatment intervention. Choline, in addition to being the precursor of acetylcholine in cholinergic neurons, is ubiquitously present in all cells. Choline also is the precursor of cellular membrane constituents such as phosphocholine, phosphatidylcholine (lecithin), sphingomyelin, and plasmalogens. Free choline also is itself a constituent of membranes. Despite considerable investigation, the regulation of choline availability to cholinergic neurons remains an enigma. The brain is unable to synthesize functionally relevant amounts of choline de novo (Blusztajn & Wurtman, 1981). Dietary choline entering the plasma has been shown by some to increase brain concentrations of acetylcholine (Cohen & Wurtman, 1975; Wecker & Schmidt, 1980) but exogenously administered choline is quickly cleared from plasma and tissues and therefore has a very limited period of availability to cross the blood-brain barrier (Wood & Allison, 1982). Dietary lecithin is cleared less quickly (Wurtman, Hirsch, & Growdon, 1977). Under normal circumstances, most choline used to synthesize acetylcholine in the neuron cycles in and out of a cholinergic, neuronal-associated choline pool. Released acetylcholine is broken down rapidly by acetylcholinesterase enzymes. While choline uptake into the neuron can proceed via a low-affinity passive reuptake site, the majority of the free choline released by the action of the acetylcholinesterase enzyme is then rapidly taken up into the cholinergic neuron via a high affinity reuptake site that is found exclusively in cholinergic neurons. Choline is thereby recycled to be available for acetylcholine resynthesis (Blusztajn & Wurtman, 1983). The precise location and functional significance of the free choline pool that is relevant to neuronal acetylcholine synthesis is poorly understood. It appears that membrane phosphatidylcholine also is an important store of choline used to support acetylcholine synthesis (Browning & Schulman, 1968). It has been suggested that in some brain regions, in the circumstance of sustained demand, availability of choline to the high affinity transport system might become a rate limiting step in acetylcholine synthesis (Blusztajn et al., 1986).

Precursor Therapy

The Influence of the High Affinity Choline Uptake System on Acetylcholine Synthesis

Against this incomplete understanding of the functional choline pool, clinical trials were undertaken to attempt to alter the nature of symptoms seen in AD. In an effort to increase available acetylcholine in AD, clinical trials were conducted to determine if supplemental oral choline precursor substances produced improvement in cholinergic system function. The hope was that improved neuronal function would be mirrored in improved cognitive functioning. The rationale underlying the trials was that provision of exogenous choline would, in vivo, result in increased intracellular choline availability and consequently increased acetylcholine synthesis. Several different approaches to increasing synthesis and release of acetylcholine have been examined (Table 12.1). Choline given alone in dosages as high as 16 gms per day, over periods of up to 12 weeks, has been evaluated in AD. Such treatment is reported to have produced minimal benefit in two double-blind studies, whereas several other studies found no benefit (Kumar & Calache, 1991). Lecithin, considered to be more likely to have a sustained availability in the brain, has been given at dosages up to 19 gms per day in AD. While one small study of lecithin suggested that acute cognitive benefit was evident and another study suggested lecithin therapy reduced the rate of cognitive decline over a 6-month study period, many other double-blind studies have reported no benefit (Kumar & Calache, 1991). A more recent meta-analysis of trials of the acetylcholinesterase inhibitor Tacrine (Cognex®) noted that a subgroup treated with combined Tacrine plus lecithin tended to be more likely to show benefit (Halford & Pearce, 1994). Further similar combined studies of precursor plus acetylcholinesterase inhibitors are needed to clarify the role, if any, of precursor augmentation in trials.

TABLE 12.1 Compounds Influencing Acetylcholine Synthesis and Release

Precursors/Reuptake Enhancers	Acetyl Group Donors	Enhancing of Activity of Choline Aceyltransferase	Promotion of ACh Release
Choline Lecithin	Acetyl-carnitine	None	DUP-996 Tacrine Glyburide Tolbutamide M2 receptor antagonists

Because of the poor outcomes observed with precursor therapy given alone, attention has focused on the functional aspects of the neuron that play a role in regulation of acetylcholine synthesis. This has led to examination of the functioning of the choline reuptake mechanisms; the availability of acetyl groups from mitochondrially derived acetyl coenzyme A; and the activity of choline acetyltransferase [ChAT].

Choline uptake, as discussed previously, can occur via a low-affinity process seen in all cells in the body or via the Na^+- dependent high-affinity choline uptake system found in cholinergic neuronal terminals. Of these two mechanisms that govern choline entry into cells, it is the high-affinity uptake system that is most evidently coupled to acetylcholine synthesis. The availability of choline, too, and the functional status of the high-affinity uptake system, is considered to be a potentially important rate-limiting step in acetylcholine formation (Blusztajn et al., 1986). Evidence for this view of the high-affinity uptake system is seen in the in vitro effects of hemicholinium-3 on acetylcholine synthesis. Hemicholinium-3 in vitro preferentially inhibits high-affinity choline uptake. The in vitro presence of Hemicholinium-3 produces decreased acetylcholine synthesis. In this pharmacologic model decreasing acetylcholine synthesis induced by Hemicholinium-3 results in a progressive and profound depletion of acetylcholine and a progressive reduction in acetylcholine release (Taylor & Brown, 1994). In view of this model, the results observed in clinical studies of dietary choline augmentation in AD were particularly disappointing. Why poor results were obtained is unclear.

At least one study has examined the quantity and activity of the high-affinity choline uptake transported in patients with AD (Slotkin et al., 1990). It has been suggested that the synthesis of the choline transporter is linked to its rate of being degraded as well as the firing rate of the neuron (Bissette, 1996). In AD, it has been shown that the synthesis of the choline transporter is upregulated and that quantitatively the amount of choline transporter found in the cortical tissues of AD patients is many times greater than is seen in non-AD control subjects (Slotkin, Nemeroff, Bissette, & Seidler, 1994). This finding has led to the suggestion that the adaptive response to acetylcholine decreases in AD, is typically maximally achieved without the addition of choline, and, therefore, added choline might be expected to have no benefit (Bissette, 1996).

Enhancing Availability of Acetyl Groups for Acetylcholine Synthesis

An alternative approach to precursor loading, which in theory could enhance acetylcholine synthesis, would be to increase the availability of acetyl groups derived from mitochondrially synthesized acetyl coenzyme A. Such acetyl groups are donated to choline in the formation of acetylcholine. Increasing acetyl group availability would require enhanced provision of the mitochondrial-secreted acetyl groups associated with acetyl coenzyme A (Tucek, 1993). Similar to choline dynamics, the transport of acetyl CoA from its site of formation in the mitochondria to the site of acetylcholine synthesis is not well understood. Similarly, the transport mechanism's role in regulation of acetyl CoA availability for acetylcholine synthesis is unclear. Experimental in vitro data suggest that in the normal brain, it does not appear that acetyl CoA availability is a factor in limiting acetylcholine synthesis. It is less clear if acetyl CoA availability could become critical if demand is significantly increased. Such conditions might include the circumstances of greatly increased acetylcholine release or reduction of acetyl CoA as a result of impaired formation by mitochondria (Perry, Perry, Tomlinson, Blessed, & Gibson, 1980; Sirviö & Riekkinen, 1992). Either situation might produce an imbalance in favor of demand over supply, and either or both could be relevant in the pathophysiology of AD. Consistent with this perspective, it is reasonable to consider in AD that the remaining healthy cholinergic neurons might be required to increase substantially their activity to compensate for cholinergic system neurodegeneration. It also is considered likely that degenerating cholinergic neurons have impaired energy production that would reduce the supply of acetyl CoA. Relevant to the preceding information, clinical studies designed to evaluate in vivo the presumed increased acetyl CoA availability produced by administration of acetyl-carnitine have been reported (Bonavita, 1986). One group initially suggested the presence of some improvement in cognitive function in AD patients following L-acetyl carnitine administration (Sans et al., 1992). Results of more recent large trials of L-acetyl carnitine have been more disappointing. In the United States, L-acetyl carnitine continues to be studied in only the youngest group of AD patients.

Modulation of Choline Acetyltransferase Activity

Another avenue to increase acetylcholine synthesis might be to alter or increase the activity of choline acetyltransferase (ChAT), the enzyme required for acetylcholine synthesis. It has been long observed that ChAT activity declines modestly with normal aging and much more significantly in AD (McGeer, 1984). However, it also has been demonstrated that there is normally a large excess of ChAT activity in the brain (Rylett & Schmidt, 1993). The available potential ChAT activity is much greater than that needed to sustain the observed maximum rate of acetylcholine synthesis. Because of this and because inhibitors of ChAT do not affect acetylcholine synthesis or reduce acetylcholine levels in vitro, it is considered unlikely that ChAT has a regulatory role in acetylcholine synthesis. Therefore, it is thought that ChAT modulation would not be an effective target for pharmacologic intervention in disorders such as AD.

Enhancing Release of Synthesized Acetylcholine

A final conceptual approach to enhancing presynaptic acetylcholine availability is attempting to augment the release of available neuronal acetylcholine. Very few clinical studies have been undertaken with the intent of examining the effects of presumed enhancement of in vivo acetylcholine release. The investigational medicine DUP-996 possesses the property in vitro of inducing release of acetylcholine, dopamine, and serotonin. DUP-996 was studied in AD in the late 1980s. Results varied from country to country and work in the United States was discontinued (Davidson & Stern, 1991). In addition to DUP-996, other agents have been studied in AD patients that induce release of acetylcholine and include the acetylcholinesterase inhibitor Tacrine. This effect of Tacrine is thought to have little if any clinical relevance to its therapeutic properties (Schwartz et al., 1991). Finally, several classes of medicines that release acetylcholine by modulation of potassium channels (such as the antidiabetic sulfonylurea class drugs glyburide and tolbutamide) have been suggested to be of value in the treatment of AD (Lavretsky & Jarvik, 1992) but, to our knowledge, have yet to be systematically studied. As noted below, it also is likely that new drug development that results in the availability of highly selective m_2 receptor antagonists will allow testing the hypothesis that increased release of acetylcholine will improve cognitive and other symptoms in AD.

Prolonging Availability of Released Acetylcholine: Cholinesterase Inhibition

A classical approach to the pharmacotherapy of central nervous system disorders such as AD, where reduced neurotransmitter availability is considered to be a significant feature of the disorder, and where this availability is reduced further by the normal process of enzymatic destruction, has been to explore the benefit of agents that inhibit neurotransmitter destruction. This is the same rational basis as of monoamine oxidase inhibitor therapy in major depression, where the focus of inhibition is to increase the availability of noradrenalin and serotonin, as well as in Parkinson's disease, where the focus of enzyme inhibition is to increase the availability of dopamine. In this regard, the characteristics of cholinesterase enzymes in humans have been a significant focus of research during the past decade.

Structural and Functional Characteristics of Cholinesterases

Once acetylcholine is released from the cholinergic synapse, it is subjected to very rapid hydrolytic metabolism by cholinesterase enzymes. There are two distinct types of cholinesterase enzymes that are responsible for acetylcholine hydrolysis: acetylcholinesterase (AchE) and butrylcholinesterase (BuChE; [pseudocholinesterase]). Quantitatively, total acetylcholinesterase activity predominates over total butrylcholinesterase in the mammalian brain. Independent of any subtype, acetylcholinesterase is one of the most active enzymes known, and its activity is the principal determinant of degradation of acetylcholine at the cholinergic synapse.

The structure-activity relationship of the different classes of cholinesterase has been subjected to considerable examination. Acetylcholinesterase and butrylcholinesterase each exist in up to six different polymeric forms.

For acetylcholinesterase, this results in acetylcholinesterase activity being associated with proteins having molecular weights ranging from 100,000 to greater than 600,000 (Silver, 1974). Despite this variation in structure, acetylcholinesterase in all its subforms is encoded by only a single distinct gene. This is similarly true of butrylcholinesterase, which also is encoded by a single gene, which is distinct from the acetylcholinesterase gene. The acetylcholinesterase gene and the butrylcholinesterase gene each produce two structurally similar classes of esterase enzymes. One class is comprised of three heteromeric proteinaceous forms characterized by one, two or three tetrameric subunits consisting, respectively, of 4, 8, and 12 elements (termed G_1^{A4}; G_2^{A8}; G_4^{A12}). These heteromeric forms are dimensionally asymmetric and possess a filamentous collagen-containing tail that in the brain is found attached to the synaptic membrane. The other class is comprised of three homomeric proteins characterized as monomeric, dimeric, and tetrameric forms (termed G_1; G_2; G_4) that are linked by a glycophospholipid to the external surface of cell membranes (Taylor, 1991). Acetylcholinesterase after synthesis is transported interneuronally in both anterograde and retrograde directions and is then secreted by the neuron (Hollunger & Niklasson, 1973).

The G class subtypes of acetylcholinesterase have not, to our knowledge, been reported to be functionally discriminable by their ability to degrade acetylcholine. It is thought that the G_4 form, which is enriched in the cholinergic presynaptic membrane, is primarily responsible for the degradation of released acetylcholine. The G_1 form is believed to be responsible for degradation activity unrelated to synaptic acetylcholine release (Arendt, Brückner, Lange, & Bigl, 1992).

Acetylcholinesterase in Normal Humans

In the human brain, with the exception of the human cerebral cortex, acetylcholinesterase is predominantly but not absolutely associated with the cholinergic system. In the human cerebral cortex, acetylcholinesterase occurs at low levels and is confined to presynaptic axons of the cholinergic system. Acetylcholinesterase is not considered to be a reliable marker of the cholinergic system because not all neuronal pathways that contain acetylcholinesterase are cholinergic. For example, acetylcholinesterase is coreleased with dopamine from some dopamine neurons, is colocalized in some neurons containing somatostatin (Nakamura & Vincent, 1985; Mesulam & Guela, 1992), and is found in some neurons in the ascending monoaminergic pathways (Smith & Cuello, 1984). Thus, while acetylcholinesterase in the human brain is predominantly associated with the cholinergic system, mapping of the relationship between acetylcholinesterase and ChAT reveals mismatching. Significantly, this mismatching is not evident when the tissue examined is restricted to the adult human cortex (Mesulam & Geula, 1992).

Cholinesterase (both acetyl-and butryl-type) activity also is measurably present in human lumbar CSF. This activity is thought to be due to the presence of CNS secreted cholinesterases that arise from the brain as well as spinal elements. Typically, 10%–20% of lumbar CSF-cholinesterase activity is associated with the butryl forms derived both from neurons and glial cells, while the remainder of lumbar CSF-cholinesterase activity is due to CNS-derived acetylcholinesterase (Brimijoins, 1983; Sirviö & Riekkinen, 1992; Atack, Perry, Bonham, & Perry, 1987). CSF-acetylcholinesterase in the human lumbar region possesses no rostral-caudal gradient (Lal et al., 1984). Because in animals electrical stimulation of the striatonigral system increases cisternal CSF-acetylcholinesterase activity (Greenfield & Smith, 1979), and because lesions of the Basal Forebrain in rats must be extensive before decreased cisternal acetylcholinesterase activity is evident (Riekkinen, Miettinen, Rummukainen, Pitkanen & Paljarvil, 1990), it is believed that CSF-acetylcholinesterase enzymes arise primarily from the striatum (substantia nigra) and spinal cord (Sirviö & Riekkinen, 1992). Despite the preceding, the true origins of lumbar CSF-acetylcholinesterase in humans remains unclear.

Many studies have examined changes in acetylcholinesterase activity in the brain and lumbar CSF in normal aging and in AD patients (Sirviö & Riekkinen, 1992). Normally, in the human brain the tetrameric secreted G_4 form predominates and is found abundantly at cholinergic synapses. In the young, healthy, normal individual, the G_1 form is found in smaller amounts than the G_4 form. While overall cholinesterase activity does not appear to decrease in many brain regions with normal aging (Sirviö & Riekkinen, 1992), the G_4 form decreases slightly in the neocortex and hippocampus. The G_1 form is not altered appreciably (Siek, Katz, Fishman, Korosi, & Marquis, 1990). This results in a slightly decreased G_4/G_1 activity ratio, but, as reviewed later in this chapter, the results of subform concentration changes in AD are much greater. Studies of the influence of aging on lumbar CSF acetylcholinesterase activity suggest that modest increases in acetylcholinesterase activity occur with aging (Sirviö & Riekkinen, 1992). The numerical ratio of $G_4:G_1$ in normal aging is about 2:1

(Organe, Giacobini, & Struble, 1992; Enz, Amstutz, Boddeke, Ginelin, & Malanowski, 1992).

Cholinesterase activity also is robustly present in human blood where butrylcholinesterase predominantly accounts for observed activity in plasma. Red blood cell-associated cholinesterase activity also is observed and is due principally to acetylcholinesterase (Yamamoto et al., 1990). Therefore, reports in cholinesterase inhibitor clinical trials of inhibition of RBC-cholinesterase activity are thought to reflect inhibition of G_4 subtype acetylcholinesterase activity (see next) (St. Clair, Brock, & Barron, 1986).

Acetylcholinesterase in Alzheimer's Disease

It has long been noted in AD that butrylcholinesterase activity in the temporal cortex is slightly increased (Perry et al., 1984) and that cortical acetylcholinesterase activity is reduced in AD. The reduction in acetylcholinesterase activity in AD is particularly evident in the temporal cortex, hippocampus, and striatum (Enz et al., 1993). The extent of acetylcholinesterase activity reduction has been related to the severity of the disease process, but reductions are not evident early in the illness, nor are the apparent losses as severe at any stage as those seen in reductions of choline acetyltransferase (Perry & Perry, 1983). Recent studies that evaluated acetylcholinesterase subtype changes in AD have concluded that it is the secreted membrane-bound G_4 form that is decreased selectively in the frontal and parietal cortex (Fishman, Siek, MacCallum, Bird, Voliler, & Marquis, 1986; Arendt et al., 1992). This regional finding likely depends in part on the stage of illness at death and on the associated neuroanatomically defined subtype of cholinergic system (Ch_{1-8}) pathology. In other studies, such declines also have been noted to include the temporal cortex, hippocampus, and striatum (Enz et al., 1993). Overall changes in acetylcholinesterase activity in AD therefore appear to be attributable to selective decreases in the G_4 subform. The selective loss of the G_4 form is profound and is believed to reflect selective loss of the membrane pool. The G_1 form is not significantly reduced. This has led to the observation in several studies of AD that the $G_4:G_1$ ratio may decrease significantly. In at least one study of AD, the $G_4:G_1$ ratio was decreased to 0.65:1 (Enz et al., 1993).

In AD, the observed pattern of relatively high G_1 and low G_4 has been suggested to be similar to that seen in the early embryonic brain (Arendt et al., 1992), where the secreted G forms, in particular, are thought by some to have a possible role during normal development and in the normal brain process of neuroplasticity (Layer & Sporns, 1987; Chubb, 1984; Layer, 1990; Robertson, Mostamand, Kageyama, Gallardok, & Yu, 1991). In AD, much of the acetylcholinesterase present in the cortex is associated within and attributable to the presence of neuritic amyloid plaques. Such plaques are a hallmark of the neuropathology of AD (Arendt et al., 1992; Friede, 1965; Joachin & Selkoe, 1992). One proposed explanation for the presence of cholinesterases in plaque is that with cholinergic neuron degeneration, a reactive plastic response occurs producing sprouting of acetylcholinesterase positive terminals (Hyman, Kromer, & Van Hoesen, 1987). In support of this is the finding that plaque formation is associated with the presence of embryonic components of the neuron's cytoskeleton (Miller & Geddes, 1990). The proposed linkage between plaque formation and embryonic activity is supported by at least one study that has suggested that it is predominantly the G_1 form of butrylcholinesterase and acetylcholinesterase that is present in the plaque in AD (Arendt et al., 1992). It also has been hypothesized that increased cholinesterase activity in the region about, or in the developing plaque itself, may have a role in AD pathogenesis (Wright, Geula, & Mesulam, 1993). This is discussed later in this chapter.

As noted previously, the form of plaque-associated acetylcholinesterase is thought to be chiefly G_1. Much of the G_1 is thought to be derived from reactive neuronal glial cell involvement in plaque formation (Arendt et al., 1992). The functional physiological characteristics of the plaque-associated acetylcholinesterases have been examined and differences from normal neuronal-associated acetylcholinesterases have been suggested to be evident (Wright, Geula, & Mesulam, 1993). Plaque-associated acetylcholinesterases have been shown in vitro to be more resistant to cholinesterase inhibitors, such as physostigmine and Tacrine than are acetylcholinesterases in normal neurons (Mesulam, Guela, & Moran, 1987). It has been reported in vitro that similar to glial cell-associated cholinesterase, plaque-associated acetylcholinesterases are much more sensitive to selective inhibition by some indolamines (serotonin [5-HT] and 5-hydroxytryptophan [5-HTP] but not L-Tryptophan) than is seen in examination of acetylcholinesterases derived from nonplaque and nonglial cell sources (Wright et al., 1993).

Studies of cholinesterases and acetylcholinesterase(s) in AD patients' lumbar CSF have produced very inconsistent results. This may in part reflect the criteria employed for definition of patients and controls (Sirviö & Riekkinen, 1992). While few studies have examined the relative contributions of the acetylcholinesterase molecular subforms to the total activity of acetylcholinesterase in lumbar CSF, those few have found no differences between controls and AD cases (Sirviö & Riekkinen, 1992). Taking all subforms of acetylcholinesterase together, total CSF acetylcholinesterase activity is often noted to have considerable overlap between AD cases and controls. However, it has been recently argued from a review of studies that acetylcholinesterase activity in lumbar CSF of AD patients is reduced (Arendt et al., 1992). Because of the extent of overlapping within and between AD patients and other populations, total CSF acetylcholinesterase activity is considered to be a poor indicator of the severity of dementia and its evaluation is not considered to be useful for the diagnosis of AD. At least one study of CSF-acetylcholinesterase subtypes in AD patients has suggested that an anomalous form of molecular acetylcholinesterase is present in CSF in patients with AD (Navaratnam, Priddle, McDonald, Esiri, Robinson, & Smith, 1991). In light of the previous discussion concerning possible physiologic differences in the pharmacologic inhibition of plaque-associated acetylcholinesterase, further studies examining acetylcholinesterase subtypes in AD are indicated. The preliminary finding of anomalous forms of acetylcholinesterase requires replication before its implications for treatment are examined formally.

As alluded to above, red blood cell acetylcholinesterase activity has emerged recently as a focus of broad interest in experimental treatment trials of AD patients. Interest in erythrocyte function in AD initially emerged in the early 1980s in association with clinical trials of the acetylcholine precursor lecithin (Butterfield, Nicholas, & Marksbery, 1985). In these early studies, the focus was on erythrocyte choline levels and transport. These were evaluated as surrogate markers of the illness, to determine if they had any predictive relationship to trials outcome in lecithin-treated individuals. The results of these early studies suggested that erythrocyte choline levels and transport might allow identification of a treatment responsive subgroup (Blass, Hanin, Barclay, Kopp, & Reding, 1985; Miller, Jenden, Cummings, Reads, & Rice Benson, 1986). These early findings have not been confirmed definitively or examined formally, to our knowledge, in large-scale trials. Subsequent reports continue to emerge periodically, such as a more recent small clinical study that noted that erythrocyte choline transport is abnormal in AD and suggested that this abnormality might serve as a diagnostic marker of the disorder (Uney,

Jones, Rebeiro, & Levy, 1992). As noted later in relation to retarding of the rate of AD's progression, further study of erythrocyte choline uptake in relation to the brain's function appears worthwhile. More recently, interest in the erythrocyte (RBC) has shifted to its acetylcholinesterase activity.

It is now common in U.S.-based Phase 2 and Phase 3 trials to evaluate the effect of oral doses of acetylcholinesterase inhibitors on the extent of peripheral RBC-acetylcholinesterase inhibition. Such studies have been rationalized because RBC-acetylcholinesterase activity is considered by some to index peripherally the central action of acetylcholinesterase agents. In this respect, RBC-acetylcholinesterase activity is considered to be a possibly practical surrogate marker of central nervous system events. The evidence for a relationship between peripheral RBC-acetylcholinesterase activity and CNS-acetylcholinesterase activity is derived from a few studies of animals and a postmortem study of humans (Hallack & Giacobini, 1989; Sherman & Messamore, 1988). The validity of RBC-acetylcholinesterase activity, applied as a peripheral surrogate marker of the central cholinergic system's functioning to index the events occurring in the CNS, remains unclear. This is particularly because synthesis of a new enzyme in the brain appears to occur with a mean half-life of 11 days compared with 1–6 days required for most peripheral tissues.

Cholinesterase-Inhibitor Therapy

The preceding background is necessary to understand the current state of treatment of AD with cholinesterase inhibitors (Table 12.2). Such treatments include use of the only current U.S. Food and Drug Administration (FDA)-approved medications, Tacrine (Cognex®), and E2020 [Donzepil Hydrochloride] (Aricept™). The history of the application of cholinesterase therapy to the treatment of cognitive symptoms of AD with medicines such as physostigmine and Tacrine has been well reviewed (Kumar & Calache, 1991). The historical rationale underlying the use of cholinesterase inhibitors has been directed at prolonging the availability in the synapse of released acetylcholine via inhibition of cholinesterase activity. This orientation to treatment is based on the goal of potentiating residual cholinergic function. The approach was considered likely to have some beneficial effect because postsynaptic acetylcholine receptors are believed to be unable to discriminate between the presence of high levels of presynaptically released acetylcholine, which is present at high levels for only

TABLE 12.2 Cholinesterase Inhibitors

Relatively Nonspecific Inhibition of Butryl/Acetylcholinesterase at Probable Effective Clinical Dosages	Uncertain Specific inhibition of Butryl/Acetylcholinesterase at Probable Effective Clinical Dosages	Relatively Specific Inhibition of Butryl/Acetylcholinesterase at Probable Effective Clinical Dosages
Physostigmine Tacrine (Cognex®) Heptyl-physostigmine	Metrifonate Galanthamine Eptastigmine	Zifrosilone ENA-713 (Exelon™) E_{2020}/donzepil hydrochloride (Aricept™)

a very brief period, and prolonged persistence of acetylcholine that has been released at much lower concentrations. Following many small studies of physostigmine (Kumar & Calache, 1991), and after two widely criticized small pilot studies of Tacrine that reported beneficial effects in AD (Summers, Majovski, Marsh, Tachiki, & Kling, 1986; Division of Neuropharmacological Drug Products, 1991), the National Institute of Aging, the National Institute of Health, the Alzheimer's Association, and Warner-Lambert (Parke-Davis) Co. supported a formal, large-scale study of Tacrine treatment. This effort led eventually to FDA approval of Tacrine for treatment of symptoms of AD. In the initial large, multicenter study, maximal dosages of 80 mg a day were ultimately employed because of problems with side effects, particularly reversible liver toxicity and other problems requiring intensive medical monitoring at higher daily dosages (Davis et al., 1992). The results of a subsequent multicenter study suggest that Tacrine at higher oral dosages (160 mg a day) is tolerated by many AD patients. This later study also suggested that cognitive benefit increased as the oral dose was increased, but, unfortunately, so did the likelihood of the patient's developing intolerable side effects (Knapp, Knopman, Solomon, Pendelbury, Davis, & Gracon, 1994). Testing of cognitive functioning in AD patients during clinical trials of cholinesterase inhibitors suggests that only a small number of objective measures are likely to demonstrate acute improvement with such therapy and that for any acetylcholinesterase therapy-responsive individuals, the benefit achieved is modest. Much of the measured cognitive benefits using the standardized instrument Alzheimer's Disease Assessment Scale-cognitive subsection

(ADAS-cog) (Rosen, Mohs, & Davis, 1984) is a result of improvement in two items: ideational praxis (indexed by a task that has the patient prepare a letter for mailing) and improvement in geographic and temporal orientation (Mohs, personal communication, 1995). Beyond a directly assessed "cognitive" benefit, Tacrine also has been shown to produce some objectively rated benefit in noncognitive domains that often are the features of AD that bring the patient to the attention of the health care system. Noncognitive benefit was present during the formal assessment of Tacrine in instruments that quantified caregiver impressions of benefit and also in quality of life measures. However, these noncognitive improvements also were only very modestly evident (Knapp et al., 1994). Such benefit is obviously very important, and the specificity of these findings to Tacrine's effects, versus a general effect of acetylcholinesterase therapy requires clarification. Tacrine and also physostigmine share problems of poor bioavailability, short elimination half-lives requiring multiple daily dosing, and dosage-limiting adverse events. Studies of Tacrine suggest that it inhibits nondiscriminately all of the butrylcholinesterase G_1, G_2, G_4 subforms of cholinesterase, and this may account for its prominent peripheral cholinergic side effect profile (Catalan, Martinez, Aragones, Miguel, Hernandez, & Cruz, 1993). New acetylcholinesterase inhibitors currently in drug development hold promise of not having these pharmacologic limitations.

In response to the apparent limited effect on symptoms of AD with Tacrine therapy, the focus on drug development has turned to the development of acetylcholinesterase selective and acetylcholinesterase subtype G_1 selective inhibitor treatments. The purpose of such new drug development has been aimed at reduction of side effects. A secondary consideration in drug development has been interest in the role of acetylcholinesterase inhibitors in reducing the rate of AD progression (discussed later). One newly available FDA-approved medicine is E_{2020}/ donzepil hydrochloride, marketed as Aricept™ (Rogers & Friedhoff, 1996), a cholinesterase inhibitor imported into the United States from Japan. Aricept™ has been shown in in vitro studies to be relatively more selective for brain cholinesterase and to be more potent than Tacrine in this regard (Rogers, Yamanishi, & Yamatsu, 1991). Aricept™'s selectivity for brain cholinesterase is likely due to its chemical characteristic of being very lipid soluble. It is reported to have a $t_{1/2\beta}$ (half-life) twice as long in older normal adults compared to younger normals. This has been explained as being caused by the larger volume of distribution with aging (Minhara et al., 1993). Aricept™ has a mean 50-hour half-life that allows it to reach steady-state levels after 2 weeks. In studies of aged normals, at higher dosages studied (10 mg per day), its chief adverse effects have been transient: nausea, weakness, dizziness, and headache (Ohnishi et al., 1993).

Clinical experience suggests that Aricept™ enjoys a true side effect advantage over its only current competitor. Clinical impression suggests that it is typically, but not always, well tolerated by the individuals who constitute the heterogeneously affected AD population. Clinical impression also leaves unclear if some patients who are switched off of Cognex® and placed on Aricept™ do equally well from the perspective of symptom reduction. Clearly these two competing compounds are different in both general chemical structure as well as in overall physiological activity, particularly beyond these differences in cholinesterase inhibition. The absence of head-to-head parallel studies, as well as the absence of reported data on the effects of switching therapies, leaves unclear if a patient who fails one of the treatments is more or less likely to respond to the other. Also unclear is if it is appropriate to switch the patient taking Cognex®, when the patient is demonstrating benefit and minimal or no clinically significant side effects, and to place them on Aricept™. Anecdotal clinical experience suggests that for some individuals Cognex® is the robustly more effective treatment. Only further focused studies will determine the answers to such questions and advise the clinician if all the data related to Cognex®, such as effects on anxiety, psychosis, and other noncognitive features are equally applicable to Aricept™.

Several other cholinesterase inhibitors are under active study in Phase 2 or 3 clinical trials in the United States or are being considered for evaluation. These include: Zifrosilone, Galanthamine, Physostigmine, Metrifonate, Eptastigmine, and SDZ-ENA 713 (Exelon™). Zifrosilone is reported to be a long-lasting, reversible-specific acetylcholinesterase inhibitor, which has a sixfold higher affinity for acetylcholinesterase than butrylcholinesterase. Single dosages of the medication preliminarily appear to have a 12–16-hour pharmacodynamic period of activity when indexed by peripheral RBC inhibition. No information concerning its beneficial or unwanted side effects in AD patients is available (Cutler et al., 1995). Galanthamine (Janssen Pharmaceuticals USA) is an alkaloid of the snow drop plant and has been used for many years in Europe as an anesthetic agent. At least one in vitro study has examined the effects of Galanthamine compared to physostigmine and Tacrine on selective inhibition of acetylcholinesterase. This study noted that Galanthamine was more selective for acetylcholinesterase over butrylcholinesterase than either Physostigmine or Tacrine. It also was reported that the rank order of acetylcholinesterase: butrylcholinesterase inhibition ratios for in vitro activity was Galanthamine, Physostigmine, Tacrine. This in vitro work suggests that Galanthamine's side-effects' profile would be better than that of Physostigmine or Tacrine. Galanthamine has been studied in Europe in patients with AD and suggested to be well tolerated and of some benefit. It is being evaluated clinically in AD patients in North America (Thomson, Zendeh, Fisher, & Kewitz, 1991). Metrifonate (Bayer Corp.), another compound currently being studied in clinical trials in the United States, is an organic phosphate and is not itself a cholinesterase inhibitor. Metrifonate has been sold for many years, in many countries around the world, as a treatment for schistosomiasis. Metrifonate is converted by metabolism into a nonreversible inhibitor of acetylcholinesterase. Its nonreversible pharmacodynamic features may offer the advantage of reducing the frequency of dosing required to maintain effective levels of inhibition of CNS acetylcholine activity. Initial reports of open examination of metrifonate in AD reflect well on support by the National Institutes of Health (NIH) for innovative ideas (Becker et al., 1990). Subsequently, the current support for development of metrifonate has been drawn primarily from industry. In the United States, metrifonate has completed its pivotal phase studies, and its new drug application is in the process of being prepared for submission for review by the FDA. Eptastigmine (Merck) is a compound that, like Zifrosilone, has undergone Phase 1 and early Phase 2 study in the United States. It has been reported to lack prominent peripheral cholinergic effects at dosages that produce centrally determined adverse effects. This suggests that it is centrally selective, and it is hoped that it will undergo an expanded formal exam (Sramek, Block, Reines, Sawin, Barchowsky, & Cutler, 1995).

SDZ-ENA 713 [Exelon™] (Novartis), is a carbamate-type cholinesterase inhibitor. It represents a possible alternative to Tacrine and Donzepil hydrochloride therapies. ENA-713 has shown promising results in the Phase 2 and 3 studies (Anand, Gharabawi, & Enz, 1996). This inhibitor has very specific inhibition of the acetylcholinesterase enzyme and a purported favorable side-effect profile. It also is interesting that ENA-713 appears to have minimal cardiovascular, hepatic, or other adverse side effects, which are typically seen with cholinesterase inhibitors that are less specifically selective for the acetylcholinesterase enzyme (Anand &

Gharabawi, 1996). ENZ-713 is suggested, from information available to date, to be well tolerated by AD patients (Kumar, 1996). It is notable that SDZ-ENA-713 is a first effort by medical chemists to develop a new generation of highly selective acetylcholinesterase inhibitors at the bench rather than by extracting compounds directly from nature or recognizing the characteristics of existing medicines developed for other purposes. Its emergence reflects interest in development of drugs selective for the CNS.

CNS selective development of medications for AD is evidently advancing as is seen in recently reported in vitro studies where the focus has been on examining the relative effects of available cholinesterase inhibitors on selective G_1 versus G_4 acetylcholinesterase inhibition. One in vitro study has reported the results of comparing heptyl-physostigmine (a derivative of physostigmine) and physostigmine on inhibition of acetylcholinesterase subtypes. In this report, heptyl-physostigmine was highly selective for the acetylcholinesterase G_1 form. Physostigmine was essentially nondiscriminatively active at both G_1 and G_4 forms (Ogane et al., 1992). Heptyl-physostigmine was received with excitement by the clinical research community as it entered Phase 2 evaluation in the United States, but it was withdrawn from clinical evaluation because of emergent cases of toxicity. Similar to heptyl-physostigmine in being differentially active at G_1 versus G_4 acetylcholinesterase subforms, SDZ ENA-713 has been shown to be potently selective for the G_1 form of acetylcholinesterase compared with its effects on the G_4 form. In the comparison of SDZ-ENA-713 to heptyl-physostigmine, Physostigmine and Tacrine, the rank order of selectivity for G_1:G_4 was noted to be SDZ-ENA-713 >> physostigmine > heptyl-physostigmine > Tacrine (Enz et al., 1993). The difference in rank order in this study from the previously mentioned report of heptyl-physostigmine may be attributable in part to different methods of preparing samples and for evaluating activity changes. SDZ-ENA-713 has been approved as a treatment of AD in Switzerland and is completing Phase 3 trials in the United States where results of efficacy and safety studies are being prepared for submission for review by the FDA.

Clearly, the current direction of drug development is to develop brain selective acetylcholinesterase inhibitors that, using the example of SDZ ENZ-713 (Exelon™), seek to reduce the altered activity of plaque-associated G_1 acetylcholinesterase and presumably result in a normalized acetylcholinesterase G_4:G_1 activity ratio in AD. The expectation of such a successful effort would be an improved side-effect profile compared to the pattern of typical side effects characteristic of earlier generation cholinesterase therapies. This ideally would have the consequence of improved dosing capability and, most important, an enhanced patient-symptom response.

Cholinergic System: Direct Receptor Modulation

As implied previously, any approach to increasing acetylcholine availability or release is thought to result in increased pre- and postsynaptic receptor stimulation. Alternative strategies to produce receptor stimulation include direct stimulation by drugs that act like acetylcholine at the receptor of interest. Such an approach is conceptualized to be a "direct" receptor agonism or antagonism, depending on any particular drug's effect when it binds to the receptor. A further focus of attempts to modify the functioning of the brain's cholinergic system has been to evaluate the effects of both agonists (to mimic) and antagonists (to block), the functioning of cholinergic system pre- and postsynaptic:muscarinic (m-ACh-r), and nicotinic (n-ACh-r) receptor systems.

Muscarinic Receptors

A very long series of experimental studies in animals, followed by the use of receptor-cloning techniques, suggests that currently there are four pharmacologically defined subtypes and five molecular, biologically defined subtypes of the muscarinic receptor (Ehlert, Roeske, & Yamamura, 1995; Mutschler, Moser, Wess, & Lambrecht, 1995). Research to date supports the view that the pharmacologically defined m-ACh-rs have a direct correspondence to the cloned m-ACh-rs and are named m_1-ACh-r; m_2-ACh-r; m_3-ACh-r; m_4-ACh-r. The fifth cloned receptor named m_5-ACh-r has not yet been pharmacologically defined (Mutschler et al., 1995). From analysis of the physiological behavior of cloned receptors that were transfected into, and induced to become functional in several different nonneuronal cell lines, and from studies of the cloned muscarinic receptors' structural characteristics, it is evident that the muscarinic receptors have membership in a single superfamily (S) of receptors. All the S receptors are characterized by containing seven transmembrane spanning regions and being linked to a cellular G protein (Ehlert et al., 1995). The terminology used in the literature to describe the linkage of the receptor to the G protein is that the receptor is "coupled" to this protein. Stimulation of any of these S subtype receptors causes the G protein to become activated. Activation of the G protein leads to a series of intracellular second messenger event cascades. The outcome of the second messenger events is a cell response (Ehlert et al., 1995). It is also suggested by much experimental data that within the muscarinic receptor subtype family, the m_1-ACh-r, m_3-ACh-r, and m_5-ACh-r show the most homology of structure and in common when stimulated, cause intracellular phosphoinositide hydrolysis. Distinct from the m_1, m_3, and m_5 receptor subgroup members, the m_2 and m_4 receptors are considered a separate pair which both share a considerable homology and are only distantly homologous with the m_1, m_3, m_5 subgroup. The m_2 and m_4 when stimulated, cause strong inhibition of intracellular adenylate cyclase activity (Ehlert et al., 1995).

The muscarinic class of receptors is very widely distributed in the human body (Lefkowitz, Hoffman, & Taylor, 1990). Unfortunately, today both in vitro and in vivo muscarinic receptor research is sharply constrained by the absence of purely selective agonists or antagonists for any of the muscarinic receptor subtypes. This technical limitation leaves somewhat unclear the true distribution of muscarinic receptor subtypes throughout the human brain and does not clarify which muscarinic receptor subtype is responsible for particular observed effects of muscarinic agonists or antagonists given to either animals or humans. As discussed later in this chapter, the pharmaceutical industry is currently attempting to develop medicines that are both highly selective for specific muscarinic receptor subtypes and particularly with respect to disorders of the brain, also very lipophilic so that at centrally active dosages, little or no peripheral activity is evident. Currently, the available descriptions of the central and peripheral distribution and physiologic effects linked to the muscarinic receptor subtypes are based almost entirely on studies of the rat and rabbit.

As reviewed next, muscarinic receptors in the human brain are believed to have an important mediating role in aspects of attention, learning, memory, and control of posture. Other features of muscarinic system function in vivo, such as regulation of sleep, while important in AD are beyond the scope of this chapter. Muscarinic receptors in the periphery in humans are believed to mediate phenomena such as heart rate, cardiovascular system relaxation; constriction of: airways, iris sphincter and ciliary muscles of the eye; and gut mobility, and lacrimal/sweat gland secretions (Ehlert et al., 1995).

Neuroanatomical Location of Central Muscarinic Receptors

In the rat, the central m_1 receptor is found predominantly on postsynaptic neurons in the cerebral cortex and hippocampus. The m_1 receptor also is localized in other brain regions. The m_1 receptor is next most prominently localized in the striatal nigral region, where almost all GABA neurons that synthesize substance P and dynorphin express m_1 (and also m_4) messenger RNA (Mavardis, Rogard, & Besson, 1995). The m_1 receptor is much more evidently present than the m_2 in the striatal muscarinic receptor population when the striatum is considered (quantitatively) as a whole. The rank density of the m_1 receptors distribution in the rat brain is: hippocampus > cortex > striatum >> midbrain > medulla-Pons >>> cerebellum (Ehlert et al., 1995). In humans, the m_1 density defined using postmortem brains from aged normal individuals has been reported to be: hippocampus > temporal cortex > frontal cortex > parietal cortex > occipital cortex = putamen > nucleus basalis (Flynn, Ferrari-DiLeo, Mash, & Levey, 1995). Because of this distribution and as discussed later, m_1-ACh-r's relative preservation in AD, selective m_1-ACh-r agonists are a focus of vigorous interest in the possible treatment of AD.

The central M_2 receptor, m_2-ACh-r, is a presynaptic acetylcholine auto receptor that when stimulated causes decreased release of acetylcholine by negative feedback. In addition to decreased acetylcholine release, stimulation of the m_2-ACh-r also results in increased tissue concentrations of acetylcholine, which is thought to reflect increased storage (Consolo, Ladinski, Vinci, Palazzi, & Wang, 1987; Sethy & Francis, 1988). M_2-ACh-r is distributed nearly uniformly in low concentrations in the rat brain (Ehlert et al., 1995). Within the brain of the rat, the ranked density distribution of the m_2-ACh-r is: midbrain = medulla-Pons > cortex = cerebellum > striatum > hippocampus (Ehlert et al., 1995). In humans, the m_2 density, using postmortem brains from aged normal individuals, has been reported to be nucleus basalis > occipital cortex > hippocampus > frontal cortex = Temporal cortex = parietal cortex > putamen (Flynn et al., 1995). The m_2 receptor is considered to have an important potential role in AD and its therapy because deficits in m_2-ACh-r correlate with both the number of senile plaques and dementia severity in patients with AD (Ball, Fishman, Hachinski, Blume, Fox, & Merskey, 1985; Aubert, Araujo, Cécyre, Robitaille, Gauthier, & Quirion, 1992).

The apparent decline in AD of the postsynaptic m_2-ACh-r population, in the presence of the relative preservation of the presynaptic m_1-ACh-r in the cortex and hippocampus, has given rise to much interest in developing m_1 agonists and presumably also m_2 antagonists as well as combined m_1 agonists/m_2 selective antagonists for trials in AD (Mash, Flynn, & Potter, 1985; Quirion et al., 1989; Shapiro et al., 1992).

The central M_3 receptor, m_3-ACh-r, is found at very low levels throughout the rat brain and currently is considered to be of greater importance in relation to side effects associated with stimuli of peripheral m_3-ACh-r's than in relation to its central effects that have been essentially unexplored (Ehlert et al., 1995). In humans, the m_3 density defined, using postmortem brains from aged normal individuals, has been noted to be characterized by only small numbers of receptors in even the most densely populated brain regions. The m_3 density has been reported as: frontal cortex = temporal = parietal cortex > occipital cortex > hippocampus > nucleus basalis >> putamen (Flynn et al., 1995).

The central M_4 receptor, m_4-ACh-r, is not yet well localized in either the rat or the human brain. In humans, the m_4 density, defined using postmortem brains from aged normal individuals [and by application of technically novel methods that require independent confirmation of their validity], has been suggested to be diffusely present in significant amounts in the brain. The rank order of m_4 density in this report was: Putamen > nucleus basalis > frontal cortex = temporal cortex = parietal cortex = hippocmpus > occipital cortex (Flynn et al., 1995). This study also noted that, in agreement with other studies, AD subjects demonstrated modest decreases in m_1-ACh-r in the frontal cortex, the temporal cortex, the parietal cortex, and the hippocampus. The authors also noted previously reported decreases in m_2 in the hippocampus, the frontal cortex, and the nucleus basilis. Unexpectedly, they reported that m_4 receptors were either unaffected or increased in the temporal, frontal, and parietal cortices. M_4-Ach-r receptors have been suggested to be involved in the release of potentially neurotoxic excitatory neurotransmitters (McKinney, Miller, & Aagaard, 1993). The authors suggested that if the observed m_4 receptor increases are compensatory to loss of m_1, they may provide a target for treatment of AD (Flynn et al., 1995).

The distribution and functional role of the central m_5 receptor, m_5-ACh-r, in the brain is poorly understood. This reflects the m_5-ACh-r's identification by cloning techniques, but the absence of published information clarifying its pharmacologic properties. In the rat, the m_5 comprises only 2% of all muscarinic receptors in the brain (Yasuda et al.,1992). In humans, the m_5 density defined, using postmortem brains from aged normal individuals, has been suggested to be similarly low, and the regional distribution has been reported to be temporal cortex > frontal cortex = parietal cortex > occipital cortex > nucleus basalis. In this study, the hippocampus and putamen were characterized as possessing very few or no m_5-ACh-r receptors (Flynn et al., 1995). The m_5 is considered to be potentially important in regard to its involvement in dopamine function, which is reflected in the messenger RNA (mRNA), for m_5 being localized in striatal nigral dopamine neurons (Mavardis et al., 1995). Unfortunately, the localization of receptors using mRNA is fraught with problems in interpretation because once synthesized, the receptors may be transported to other sites both pre- and postsynaptically. Where receptors are located is considered to be the key to understanding their functional role and possible synaptic interactions (Hersch, Gutekunst, Rees, Hellman, & Levey, 1994).

Peripheral Muscarinic Receptors

A principal issue in cholinomimetic treatment of conditions such as AD is the determinants of treating emergent side effects arising from the effects of stimulation of peripherally located receptors and the stimulation-related consequent induction of changes in peripheral tissue function. For the muscarinic receptor system, prediction of side effects is believed to be most related to the distribution and normal functional role of the muscarinic receptors in peripheral tissues. In the periphery, m_1-ACh-r is found principally in association with peripheral sympathetic ganglia, where it likely has a role in the mediation of vagal-induced broncho constriction, gastric acid secretion, and via peripheral ganglion stimulation, increases in heart rate and blood pressure. Peripheral m_2-ACh-r is found in very high concentrations in the heart, where its stimulation produces bradycardia (Mutschler et al., 1995), and in the smooth muscle, where its activation indirectly modulates smooth muscle contractions by inhibiting relaxation (Ehlert et al., 1995). The peripheral m_3-ACh-r is found in the highest concentration in exocrine glands, where its stimulation results in salivation, lacrimation, and sweating (Ehlert et al., 1995; Mutschler et al., 1995). The peripheral m_3-ACh-r also is found in low amounts in smooth muscles, where it has the important functional role of triggering contractions of the intestinal smooth muscles (Ehlert et al., 1995) and inducing urinary bladder contractions (Mutschler et al., 1995). Thus muscarinic agonists, which have a relatively low selectivity for m_1 and m_3 and the brain, are expected to produce potential side effects such as diarrhea, among other physiologic responses to peripheral receptor stimulation. With respect to peripheral effects of the m_4-ACh-r and m_5-ACh-r, these are believed to occur in very low amounts in the periphery. Little is understood concerning the effects of peripheral stimulation of these receptors (Ehlert et al., 1995; Mutschler et al., 1995).

Central Muscarinic Receptor Functions

Much of the interest in the functioning of the brain's muscarinic receptor systems has its history in the use of receptor antagonists to block brain muscarinic receptors in animals and humans in attempts to mimic or model the cognitive dysfunction observed in patients with dementia. Typically, the medication employed has been the antimuscarinic drug scopolamine (Hyoscine®), which acts at m-ACh-r's as a competitive inhibitor of acetylcholine binding and has potent effects on human memory, as reviewed later (Aigner & Mishkin, 1993; Buresova & Bures, 1983; Broks, Preston, Traub, Poppelton, Ward, & Stahi, 1988; Christensen, Maltby, Jorm, Creasey, & Broe, 1992). Scopolamine models of AD have been extensively researched in humans since the time of the earliest studies showing scopolamine-induced cognitive deficits were reversed by the acetylcholinesterase inhibitor Physostigmine (Drachman & Leavitt, 1974). Scopolamine's clinical use in psychiatry predates its application in modeling dementia as is evident from the literature of Kraepelin (1899) and Bleuler (1916), where it was recommended to induce sleep as a treatment of acute states of agitation such as occurs in mania (Spiegel, 1989). Scopolamine typically causes sleepiness, body fatigue, and euphoria (Spiegel, 1989). Recently, the m-ACh-r subtype binding characteristics of scopolamine in cells expressing the cloned m-ACh-rs have been reported. Scopolamine reversibly binds to the m-ACh-r subtypes with the differential potency of: m_3-ACh-r > M_4-ACh-r > m_1-ACh-r > m_2-ACh-r = m_5-ACh-r. (Bolden, Cusak, & Richelson, 1992). Scopolamine is less specifically potent at blocking m_1-ACh-r than is either benzotropine, biperiden, or trihexyphenidyl (Richelson, 1995). The clinical properties of scopolamine are thought to be associated with its receptor-binding profile. This is evident in that in contrast to many other anticholinergics, it is not used in treatment of extrapyramidal side effect of neuroleptics (Mavardis et al., 1995). In young healthy normals, scopolamine produces a deficit in information learned during exposure to scopolamine (anterograde memory impairment) but not to information memorized prior to exposure to scopolamine (Ghoneim & Mewalt, 1975). Thus it does not produce the dense retrograde memory problem seen particularly in the later stages of AD. Many studies of scopolamine's effects in normal humans have confirmed that scopolamine, even at very low dosages, substantially impairs tasks requiring the movement or storage of information into long-term memory. Scopolamine has been reported to have no effect in young humans on cognitive functions such as constructional praxis or verbal fluency (Mohs, Johns, Dunn, Sherman, Rosen, & Davis, 1986), or on attention as indexed by the digits-backward task of the WAIS (Christensen et al., 1992). A more recent study examining scopolamine's effects on young adult humans concluded that the scopolamine modeling in young adults may be useful for induction of the typical changes seen in cognitive functions of AD patients early in the course of their illness, but not for induction of the changes in cognitive functions in the moderate or severe stages of AD (Christensen et al., 1992). Scopolamine challenge studies also have been conducted in the elderly normals and in individuals with AD (Sunderland, Tariot, Cohen, Weingartner, Mueller, & Murphy, 1987; Huff, Mickel, Corkin, & Growdon, 1988). In these studies both the elderly normal and AD affected groups were seen to be more sensitive to the effects of scopolamine than was seen in younger individuals. It has been pointed out that the principal difficulties with the scopolamine model are: its nonselective receptor antagonism, the fact that specific receptor subtypes are distributed variably throughout many brain structures, and that at each receptor on each structure, the degree of scopolamine's effect also is influenced by the extent to which it antagonizes the release of acetylcholine (Reiner & Fibiger, 1995). Despite these limitations, modeling of dementia in animals and humans by utilizing scopolamine remains a main method in drug development for the evaluation of compounds expected to reverse cognitive symptoms of dementia. Nonspecific muscarinic receptor antagonists other than scopolamine also have been of interest in AD research. Recently, the nonspecific muscarinic antagonist tropicamide was reported to possibly allow identification of patients with AD by eyedrop application and measurement of the pupillary response (Scinto, Daffner, & Dressler, 1994). This study has been criticized in part because of the methods employed to measure pupillary change. A more recent study failed to replicate the initial report (Loupe et al., 1996). Tropicamide eyedrop testing for diagnosis of AD remains experimentally interesting but should not be used clinically at the present.

Central Muscarinic Receptor Functions: Muscarinic ACh-R Agonist Therapies in Alzheimer's Disease

Interest in the potential utility of muscarinic receptor agonist effects on memory functions emerged in the literature with an initial study of the m-ACh-r agonist RS-86 (Hollander et al., 1978). See Table 12.3. Subsequently, pilocarpine, arecoline, bethanechol, and oxotremorine have been examined in AD (Gray, Enz, & Spiegel, 1989), with occasionally promising results such as improvement in recognition memory with arecoline and improved alertness with intracerebroventricular bethanechol infusion (Penn et al., 1988). All these agonists share the characteristic of being relatively nonselective for m-ACh-r subtypes. For example, both arecoline and RS-86 show no difference in vitro for m_1, m_2, m_3, m_4, or m_5-ACh-r affinities. Pilocarpine is characterized as having muscarinic receptor affinities of $m_1 = m_3$-$m_5 > m_2 = m_4$. Oxotremorine is characterized as having muscarine receptor affinities of $m_1 = m_2 = m_5 > m_3 = m_4$ (Schwarz, Davis, Jaen, Spencer, Tecle, & Thomas, 1993). Each of the aforementioned medications is substantially limited by some aspect of its pharmacologic properties such as either requiring continuous IV infusion to attain effective brain levels (arecoline), having limited ability to cross the blood-brain barrier (bethanechol), having unexpectedly severe side effects such as depression (oxotrimorine), or having inadequate lipophilicity so that effective brain concentrations were difficult to achieve without evident and occasionally severe peripheral side effects (RS-86) (Davis, Hollander, Davidson, Davis, Mohs, & Horvath, 1987) (Davis et al., 1993). Typical centrally determined side effects of these medicines include tremor, hypothermia and chills, and peripheral side effects include diarrhea, lacrimation, salivation, and cardiovascular system changes.

A new generation of purportedly more selective m_1-ACh-r agonists or pharmacologically advantaged nonspecific muscarinic agonist agents are currently either in preclinical development or in clinical trials in humans

TABLE 12.3 Cholinergic Direct Receptor Agonists

Muscarinic Receptors		Nicotinic Receptors
Nonspecific for M_1	*Relatively M_1 Specific*	Nicotine
RS-86	Xanomeline®	ABT-418
Pilocarpine		Metanicotin®
Arecoline		
Bethanechol		
Oxotremorine		
CI-979		

for possible treatment of AD. CI-979 (Parke-Davis) is a muscarinic agonist which recently was examined in phase II clinical trials in the United States. It is derived from the naturally occurring alkaloid arecoline (Toja et al., 1991). It has been demonstrated to reverse Basal Forebrain lesions in rats and binds nonspecifically like RS-86 to m_1-ACh-r = m_2-ACh-r = m_3-ACh-r = m_4-ACh-r (Davis, Doyle, Carroll, Emmerling, & Jaen, 1995). In trials in AD patients, CI-979 produced in some patients typical muscarinic agonist side effects, including diaphoresis, chills, nausea, abdominal pain, diarrhea, dizziness, postural hypotension, hypersalivation, lacrimation, and urinary frequency. It is noteworthy that Parkinsonian symptoms such as bradykinesia, cogwheeling, gait changes, tremor, and pill rolling also have been reported and that these may reflect the effects of muscarinic agonism in altering dopamine availability (Sramek et al., 1995). This effect may reflect action on m_5 receptors located on the dopamine neuron, as described previously. CI-979 side effects are presumed to reflect primarily its pattern of agonism of both central and peripheral muscarinic receptor subtypes at the dosages given. As noted for the acetylcholinesterase inhibitors, and also for other m_1 agonists (see the next discussion), there also is some suggestive evidence that AD patients may tolerate higher dosages of CI-979 than normal healthy individuals (Sramek, Sedman, Reece, Hourani, Brockbrader, Cutler, et al., 1995). The nature and extent of cognitive improvement experienced by AD patients who received dosages of CI-979 that were not so likely to cause the aforementioned side effects has not been reported, and recently CI-979 was withdrawn from further clinical development.

A further m_1-ACh-r agonist which has been undergoing clinical trials in the United States is Xanomeline® (Eli-Lilly). Based on studies in rats, this medicine has reported greater selectivity for the m_1-ACh-r than for the m_2-ACh-r and may have no affinity for the m_3-ACh-r (Shannon et al., 1994). Such selectivity is expected to minimize side effects such as salivation, lacrimation, and gastrointestinal activity (Bymaster et al., 1994). Early experience in the normal elderly suggests it is well tolerated (Eckols, Bymaster, Mitch, Shannon, Ward, & Delapp, 1995). The initial report of Xanolemine®'s effects in patients with AD suggested the presence of improvement in cognitive function as measured by standard clinical trial measures appropriate for the AD population. A robust response of behaviors typically found to be disturbing to caregivers was also noted. However, over 10% of the study subjects experienced syncope, defined as a loss of consciousness and muscle tone at the highest dose employed in the trial (Bodick et al., 1997).

Xanomeline®'s clinical trials-related development is currently underway with a formulation for delivering the medicine that has been revised in the hopes of improving the benefit: side effect ratio. As with CI-979, Xanomeline® has been suggested to be better tolerated at higher dosages by patients with AD than by normal healthy elderly (Cutler, Sramek, & Veroff, 1994). This suggestion of better tolerance of higher dosages of drugs by AD patients than healthy normal elderly is considered to be counterintuitive by some, and requires clarifying research to determine if this observation is sustained in the face of independent examination. Such an observation could, for example, simply reflect the AD patient's reduced ability to report side effects. Alternately, as discussed later in this chapter, alterations in m_1 receptor functioning have been suggested to be present in AD, and this tolerance of higher dosages may reflect greater m_1 dysfunction in any particular AD subject. Several other m_1 selective medicines also are being considered for, or are actively being evaluated in, clinical trials in the United States. This includes a compound being developed by Smith-Kline-Beecham, but no information is available concerning its muscarinic receptors profile, beneficial effects on symptoms, or side effects in humans (Jenkens et al., 1992). Thus it remains to be seen to what extent symptoms of AD are acutely ameliorated with the m_1 agonist approach and to what extent the wizards of medical chemistry are able to construct medications that have selective central effects, thereby allowing adequate dosages for central benefit without significant presentations of peripheral side effects. Of notable concern regarding the potential limits of m_1 receptor agonist therapy in AD is the report that in AD the m_1 receptor system may be "uncoupled" from the G protein (Flynn, Weinstein, & Mash, 1991). It also has been observed that there are changes in the G protein-mediated second messenger transduction of signaling in AD (Joseph, Cutler, & Roth, 1993). Stimulation by a drug might result in an altered response in the receptor m_1-associated effector cascade of second messenger events that normally occurs after m_1 receptor binding (Flynn, Weinstein, & Mash, 1991). If the uncoupling noted in the in vitro studies is the rule rather than the exception in affected brain regions in vivo, then m_1 agonist binding would be expected to have significantly less effect than would otherwise be anticipated. Further support for this possible concern is the more recent report of altered immunoreactivity of the m_1 receptor population in the brains of AD patients evaluated after death. In this report, the authors provided further evidence that the m_1 receptor may be altered in AD (Flynn et al., 1995). As with all efforts in new drug development, the "proof of the concept" of m_1 agonism therapy will require careful study in the clinical arena.

Nicotinic Cholinergic System Receptor Agonism

Nicotinic Receptors

Until recently, the nicotine cholinergic receptor (n-ACh-r) system held little interest outside of its obvious relevance to the study of tobacco dependence. Nicotinic system research also has been hampered by the availability of suitable ligands needed to study nicotinic receptors in human tissue and by a lack of interest in developing better nicotine ligands in part because of the association between tobacco use and its deleterious health effects (Arneric & Williams, 1994). Thus, while n-ACh-r was the earliest neurotransmitter receptor to be characterized, comparatively little is known concerning its attributes in the mammalian CNS (Watson, Roeske, & Yamamaura, 1987) and particularly in man (Arneric, Sullivan, & Williams, 1995). In muscle, n-ACh-r is a pentameric structure comprised of five subunit proteins named α (alpha), β (beta), γ (gamma), δ (delta), and ε (epsilon) (Changeux, Galzi, Devillers-Thiery, & Betrand, 1992). In nonhuman species, many subunit genes regulating the expression of the subunit proteins have been identified. It appears for neuronal genes that at least seven code for α subunits (α 2–α 8) (Sargent, 1993). It is believed that various combinations of subunits will be found and that many functional subtypes of n-ACh-r exist in the brain (Changeux et al., 1992). The belief in the likely presence of many functional central nicotine receptor subtypes, arising from different combinations of types of subunits, is supported by studies of muscle n-ACh-r. These muscle studies have shown that the binding sites for cholinergic ligands are located at the junction of α and β subunits and δ and ε subunits (Changeux et al., 1992). It is against this still preliminary but evolving background of neuronal nicotinic receptor pharmacology that selective nicotinic receptor drugs are being developed, some with a potential for treatment of cognitive disorders in humans.

Central Nicotinic Receptors Functions in Normal Humans

The interest in nicotinic agonist treatment of human memory disorders arises from several lines of research, both in animals and humans, which implicate nicotinic brain system changes in abnormal cognitive functions. Animal studies suggest that nicotine administration increases vigilance, improves learning and memory, and produces resistance to behavioral extinction (Gray, Mitchell, Joseph, Grigoryan, Dawes, & Hodges, 1994). These properties of nicotine may be due to its stimulation of presynaptic n-ACh-rs, whereby nicotine facilitates the release of neurotransmitters such as acetylcholine, dopamine, serotinin, GABA, and glutamate (Gray et al., 1994; Wonnacotts, Irons, Rapier, Thorne, & Lunt, 1990). To date, only limited attention has been focused on the role of nicotinic receptor stimulation in cognition in normal humans. It has been demonstrated in humans that nicotine enhances attention and vigilance, rapid information processing, and some memory functions (Warburton, 1992; Wesnes & Warburton, 1983), and that nicotine has the opposite effect on rapid human information processing than that of the muscarinic antagonist scopolamine (Wesnes & Warburton, 1984). It also has been demonstrated in normal humans that the antihypertensive drug mecamylamine, a noncompetitive antagonist of n-ACh-r, impairs some cognitive functions (Newhouse, Potter, Corwin, & Lennox, 1994). These data support the view that nicotinic receptor modulation produces some cognitive effects in humans that are believed to be similar to the behavioral effects observed in nonhuman studies. By extension, it also is thought that similar underlying neurobiologic mechanisms that account for effects in lower animal species may be involved in these effects in man.

Nicotinic Receptor Changes in Alzheimer's Disease

Interest in nicotinic system modulation in AD is derived from neuropathologic and in vivo imaging studies, suggesting that it has importance in disorders of cognition. Autoradiography and kinetic analysis of the binding of (^{3}H)-nicotine to postmortem brain revealed that substantial reductions in nicotine binding were present in the cortices of individuals with AD, relative to age-matched controls (Whitehouse et al., 1986; Aubert et al., 1992). This finding has been independently confirmed by several other groups, and it also has been demonstrated that while decreased nicotine binding in the hippocampus occurs with normal neurological aging, reductions are substantially greater in AD (Perry et al., 1987; Aubert et al., 1992). Further heightening the interest in the nicotinic system in AD was the finding, using postmortem tissues, that the highest concentration of n-ACh-r receptors in the human brain are in the Basal Forebrain (Shimohama, Taniguchi, Fujinara, & Kameyama, 1985). As reviewed previously, the Basal Forebrain projects to the hippocampus and the cerebral cortex, two regions involved in learning and memory (Sahakian, Jones, Levy, Gray, & Warburton, 1989). Animal studies have shown that the Basal Forebrain Cholinergic system is involved in the coordination or regulation of components of CNS functions such as attention and arousal to normal stimuli (Arneric et al., 1995). It has been suggested that the loss of the Basal Forebrain system may be responsible for the decreased attentional activity of the AD patient (Sahakian et al., 1989; Warburton, 1992).

Nicotinic Receptor Agonist Therapies in Alzheimer's Disease

To date, we are aware of only a few small studies of the acute effects of nicotine on cognitive functions in patients with AD. In one study, patients were given nicotine intravenously, and improvement in verbal recall was noted (Newhouse et al., 1988). In a second study, patients were given subcutaneous nicotine injections that caused a dose-related improvement in some aspects of attention and rapid information processing, but not in attention as indexed by the digit-span test (Jones, Sahakian, Levy, Warburton, & Gray, 1992). It has been suggested of this latter study that side effects of nausea and dizziness may not have allowed maximal nicotine efficacy to be determined (Arneric & Williams, 1994).

One approach to identifying determinants of response to trials of therapies such as nicotine has been to examine, using proton emission tomography (PET), in vivo changes in regional cerebral blood flow (r-CBF) and receptor densities in the human brain. Animal studies suggest that cholinergic neurons of Basal Forebrain origin are involved intimately in the neurogenic control of cortical CBF and that CBF is significantly increased when the Basal Forebrain is stimulated (Linville, Williams, Raskiewicz, & Arneric, 1993). We are unaware of any CBF studies of the effects of nicotinic agonism on AD. With respect to in vivo characterizations of nicotinic receptors in AD patients, a single series of studies examining (S) (-)- ^{11}C-nicotine in a small number of AD patients at various stages of their illness has been reported (Nordberg, 1993). In this report, the authors observed a consistent and marked loss of cortical nicotinic receptors. The most evident decline in (S) (-)- ^{11}C-nicotine binding occurred in the frontal and temporal cortex of AD patients when compared to controls. The authors noted further that a positive correlation was present between the patients' Mini-Mental State Score and the extent of uptake of (S) (-)- ^{11}C-nicotine into the temporal cortex. These authors also reported on five AD subjects in whom they had evaluated n-ACh-r binding using (S)(-)- ^{11}C-nicotine and also brain glucose metabolism using ^{18}F-fluor-deoxy-glucose. Each AD patient was evaluated prior to and then after 3 months of Tacrine (Cognex®) treatment. The authors observed that Tacrine increased (S)-(-)- ^{11}C-nicotine uptake and glucose metabolism, and that the increases approximately paralleled the observed improvement in neuropsychological test performance. The most significant effects were found early on in the course of illness (Nordberg, 1993). Obviously, the tantalizing suggestion of improvement requires many more than the few patients reported on before any valid conclusion about the nicotinic system can be formulated.

At the present, the chief barrier to evaluation of n-ACh-r agonist therapy of AD is the low dosages of nicotine (such as the low dosages provided by nicotine patches) that are safely tolerated. ABT-418 (Abbott Lab) (Arneric et al., 1994) a selective activator of n-ACh-rs has been reported in preliminary studies in humans to be well tolerated over a broad dose range (Arneric et al., 1995) but more recently has been withdrawn from clinical development. Others also have more recently reported a new class of nicotine agonists that appear to be selective for central nicotine receptor subtypes. The analog metanicotin (R. J. Reynolds Co.) (Lippiello et al., 1996) displayed significant effects in antagonizing the cognitive defects produced by a model of cholinergic deficits in rats without producing significant peripheral side effects. These or some other such medicine, if successfully developed for use in man, might allow clarification of the role of nicotinic agonism in the treatment of AD and appear to offer an exciting new area of investigation.

Reducing the Rate of Progression of AD

It is considered likely that a primary factor in the evolution of AD is that amyloid precursor protein (APP) undergoes abnormal cellular processing (Joachin & Selkoe, 1992). Under normal circumstances, APP is thought to be principally metabolized to a soluable sulfated end product, which is considered to be involved in neuronal cell growth and the maintenance of synapses (Robakis, Vassilacopoulou, Efthimiopoulos, Sambamurti, Refold, & Shioi, 1993; Mattson, Cheng, Culwell, Esch, Lieberburg, & Rydel, 1993). In AD, abnormal processing of APP is believed to result in the formation of significantly greater than normal amounts of the insoluble end product of APP processing, β-amyloid peptide (β/A_4). The excess β/A_4 is then continuously deposited into and contributes to expansion of the developing plaque (Joachin & Selkoe, 1992). In-vivo examination of the processing of APP suggests that increased acetylcholine-like activity, mediated via muscarinic receptor agonism, reduces β/A_4 production (Emmerling, Moore, Doyle, Carroll, & Davis, 1995). It is therefore considered theoretically possible that either inhibition of cholinesterase's (including that in plaque) or cholinomimetic direct receptor modulation therapy may reduce the rate of β/A_4 deposition and thereby the rate of AD-related progressive neurodegeneration (Emmerling et al., 1995).

Acetylcholine is the principal endogenous agonist compound for muscarinic receptors. As noted previously, any means by which acetylcholine levels are increased in the synapse has in effect potential to produce enhanced muscarinic receptor agonism. This is presumed to be the effect of both precursor and acetylcholinesterase-inhibitor therapy. In this regard, several studies and at least one review of early precursor therapy trials have suggested that some patients appear to experience a less rapidly progressive illness when treated with lecithin (Boyd, White, Blackwood, Glen, & McQuenn, 1977; Dysken, 1987; Dysken, Fovall, & Harris, 1982; Levy, Little, Chuaqui, & Reith, 1983). More recently reported data that examined results of several small 1-year studies of various acetylcholinesterase inhibitors suggested that acetylcholinesterase inhibitors also may slow progression (Giacobini, 1994). The intent of the aforementioned studies, which were reviewed by Giacobini for possible influences on disorder progression, were to evaluate acute symptomatic benefit, not to observe slowing of progression. It remains uncertain if the design of these trials allows for the meaningful interpretation of the studies for purposes beyond their original intent. This possible effect of precursor or cholinesterase therapy on reducing the rate of AD progression has not yet been reported as having been formally evaluated in prospective trials employing the clinical trials designs necessary to avoid the confound of the influence of acute symptom improvement on measurement of long-term therapy outcome (Gershon et al., 1994).

In vitro data support the view that m_1-ACh-r agonist therapy should be of considerable interest in regard to its potential to reduce the rate of deposition of the B/A_4 protein in AD and thereby in theory reduce the rate of neurodegeneration-related progression of the illness. In vitro cell studies, employing both CI-979 and Xanomeline®, have demonstrated that for transfected cells possessing the cloned receptor m_3-ACh-r and/

or m_1-ACh-r, treatment with muscarinic agonists causes: an increase in secretion of the soluble APP (for Xanomeline® in a dose-dependent fashion); a decrease in intracellular levels of APP; and a decreased production and release of the B/A_4 protein. The production and release of B/A_4, which under normal circumstances is produced in trace rather than large amounts and is believed in trace amounts to be unable to aggregate and produce neurotoxicity, is considered by many basic scientists to be the best hope for the foreseeable future to allow effective intervention in the disorder progression (Emmerling et al., 1995; Eckols et al., 1995; Yankner, Duffy, & Kirschner, 1990). The logic supporting this hope is that if a change in APP processing occurs in vivo because of muscarinic agonist influences, B/A_4 deposition would be expected to be decreased. If B/A_4 deposition is a primary cause of disorder progression in AD patients, then long-term trials designed specifically to examine the change in rate of progression of the disorder in patients should be able to reveal this. Presumably, because trial design requirements to show symptomatic improvement are different from those required to show reduction in the rate of disorder progression, cholinomimetic therapy trials examining the effects on the rate of progression will follow evidence of efficacy and safety in the use of proposed treatments in shorter term acute symptomatic therapy.

Another focus of interest specific to neuroprotective mechanisms is the role of the nicotinic system in AD. Indirect evidence from epidemiologic studies suggests that nicotinic receptor stimulation may have a neuroprotective role in the evolution of AD. Several epidemiologic studies, which controlled for the obvious major confounding factors such as differential rates of early deaths in smokers versus nonsmokers, have purported that tobacco smokers and previous smokers have a reduced risk for developing AD compared to nonsmokers (Van Dui & Hoffman, 1991; Van Dui & Hofman, 1992; Ford, Mefrouche, Friedland, & Debanne, 1996; Smith & Giacobini, 1992). Although it may be shown eventually that this apparent neuroprotective effect is due to the operation of some other factor, nicotine agonism has demonstrated the ability to inhibit presynaptic neuronal loss following Basal Forebrain lesions in animals. To allow for the purported neuroprotective actions of nicotine use, it has been suggested that nicotine, by means of a receptor-mediated activation of gene transcription factors, elicits nerve growth factor production that may act to restore nerve function (Arneric et al., 1995). As with precursor supplementation, cholinesterase inhibition, and muscarinic agonist therapies, the determination of the possible effects of nicotinic agonism on AD progression also will require clinical trials that are designed differently than those necessary to demonstrate short-term symptomatic improvement (Gershon et al., 1994). Because of the expected nature of the progress of the disorder and the localization of many of the muscarinic and nicotinic postsynaptic receptors on noncholinergic neurons, such trials should include not only a careful evaluation of cognitive functions but also measures of the psychopathologic symptoms that are pervasively evident in AD and were notably present in the initial case described by Dr. Alzheimer (1907).

Nonpharmacologic Treatment Strategies: Nerve Growth Factor, Fetal Neuronal Transplants, and Gene Therapy

The obvious loss of cholinergic cells is a cardinal feature of AD, and recognition of this has resulted in interest in nonpharmacologic therapy strategies such as use of nerve growth factors (NGF) (Olson et al., 1994) and fetal neuronal transplants to stimulate new or to supportively maintain neuronal growth and to thereby replace dead neurons. Today, understanding the limits of NGF-based therapies and the possible effective and general use of an NGF-based approach to treatment, awaits advances in development, and careful examination, of medicines that are able to mimic or stimulate NGF activity. Effective use of fetal transplants will require a significantly improved understanding of the pathophysiology of the disorder. For example, at least one follow-up report of the postsurgical mental states of experimental patients following fetal neuronal transplantation offers a less than optimistic picture (Starkoval, Mrna, & Bartosova, 1993). Given the developing understanding of the predisposing genetic vulnerability of some individuals to developing Alzheimer's disease, it is expected that approaches to modifying genetic predisposition will eventually be attempted. Such efforts also await future basic discoveries concerned with the role of gene expression in the pathophysiology of AD.

FUTURE DIRECTION FOR DEVELOPING CHOLINERGIC THERAPIES

As is evident from this chapter, cholinergic drugs, especially cholinesterase inhibitors, are the only group of compounds that, to date, have shown promise consistently in the treatment of symptoms of Alzheimer's disease.

The cholinesterase inhibitors Aricept™ and Cognex® that have been approved by the FDA (Food & Drug Administration), and novel acetylcholinesterase inhibitors (such as ENA-713, metrifonate), which are not yet available in the United States for routine prescribing, have already shown modest ability to enhance cognitive function in Alzheimer's disease patients treated in Phase 1 and Phase 2 trials.

It will be interesting to evaluate the effectiveness of choline/lecithin with these acetylcholinesterase inhibitors and as well, the new generation of muscarinic/nicotinic agonist, for their ability to attenuate the progression of this illness. This would be particularly important in evaluation of their potential role in the at-risk patient who has equivocal symptoms of the disease. The data concerning acetylcholinesterases inhibitors and muscarinic agonists's effects on APP processing are possibly demonstratable in vivo in man, utilizing well-designed studies. The cost of prospective studies designed to examine delay of progression would not be appreciably greater than looking at the effects of treatment of high cholesterol levels on the development of myocardial infarctions. The study of acetylcholinesterase inhibitors in combination with drugs that modulate other neurotransmitter systems (NE, 5-HT, DA enhancers) would seem to be important in light of the overwhelming evidence that these systems are also affected in this disorder (Kennedy & Whitehouse, 1993). This may be particularly relevant to the use of serotonin reuptake inhibitors to increasing levels of serotonin in vivo in light of the in vitro data suggesting that the G_1 subtype of the plaque-associated acetylcholinesterase enzyme is preferentially inhibited by serotonin and that this enzyme is relatively resistant to inhibition by some pharmacologic agents that act as acetylcholinesterase inhibitors. The use of antioxidants (such as Vitamin E), estrogen, anti-inflammatory medications and nerve growth factors (as they become available) in combination with cholinergic system modulating medications, also needs to be explored. In closing, it must be stated that until the pathophysiology giving rise to AD is clarified, a method of identifying preonset of the disorder (early presymptomatic) individuals at risk and an effective intervention is developed for treatment, cholinominetic therapy will remain a central mainstay for the AD patient.

REFERENCES

Aigner, T. G., & Mishkin, M. (1993). Scopolamine impairs recall of one trial stimulus-reward associations in monkeys. *Behavioral Brain Research 54*, 133–136.

Alzheimer, A. (1907). Über eine eigenartige Erkrankung der Hirnrinde Aug. Z. *Psychiatric Psychische Gerichtliche Medizin, 64*, 146.
Anand, R., Gharabawi, G., & Enz, A. (1996). Efficacy and safety results of the early phase studies with Exelon™ (ENA-713) in Alzheimer's disease: An overview. *Journal of Drug Development and Clinical Practice*. (In press).
Anand, R., & Gharabawi, G. (1996). Clinical development of Exelon™ (ENA-713): The Adena® Programme. *Journal of Drug Development and Clinical Practice*. (In press).
Arendt, T., Brückner, M. K., Lange, M., & Bigl, V. (1992). Changes in acetylcholinesterase and butrylcholinesterase in Alzheimer's disease resemble embryonic development—A study of molecular forms. *International Neurochemistry, 21*, 381–396.
Arneric, S. P., & Williams, M. (1994). Nicotinic agonists in Alzheimer's disease: Does the molecular diversity of nicotine receptors offer the opportunity for developing CNS-selective cholinergic channel activators? In G. Racagni, N. Brunello, & S. Z. Langer (Eds.), Recent advances in the treatment of neurodegenerative disorders and cognitive dysfunction, *Int. Acad. Biomed. Drug. Res., 7*, pp. 58–70, Basel: Karger.
Arneric, S. P., Sullivan, J. P., Briggs, C., Donnelly-Roberts, D., Anderson, D. J., Raskiewicz, J. L., Hughes, M. L., Cadman, E. D., Adams, P., & Garvey, D. S. (1994). A novel cholinergic ligand with cognitive enhancing and anxiolitic activity. *Journal of Pharmacology Experimental Therapy, 270*(1), 310–318.
Arneric, S. P., Sullivan, J. P., & Williams, M. (1995). Novel Targets for Central Nervous System Therapeutics. In F. E. Bloom & D. J. Kupfer (Eds.), *Psychopharmacology: The fourth generation of progress* (pp. 95–110). New York: Raven Press.
Atack, J. R., Perry, E. K., Bonham, J. R., & Perry, R. H. (1987). Molecular forms of acetylcholinesterase and butrylcholinesterase in human plasma and cerebro spinal fluid. *Journal of Neurochemistry, 48*, 1845–1850.
Aubert, I., Araujo, D. M., Cécyre, D., Robitaille, Y., Gauthier, S., & Quirion, R. (1992). Comparative alterations of nicotinic and muscarinic binding sites in Alzheimer's and Parkinson's diseases. *Journal of Neurochemistry, 58*, 529–541.
Ball, M. J., Fishman, M., Hachinski, V., Blume, W., Fox, H., & Merskey, H. (1985). A new definition of Alzheimer's disease: A Hippocampal dementia. *Lancet, 1*, 14–16.
Becker, R. E., Colliver, J., Elble, R., Feldman, E., Giacobini, E., Kumar, V., Mark Wells, S., Moriearty, P., Parks, R., Shilcutt, S. D., Unni, L., Vicaris, M., Womack, C., & Zec, R. (1990). Effects of metrifonate, a long acting cholinesterase inhibitor, in Alzheimer's disease: Report of an open trial. *Drug Developmental Research, 19*, 425–434.

Bissette, G. (1996). Chemical messengers. In E. W. Busse & D. G. Blazer, *Textbook of geriatric psychiatry* (pp. 73–94). Washington, DC: The American Psychiatric Press.

Blass, J. P., Hanin, I., Barclay, L., Kopp, U., & Reding, M. J. (1985). Red blood cell abnormalities in Alzheimer's disease. *Journal of the American Geriatrics Society, 33*(6), 401–405.

Bleuler, E. (1916). *Lehrbuch der Psychiatrie*. Berlin: Springer.

Blusztajn, J. K., & Wurtman, R. T. (1983). Choline and cholinergic neurons. *Science, 221*, 614–620.

Blusztajn, J. K., Holbrook, P. G., Liscovitch, M., Maire, J. C., Mauron, C., Richardson, I. U., Tacconi, M., & Wurtman, R. J. (1986). Pathogenesis: Possible role of choline phospholipids. In T. Crook, R. Bartus, S. Ferris, & S. Gershon (Eds.), *Treatment development strategies for Alzheimer's disease* (pp. 539–552). Madison, CT: Mark Powley Associates.

Blusztajn, J. K., & Wurtman, R. J. (1981). Choline biosynthesis by a preparation enriched in synaptosomes from rat brain. *Nature, 290*, 417–418.

Bodick, N. C., Offen, W. W., Levey, A. L., Cutler, N. R., Gauthier, S. G., Satlin, A., Shannon, H. E., Tollefson, G. D., Rasmussen, K., Bymaster, F. P., Hurley, D. J., Potter, W. Z., & Paul, S.M . (1997). Effects of Xanomeline, a selective muscarinic receptor agonist, on cognitive function and behavioral symptoms in Alzheimer's disease. *Archives of Neurology, 54*(4), 465–473.

Bolden, C., Cusak, B., & Richelson, E. (1992). Antagonism by antimuscarinic and neuroleptic compounds and the five cloned human muscarinic receptors expressed in chinese hamster ovary cells. *Journal of Pharmacology Experimental Therapy, 260*, 576–580.

Bonavita, E. (1986). Study of the efficacy and tolerability of L-acetylcarnitine therapy in the senile brain. *International Journal of Clinical Pharmacology, Therapy and Toxicology, 24*, 511–516.

Boyd, W., White, J., Blackwood, G., Glen, I., & McQuenn, J. (1977). Clinical effects of choline in Alzheimer's disease. *Journal of Gerontology, 374*, 4–9.

Brimijoin, S. (1983). Molecular forms of acetylcholinesterase in brain, nerve, muscle: Nature, localization, and dynamics. *Progress in Neurobiology, 21*, 291–322.

Broks, P., Preston, G. C., Traub, M., Poppelton, P., Ward. C., & Stahi, S. M. (1988). Modeling dementia: Effects of scopolamine on memory and attention. *Neuropsychologia, 26*, 685–700.

Browning, E. T., & Schulman, M. P. (1968). ^{14}C-Acetylcholine synthesis by cortex slices of rat brain. *Journal of Neurochemistry, 15*, 1391–1405.

Buresova, O., & Bures, J. (1982). Radial maze as a tool for assessing the effects of drugs on the working memory for rats. *Psychopharmacology, 77*, 268–271.

Butterfield, D. A., Nicholas, M. M., & Markesbery, W. R. (1985). Evidence for an increased rate of choline efflux across erythrocyte membranes in Alzheimer's disease. *Neurochemical Research, 10*, 909–918.

Bymaster, F. D., Wong, D. T., Mitch, C. H., Ward, J. S., Calligaro, D. O., Schoepp, D. D., Shannon, H. E., Sheardown, M. J., Olesen, P. H., & Suzdak, P. D. (1994). Neurochemical effects of the M_1 muscarinic agonist Xanomeline (LY246708/NNC11-0232). *Journal of Pharmacology and Experimental Therapeutics, 269*(1), 282–289.

Catalan, R. E., Martinez, A. M., Aragones, M. D., Miguel, B. G, Hernandez, F., & Cruz, E. (1993). Tetrahydroaminoacridine affects the cholinergic function of blood-brain barrier. *Life Science, 53*, 1165–1172.

Changeux, J. P., Galzi, J. L., Devillers-Thiery, A., & Betrand, D. (1992). The functional architecture of the acetylcholine nicotinic receptor explored by affinity labeling and site directed mutagenesis. *Quarterly Reviews of Biophysics, 25*, 395–432.

Christensen, H., Maltby, N., Jorm, A. F., Creasey, H., & Broe, G. A. (1992). Cholinergic 'blockade' as a model of the cognitive deficits in Alzheimer's disease. *Brain, 115*, 1681–1699.

Chubb, I. W. (1984). Acetylcholinesterase-multiple functions. In M. Brzin, T. Kiauta, & E. A. Barnard (Eds.), *Cholinesterase—Fundamental and applied aspects* (pp. 345–359). Berlin: Walter de Gruyter.

Cohen, E. L., & Wurtman, R. J. (1975). Brain acetylcholine: Increase after systemic choline administration. *Life Science, 16*, 1095–1099.

Consolo, S., Ladinski, H., Vinci, R., Palazzi, E., & Wang, J. X. (1987). An in vivo pharmacological study on muscarinic receptor subtypes regulating cholinergic neurotransmission in rat striatum. *Biochemical Pharmacology, 36*, 3075–3077.

Cutler, N. R., Seifert, R. D., Schleman, M. M., Sramek, J. J., Szylleyko, O. J., Howard, D. R., Barchowsky, A., Wardle, T. S., & Blass, E. P. (1995). Acetylcholinesterase inhibition by Zifrosilone: Pharmacokinetics and pharmacodynamics. *Clinical Pharmacology and Therapeutics, 58*, 54–61.

Cutler, N. R., Sramek, J. J., & Veroff, A. E. (1994). Finding the dose: The bridging study. In N. R. Cutler, J. J. Sramek, & A. E. Veroff (Eds.), *Alzheimer's disease: Optimizing drug development strategies* (pp. 139–157). New York: John Wiley & Sons, Inc.

Dale, H. H. (1914). The action of certain esters of choline and their relation to muscarine. *Journal of Pharmacology, 6*, 147–190.

Davis, K. L., Hollander, E., Davidson, M., Davis, B. M., Mohs, R. C., & Horvath, T. B. (1987). Induction of depression with Oxotremorine in patients with Alzheimer's disease. *American Journal of Psychiatry, 144*, 468–471.

Davidson, M., & Stern, R. G. (1991). The treatment of cognitive impairment in Alzheimer's disease: Beyond the cholinergic approach. *Psychiatric Clinics of North America, 14*, 461–482.

Davis, K. L., et al. (1992). A double-blind, placebo-controlled multicenter study of Tacrine for Alzheimer's disease. *New England Journal of Medicine, 327*, 1253–1259.

Davis, R., Raby, C., Callahan, M. J., Lipinski, W., Schwartz, R. Dudley, D. T., Lauffer, D., Reece, P., Jaen, J., & Tecle, H. (1993). Selective muscarinic antagonists: Potential therapeutic agents for Alzheimer's disease. In A. C. Cuello (Ed.), *Progress in Brain Research, 98,* pp. 439–445.

Davis, R. E., Doyle, P. D., Carroll, R. T., Emmerling, M. R., & Jaen, J. (1995). Cholinergic therapies for Alzheimer's disease: Palliative or disease altering. *Arzeneimittel-Forschung, 45*(3A) 425–431.

Decker, M. W., & McGaugh, J. L. (1991). The role of interactions between the cholinergic system and other neuromodulatory systems in learning and memory. *Synapse, 7,* 151–168.

Division of Neuropharmacological Drug Products, Office of New Drug Evaluation (I), Center for Drug Evaluation and Review. (1991). An interim report from the FDA. *New England Journal of Medicine, 324,* 349–352.

Drachman, D. A., & Leavitt, J. (1974). Human memory and the cholinergic system: A relationship to aging? *Archives of Neurology, 30*(2), 113–121.

Dysken, M. (1987). A review of recent clinical trials on the treatment of Alzheimer's dementia. *Psychiatric Annuals, 17,* 78–191.

Dysken, M., Fovall, P., & Harris, C. (1982). Lecithin administration in Alzheimer's dementia. *Neurology, 32,* 1203–1204.

Eckols, K., Bymaster, F. D., Mitch, C. H., Shannon, H. E., Ward, J. S., & Delapp, N. W. (1995). The muscarinic M_1 agonist Xanomeline increases soluble amyloid precursor protein release from chinese hamster ovary-M_1 cells. *Life Science, 57*(12), 1183–1190.

Ehlert, F. J., Roeske, W. R., & Yamamura, H. I. (1995). Molecular biology, pharmacology and brain distribution of subtypes of the muscarinic receptor. In F. E. Bloom & D. J. Kupfer (Eds.), *Psychopharmacolgy: The fourth generation of progress* (pp. 111–124). New York: Raven Press.

Emmerling, M. R., Moore, C. J., Doyle, P. D., Carroll, R. T., & Davis, R. E. (1995). Cell surface receptor mediated control of amyloid precursor protein secretion: Involvement of pleiotropic signal transduction cascades. In I. Hanin (Ed.), *Alzheimer's and Parkinson's diseases: Recent developments. Advances in Behavioral Biology, 44,* 131–139.

Enz, A., Amstutz, R., Boddeke, H., Ginelin, G., & Malanowsk, J. (1993). Brain selective inhibition of acetylcholinesterase: A novel approach to therapy for Alzheimer's disease. In Cuello (Ed.), *Progress in Brain Research, 98,* pp.431–438, Elsevier Science Publishers. B.V.

Etienne, P., Robitaille, Y., Wood, P., Gauthier, S., Nair, N. P., & Quirion, R. (1986). Nucleus basalis neuronal loss, neuritic plaques and choline acetyl-transferase activity in advanced Alzheimer's disease. *Neuroscience, 19*(4), 1279–1291.

Fibiger, H. C., & Vincent, S. R. (1987) Anatomy of central cholinergic neurons. In Hymeltzer (Ed.), *Psychopharmacology: The third generation of progress* (pp. 211–218). New York: Raven Press.

Fishman, E. B., Siek, G. L., MacCallum, R. D., Bird, E. D., Volicer, L., & Marquis, J. K. (1986). Distribution of the molecular forms of acetylcholinesterase in human brain: Alterations of dementia of the Alzheimer's type. *Annals of Neurology, 19*, 246–252.

Flynn, D. D., Ferrari-DiLeo, G., Mash, D. C., & Levey, A. I. (1995). Differential regulation of molecular subtypes of muscarinic receptors in Alzheimer's disease. *Journal of Neurochemistry, 64*, 1888–1891.

Flynn, D. D., Weinstein, D. A., & Mash, D. C. (1991). Loss of high-affinity agonist binding to M_1 muscarinic receptors in Alzheimer's disease: Implication for the failure of cholinergic replacement therapies. *Annals of Neurology, 29*(3), 256–262.

Ford, A. B., Mefrouche, Z., Friedland, R. P., & Debanne, S. M. (1996). Smoking and cognitive impairment: A population-based study. *Journal of the American Geriatrics Society, 44*(8), 905–909.

Friede, R. L. (1965). Enzyme histochemical studies of senile plaques. *Journal of Neuropathology and Experimental Neurology, 24*, 477–491.

Gershon, S., Ferris, S. H., Kennedy, J. S., Kurtz, N. M., Overall, J. E., Pollock, B. G., Reisber, B., & Whitehouse, P. J. (1994). Methods for the evaluation of pharmacologic agents in the treatment of cognitive and other deficits in dementia. In R. F. O'Brien & D. S. Robinson, *Clinical evaluation of psychotropic drugs: Principles and guidelines*. New York: Raven Press.

Geula, C., Shatz, C. R., & Mesulam, M-M. (1993). Differential localization of NADPH—diaphorase and calbindin-D28K within the cholinergic neurons of the basal forebrain, striatum, and brain stem in the rat, monkey, baboon and human. *Neuroscience, 54*(2), 461–476.

Ghoneim, M. M., & Mewalt, S. P. (1975). Effects of Diazepam and Scopolamine on storage retrieval and organizational process in memory. *Psychopharmacologia (Berlin), 44*, 257–262.

Giacobini, E. (1994). Cholinomimetic therapy of Alzheimer's disease: Does it slow down deterioration. In G. Racagini, N. Brunello, & Z. S. Langer (Eds.), Recent advances in the treatment of neurodegenerative disorders and cognitive dysfunction. *International Academy Biomedical Drug Research, 7*, 51–57, Basel: Karger.

Gray, J. A., Mitchell, S. N., Joseph, M. H., Grigoryan, G., Dawes, M. A., & Hodges, H. (1994). Neurochemical mechanisms mediating the behavioral and cognitive effects of Nicotine. *Drug Development and Research, 31*, 3–17.

Gray, J. A., Enz, A., & Spiegel, R. (1989). Muscarinic agonists for senile dementia: Past experience and future trends. *Trends in Pharmacological Sciences, 12*, Suppl., 85–88.

Greenfield, S. A., & Smith, A. D. (1979). The influence of electrical stimulation of certain brain areas on the concentration of acetylcholinesterase on rabbit cerebrospinal fluid. *Brain Research, 177*, 445–459.

Halford, N. H., & Peace, K. (1994). The effect of tacrine and lecithin in Alzheimer's disease. A population pharmacodynamic analysis of five clinical trials. *European Journal of Clinical Pharmacology, 47*(1), 17–23.

Hallack, M., & Giacobini, E. (1989). Physostigmine, tacrine and metrifonate: The effect of multiple dosages on acetylcholine in rat brain. *Neuropsychopharmacology, 28,* 199–206.

Hersch, S. M., Gutekunst, C-A., Rees, H. D., Hellman, C. J., & Levey, A. I. (1994). Distribution of m_1-m_4 muscarinic receptor proteins in the rat striatum: Light and electron microscopic immunocytochemistry using subtype-specific antibodies. *Journal of Neuroscience, 14,* 3351–3363

Hollander, E., Davidson, M., Mohs, R. C., Horvath, T. B., Davis, B. M., Zemishlany, Z., & Davis, K. L. (1978). RS-86 in the treatment of Alzheimer's disease. *Biological Psychiatry, 22,* 1067–1078.

Hollunger, E. G., & Niklasson, B. H. (1973). The release and molecular state of mammalian brain acetylcholinesterase. *Journal of Neurochemistry, 20,* 821–836.

Huff, F. J., Mickel, S. F., Corkin, S., & Growden, J. H. (1988). Cognitive functions affected by Scopolamine in Alzheimer's disease and normal aging. *Drug Developmental Research, 12,* 271–278.

Hyman, B. T., Kromer, L. J., & Van Hoesen, G. W. (1987). Reinnervation of the hippocampal preforant pathway zone in Alzheimer's disease. *Annals of Neurology, 21,* 259–267.

Jenkins, S. M., Wadsworth, H. J., Bromidge, S., Orlek, B. S., Wyman, P. A., Riley, G. J., & Hawkins, J. (1992). Substituent variation in azabicyclic triazole- and tetrazole-bases muscarinic receptor ligands. *Journal of Medical Chemistry, 35,* 2392–2406.

Joachim, C. L., & Selkoe, D. J. (1992). The seminal role of β-amyloid in the pathogenesis of Alzheimer's Disease. *Alzheimer's Disease and Associated Disorders, 6,* 7–34.

Jones, G. M. M., Sahakian, B. J., Levy, R., Warburton, D. M., & Gray, J. A. (1992). Effects of acute subcutaneous nicotine on attention, information processing and short term memory in Alzheimer's Disease. *Psychopharmacology, 108,* 485–494.

Joseph, J. A., Cutler, R., & Roth, G. S. (1993). Changes in G protein-mediated signal transduction in aging and Alzheimer's disease. *Annals of the New York Academy of Science, 695,* 42–45.

Kennedy, J. S., & Whitehouse, P. (1993). Alzheimer's disease. In L. Barclay (Ed.), *Clinical Geriatric Neurology* (pp. 76–89). Malvern, PA: Lea and Febiger.

Knapp, M. J., Knopman, D. S., Solomon, P. R., Pendelbury, W. W., Davis, C. S., & Gracon, S. I. (1994). A 30-week randomized controlled trial of high-dose Tacrine in patients with Alzheimer's disease. *JAMA, 271,* 985–991.

Kordower, J. H., & Mufson, E. J. (1990). Galanin-like immunoreactivity within the primate basal forebrain: Differential straining patterns between humans and monkeys. *Journal of Comparative Neurology, 294*(2), 281–292.

Kosik, K. S. (1992). Alzheimer's disease: A cell biological perspective. *Science* *256*(5058), 780–783.

Kraepelin, E. (1899). Psychiatric. Bd. I: *Allgemeine Psychiatrie*. Germany: Leipzig.

Kumar, V. (1996). ENA-713. Abstract presented to CINP.

Kumar, V., & Calache, M. (1991). Therapeutic review: Treatment of Alzheimer's disease with cholinergic drugs. *International Journal of Clinical Pharmacology, Therapy and Toxicology, 29*, 23–37.

Lal, S., Wood, P. L., Kiely, M. E., Etienne, P., Gauthier, S., Stratford, J., Ford, R. M., Dastoor, D., & Nair, N. V. P. (1984). CSF acetylcholinesterase in dementia and in sequential samples of lumbar CSF. *Neurobiology of Aging, 5*, 269–274.

Lavretsky, E. P., & Jarvik, L. F. (1992). A Group of potassium-channel blockers—Acetylcholine releasers: New potentials for Alzheimer's disease? A review. *Journal of Clinical Psychopharmacology, 12*, 110–118.

Layer, P. G., & Sporns, O. (1987). Spatiotemporal relationship of embryonic cholinesterases with cell proliferation in chick brain and eye. *Proceedings of the National Academy of Science, USA, 84*, 284–288.

Layer, P. G. (1990). Cholinesterase preceding major tracts in vertebrate neurogenesis. *Bioessays, 12*, 415–420.

Leftkowitz, R. J., Hoffmann, B. B., & Taylor, P. (1990). Neurohormonal transmission: The autonomic and somatic motor systems. In A. G. Gilman, T. N. Rall, A. S. Nies, & P. Taylor (Eds.), *The Pharmacological Basis of Therapeutics* (pp. 84–121). New York: Pergamon Press.

Levy, R., Little, A., Chuaqui, P., & Reith, M. (1983). Early results from double-blind, placebo-controlled trial on high-dose phosphatidylcholine in Alzheimer's disease. *Lancet, 576*, 986–987.

Linville, D. G., Williams, S., Raskiewicz, J. L., & Arneric, S. P. (1993). Nicotinic agonists modulate basal forebrain (BF) control of cortical cerebral blood flow in anesthetized rats. *Journal of Pharmacology and Experimental Therapeutics, 267*, 440–461.

Lippiello, P. M., Bencherif, M., Gray, J. A., Peters, S., Grigoryan, G., Hodges, H., & Collins, A. C. (1996). RJR-2403: A nicotinic agonist with CNS selectivity II. In vivo characterization. *Journal of Pharmacology and Experimental Therapeutics, 279*(3), 1422–1429.

Loupe, D. N., Newman, N. J., Green, R. C., Lynn, M. J., Williams, K. K., Geis, T. C., & Edelhauser, H. F. (1996). Pupillary response to tropicamide in patients with Alzheimer's disease. *Ophthalmology, 103*, 495–503.

Mash, D. C., Flynn, D. D., & Potter, L. T. (1985). Loss of M_2 muscarinic receptors in the cerebral cortex in Alzheimer's disease and experimental cholinergic denervation. *Science, 228*, 1115–1117.

Mattson, M. P., Cheng, B., Culwell, A. R., Esch, F. S., Lieberburg, J., & Rydel, R. E. (1993). Evidence for excitoprotective and interneuronal calcium-regulating roles for secreted forms of the β-amyloid precursor protein. *Neuron, 10,* 243–254.

Mavardis, M., Rogard, M., & Besson, M. J. (1995). Chronic blockade of muscarinic cholinergic receptors by systemic trihexyphenidyl (Artane®) administration modulates but does not mediate the dopaminergic regulation of striatal prepopeptide messenger RNA expression. *Neuroscience, 66,* 37–53.

McGeer, P. L. (1984). Aging, Alzheimer's disease, and the cholinergic system. *Canadian Journal of Physiology and Pharmacology, 62,* 741–751.

McKinney, M., Miller, J. H., & Aagaard, P. J. (1993). Pharmacological characterization of the rat hippocampal muscarinic autoreceptor. *Journal of Pharmacology and Experimental Therapeutics, 264*(1), 74–78.

Mesulam, M-M., & Geula, C. (1988). Acetylcholinesterase-rich pyramidal neurons in the human neocortex and hippocampus: Absence at birth, development during the life span, and dissolution in Alzheimer's disease. *Annals of Neurology, 24,* 765–773.

Mesulam, M-M., & Guela, C. (1992). Overlap between acetylcholinesterase-rich and choline acetyltransferase-positive (cholinergic) axons in human cerebral cortex. *Brain Res, 577,* 112–120.

Mesulam, M-M., Guela, C., & Moran, A. (1987). Anatomy of cholinesterase inhibition in Alzheimer's disease: Effect of physostigmine and tetrahydroaminoacridine on plaque and tangles. *Annals of Neurology, 22,* 683–691.

Mesulam, M-M., Mufson, E. J., Levey, A. I., & Wainer, B. H. (1983). Cholinergic enervation of cortex by the basal forebrain: Cytochemistry and cortical connections of the septal area, diagonal band nuclei, nucleus basalis (substantia innominata), and hypothalamus in the rhesus monkey. *Journal of Comparative Neurology, 214*(2), 170–197.

Mesulam, M-M. (1988). Central cholinergic pathways: Neuroanatomy and some behavioral implications. In M. Avoli, T. A. Reader, R. W. Dykes, & P. Gloor (Eds.), *Neurotransmitters and cortical function* (pp. 237–260). New York: Plenum Press.

Mesulam, M-M. (1995). Structure and function of cholinergic pathways in the cerebral cortex, limbic system, basal ganglia, and thalamus of the human brain. In F. E. Bloom & D. J. Kupfer (Eds.), *Psychopharmacology: The fourth generation of progress* (pp. 135–146). New York: Raven Press.

Miller, B. L., Jenden, D. J., Cummings, J. L., Reads, S., Rice, K., & Benson, D. F. (1986). Abnormal erythrocyte choline and influx in Alzheimer's disease. *Life Science, 38,* 485–490.

Miller, F. D., & Geddes, J. W. (1990). Increased expression of the major alpha-tubulin mRNA, T alpha 1, during neuronal regeneration, sprouting, and in Alzheimer's disease. *Progress in Brain Research, 86,* 321–330.

Mihara, M., Ohnishi, A., Tomono, Y., Hasegawa, J. Shimamura, Y., Yamazaki, K., & Morishita, N. (1993). Pharmacokinetics of E2020, a new compound

for Alzheimer's Disease, in healthy male volunteers. *International Journal of Clinical Pharmacology, Therapy and Toxicology, 31*, 223–229.
Mohs, R. C., Johns, C. A., Dunn, D. A., Sherman, N. A., Rosen, W. G., & Davis, K. L. (1986). Anticholinergic dementia as a model of Alzheimer's disease. In L. W. Poon (Ed.), *Handbook for Clinical Memory Assessment of Older Adults* (pp. 403–408). Washington, DC: American Psychological Association.
Mohs, R. C. (1995). Personal communication.
Mufson, E. J., Bothwell, M., Hersch, L. B., & Kordower, J. H. (1989). Nerve growth factor receptor immunoreactive profiles in the normal, aged human basal forebrain: Colocalization with cholinergic neurons. *Journal of Comparative Neurology, 285*(2), 196–217.
Mutschler, E., Moser, U., Wess, J., & Lambrecht, G. (1995). Muscarinic receptor subtypes—pharmacological, molecular biological and therapeutic aspects. *Pharmaceutica Acta Helvetiae, 69*, 243–258.
Nakamura, S., & Vincent, S. R. (1985). Acetylcholinesterase and somatostatin immunoreactivity coexist in human neocortex. *Neuroscience Letter, 61*, 183–187.
Navaratnam, D. S., Priddle, J. D., McDonald, B., Esiri, M. M., Robinson, J. R., & Smith, A. D. (1991). Anomalous molecular form of acetylcholinesterase in cerebrospinal fluid in histologically diagnosed Alzheimer's disease. *Lancet, 337*, 447–450.
Newhouse, P. A., Sunderland, T., Tariot, P. N., Blumhardt, L. L., Weingartner, H., Mellow, A., & Murphy, D. L. (1988). Intravenous nicotine in Alzheimer's disease: A pilot study. *Psychopharmacology, 95*, 171–175.
Newhouse, P. A., Potter, A., Corwin, J., & Lennox, R. (1994). Modeling the nicotinic receptor loss in dementia using the nicotinic antagonist mecamylamine: Effects on human cognitive functioning. *Drug Development and Research, 31*, 71–79.
Nordberg, A. (1993). In vivo detection of neurotransmitter changes in Alzheimer's disease. *Annals of the New York Academy of Sciences, 695*, 27–33.
Ogane, N., Giacobini, E., & Struble, R. (1992). Differential inhibition of acetylcholinesterase molecular forms in normal and Alzheimer's disease brain. *Brain Research, 589*, 307–312.
Ohnishi, A., Mihara, M., Kamakura, H., Tomono, Y., Hasegawa, J., Yamazaki, K., Morishita, N., & Tanaka, T. (1993). Comparison of the pharmacokinetics of E2020, A new compound for Alzheimer's disease in healthy young and elderly subjects. *Journal of Clinical Pharmacology, 33*, 1086–1091.
Olson, L., Backman, L., Ebendal, T., Eriksdorfer-Jonhagen, M., Hoffer, B., Humpel, C., Freedman, R., Giacobini, M., Meyerson, B., Nordberg, A., et al. (1994). Role of growth factors in degeneration and regeneration in the central nervous system; Clinical experiences with NGF in Parkinson's and Alzheimer's diseases. *Journal of Neurology, 242 (1 suppl. 1)*, s12–15.

Ownman, C., Fuxe, K., Jason, A. M., & Kahrstrom, J. (1989). Studies of protective actions of nicotine on neuronal and vascular functions in the brain of rats: Comparison between sympathetic noradrenergic and meso-striatal dopaminergic fiber system, and the effect of dopamine agonists. *Progress in Brain Research, 79,* 267–276.

Penn, R. D., Martin, E. M., Wilson, R. S., Fox, J. S., & Savoy, S. M. (1988). Intraventricular Bethanechol infusion for Alzheimer's disease: Results of a double-blind and escalating-dose trials. *Neurology, 38,* 219–222.

Perry, E. K., & Perry, R. H. (1983). Acetylcholinesterase in Alzheimer's disease. In B. Reisberg (Ed.), *Alzheimer's disease: The standard reference* (pp.93–99). New York: The Free Press.

Perry, E. K., Atack, J. R., Perry, R. H., Hardy, J. A., Dodd, P. R., Edwardson, J. A., Blessed, G., Tomlinson, B. E., & Fairbairn, A. F. (1984). Intralaminar neurochemical distributions in human mid-temporal cortex: Comparison between Alzheimer's disease and the normal. *Journal of Neurochemistry, 42,* 1402–1410.

Perry, E. K., Perry, R. H., Smith, C. J., Dick, D. J., Candy, J. M., Edwardson, J. A., Fairbairn, A., & Blessed, G. (1987). Nicotinic receptor abnormalities in Alzheimer's and Parkinson's diseases. *Journal of Neurology and Neurosurgical Psychiatry, 50,* 806–809.

Perry, E. K., Perry, R. H., Tomlinson, B. E., Blessed, G., & Gibson, P. (1980). Coenzyme A-acetylizing enzymes in Alzheimer's disease: Possible cholinergic "compartment" of pyruvate dehydrogenase. *Neuroscience Letter, 18,* 105–110.

Quirion, R., Aubert, I., Lapchax, P. A., Schaum, H. P., Trolis, S., Gauthier, S., & Araujo, D. M. (1989). Muscarinic receptor subtypes in human neurodegenerative disorders: Focus on Alzheimer's disease. *Trends in Pharmacological Science, 10,* suppl. 80–84.

Riekkinen, P., Jr., Miettinen, R., Rummukainen, J., Pitkanen, A., & Paljarvil, R. (1990). The effects of lesioning the basal forebrain neurons on CSF AChE activity. *Neuroscience Research Communication, 6,* 37–43.

Reiner, P. B., & Fibiger, H. C. (1989). Functional Heterogeneity in central cholinergic systems. In F. E. Bloom & D. L. Kupfer (Eds.), *Psychopharmacology: The Fourth Generation of Progress* (pp. 147–155). New York: Raven Press.

Richelson, E. (1995). Cholinergic transduction. In F. E. Bloom & D. L. Kupfer (Eds.), *Psychopharmacology: The Fourth Generation of Progress* (pp. 125–134). New York: Raven Press.

Robakis, N. K., Vassilacopoulou, D., Efthimiopoulos, S., Sambamurti, K., Refolo, L. M., & Shioi, J. (1993). Cellular processing and proteoglycan nature of amyloid precursor proteins. *Annals of the New York Academy of Science, 695,* 132–138.

Robertson, R. T., Mostamand, F., Kageyama, G. H., Gallardok, A., & Yu, J. (1991). Primary auditory cortex in the rat: Transient expression of acetylcholinesterase activity in developing geniculocortical projections. *Developmental Brain Research, 58,* 81–95.

Rogers, S. L., & Friedhoff, L. T. (1996). The efficacy and safety of donzepil in patients with Alzheimer's disease: Results of a U.S. multicenter, randomized, double-blind, placebo-controlled trial. The donzepil study group. *Dementia, 7*(6), 293–303.

Rogers, S. L., Yamanishi, Y., & Yamatsu, I. (1991). E2020: The pharmacology of piperidine cholinesterase inhibition. In R. Becker & E. Giacobini (Eds.), *Cholinergic basis for Alzheimer's therapy* (pp. 314–320). Boston: Birkhäuser.

Rosen, W. G., Moh, R. C., & Davis, K. L. (1984). A new scale for Alzheimer's disease. *American Journal of Psychiatry, 141,* 356–1364.

Rylett, R. J., & Schmidt, B. M.(1993). Regulation of the synthesis of acetylcholine. In A. C. Cuello (Ed.), *Progress in brain research, 98,* 161–166. Elsevier Science Publishers B.V.

Sahakian, B., Jones, G., Levy, R., Gray, J., & Warburton, D. (1989). The effects of nicotine on attention, information processing, and short-term memory in patients with dementia of the Alzheimer type. *British Journal of Psychiatry, 154,* 797–800.

Sans, M., Bell, K., Cote, L., Dooneief, G., Lawton, A., Legler, L., Marder, K., Naini, A., Stern, Y., & Mayeux, R. (1992). Double-blind parallel design pilot study of acetyl levocarnitine in patients with Alzheimer's disease. *Arch Neurol, 49,* 1137–1141.

Sargent, P. B. (1993). The diversity of neuronal nicotinic acetylcholine receptors. *Annual Review of Neuroscience, 16,* 403–443.

Schwarz, R. D., Davis, R. E., Grazon, S., Hoover, T., Moos, W. H., & Pavia, R. (1991). Meeting report: Next generation Tacrine. *Neurobiology in Aging, 12,* 185–187.

Scinto, L. F., Daffner, K. R., Dressler, D., Ransil, B. I., Rentz, D., Weintraub, S., Mesulam, M., & Potter, H. (1994). A potential non-invasive neurobiological test for Alzheimer's disease. *Science, 266*(5187), 1051–1054.

Sethy, V. H., & Francis, J. N. (1988). Regulation of brain Acetylcholine concentrations by muscarinic receptors. *Journal of Pharmacology Experimental Therapy, 248,* 243–248.

Shannon, H. E., Bymaster, F. P., Calligaro, D. O., Greenwood, B., Mitch, C.H., Sawyer, B. D., Ward, J. S., Wong, D. T., Olesen, P. H., Sheardown, M.J., et al. (1994). Xanomeline: A novel muscarinic receptor agonist with functional selectivity for m_1 receptors. *Journal of Pharmacology and Experimental Therapeutics, 269*(1), 271–281.

Shapiro, G., Floersheim, P., Boelsterli, J., Amstutz, R., Bolliger, G., Gammenthaler, H., Gmelin, G., Supavilai, P., & Walkinshaw, M. (1992). Muscarinic activity of the thiolactone, lactam, lactol and thiolactol analogues of pilocarpine and a hypothetical model for the binding of agonists to the M_1 receptor. *Journal of Medicinal Chemistry, 35*(1), 15–27.

Sherman, K. A., & Messamore, E. (1988). Blood cholinesterase inhibition as a guide to the efficacy of putative therapies for Alzheimer's dementia: Comparison of the Tacrine and physostigmine. In E. Giocobini & R. Becker (Eds.), *Current research in Alzheimer's therapy* (pp. 73–86). New York: Taylor and Francis International.

Shimohama, S., Taniguchi, T., Fujinara, M., & Kameyama, M. (1985). Biochemical characterization of the nicotinic cholinergic receptors in human brain: Binding of (-)- [3H] Nicotine. *Journal of Neurochemistry, 45*, 604–610.

Siek, G. C., Katz, L. S., Fishman, E. B., Korosi, T. S., & Marquis, J. K. (1990). Molecular forms of acetylcholinesterase in subcortical areas of normal and demented (Alzheimer-type) patients. *Biological Psychiatry, 27*, 573–580.

Silver, A. (1974). *The biology of cholinesterases*. Amsterdam: North-Holland.

Sirviö, J., & Riekkinen, P. J. (1992). Brain and cerebrospinal fluid cholinesterases in Alzheimer's disease, Parkinson's disease and aging. A critical review of clinical and experimental studies. *Journal of Neurology Transom., [P-D Sect]4*, 337–358.

Slotkin, T. A., Nemeroff, C. B., Bissette, G., & Seidler, F. (1994). Overexpression of the high affinity choline transporter in cortical regions affected by Alzheimer's disease. Evidence from rapid autopsy studies. *Journal of Clinical Investment, 94*, 696–702.

Slotkin, T. A., Seidler, F. J., Crain, B. J., Bell, J. M., Bissette, G., & Nemeroff, C. B. (1990). Regulatory changes in presynaptic cholinergic function assessed in rapid autopsy material from patients with Alzheimer's disease: Implication for etiology and therapy. *Proceedings of the National Academy of Sciences, USA, 87*, 2452–2455.

Smith, A. D., & Cuello, A. C. (1984). Alzheimer's disease and acetylcholinesterase-containing neurons. *Lancet, 1*, 513.

Smith, C. J., & Giacobini, E. (1992). Nicotine, Parkinson's and Alzheimer's Disease. *Review of Neuroscience, 3*, 25–42.

Spiegel, R. (Ed.). (1989). *Psychopharmacology: An introduction (Edition 2)*. New York: John Wiley & Sons.

Sramek, J. J., Block, G. A., Reines, S. A., Sawin, S. F., Barchowsky, A., & Cutler, N. R. (1995). A multiple-dose safety trial of eptastigmine in Alzheimer's disease with pharmacodynamic observations of red blood cell Cholinesterase. *Life Sciences, 56*, 319–326.

Sramek, J. J., Sedman, A. J., Reece, P. A., Hourani, J., Bockbrader, H., & Cutler, N. R. (1995). Safety and tolerability of CI-979 in patients with Alzheimer's disease. *Life Sciences, 57*(5), 503–510.

St. Clair, D. M., Brock, D. J. H., & Barron, L. (1986). A monoclonal antibody assay technique for plasma and red cell acetylcholinesterase activity in Alzheimer's disease. *Journal of Neurological Science, 73*(2), 169–176

Starkova, L., Mrna, B., & Bartosova, S. (1993). Neurotransplantation—a new method of treatment in psychiatry? *Acta Universitatis Palackianae Oldmulensis Facultatis Medicae, 136*, 33–35.

Summers, W. K., Majovski, L. V., Marsh, G. M., Tachiki, K., & Kling, A. (1986). Oral tetrahydoraminoacridine in long-term treatment of senile dementia, Alzheimer's type. *New England Journal of Medicine, 315*, 1241–1245.

Sunderland, T., Tariot, P. N., Cohen, R. M., Weingartner, H., Mueller, E. A., & Murphy, D. L. (1987). Anticholinergic sensitivity in patients with dementia of the Alzheimer type and age-matched controls. *Arch Gen. Psychiatt., 44*, 418–426.

Taylor, P., & Brown, J. H. (1994). Acetylcholine. In G. J. Siegel, B. W. Agranoff, R. W. Albers, & P. B. Molinoff (Eds.), *Basic Neurochemistry: Molecular, Cellular and Medical Aspects* (5th edition, pp.231–260). New York: Raven Press.

Taylor, P. (1991). The cholinesterases. *Journal of Biological Chemistry, 266*, 4025–4028.

Thomson, T., Zendeh, B., Fisher, J. P., & Kewitz, H. (1991). In-vitro effects of various cholinesterase inhibitors on acetyl-and butrylcholinesterase of healthy volunteers. *Biochemical Pharmacology, 41*, 139–141.

Toja, E., Bonetti, C., Butti, A., Hunt, P., Fortin, M., Barzaghi, F., Formento, M. L., Maggioni, A., & Nencioni, A. (1991). 1-Alkyl-1, 2, 5, 6-tetrahydropyridine-3 carboxaldehyde-O-alkyl-oxamines: A new class of potent orally active muscarinic agonists related to arecoline. *European Journal of Medicine and Chemistry, 26*, 853–868.

Tucek, S. (1993). Short-term control of the synthesis of Acetylcholine. *Progress in Biophysics and Molecular Biology, 60*, 59–69

Uney, J. B., Jones, G. M., Rebeiro, A., & Levy, R. (1992). The effect of long-term high dose lecithin on erythrocyte choline transport in Alzheimer's patients. *Biology and Psychology, 31*, 630–633.

Van DuiJN, C. M., & Hofman, A. (1991). Relation between nicotine intake and Alzheimer's disease. *British Medical Journal, 302*, 1491–1494.

Van DuiJN, C. M., & Hofman, A. (1992). Risk factors for Alzheimer's disease: The Euroderm collaborative re-analysis of case-control studies. *Neuroepidemiology, 11 (Suppl. 1)*, 106–113.

Warburton, D. M. (1992). Nicotine as a Cognitive Enhancer. *Progress in Neuropsychopharmacological Biology and Psychiatry, 16*, 181–191.

Watson, M., Roeske, W. R., & Yamamura, H. I. (1987). Cholinergic receptor heterogeneity. In H. Y. Meltzer (Ed.), *Psychopharmacology: The third generation of progress* (pp. 241–248). New York: Raven Press.

Wecker, L., & Schmidt, D. E. (1980). Neuropharmacological consequences of choline administration. *Brain Research, 184*, 234.

Wesnes, K., & Warburton, D. M. (1984). Effects of Scopolamine and Nicotinine on human rapid information processing performance. *Psychopharmacology, 82*, 147–150.

Wesnes, K., & Warburton, D. M. (1983). Smoking, nicotine and human performance. *Pharmacological Therapy, 21*, 189–208.

Whitehouse, P. J., Price, D. L., Clark, A. W., Coyle, J. T., & Delong, M. R. (1981). Alzheimer disease: Evidence for selective loss of cholinergic neurons in the nucleus basalis. *Annals of Neurology, 10*(2), 122–126.

Whitehouse, P. J., Price, D. L., Struble, R. G., Clark, A. W., Coyle, J. T., & Delong, M. R. (1982). Alzheimer's disease and senile dementia: Loss of neurons in the basal forebrain. *Science, 215*, 1237–1239.

Whitehouse, P. J., Martino, A. M., Antuono, P. G., Lowenstein, P. R., Coyle, J. T., Price, D. L., & Kellar, K. J. (1986). Nicotine acetylcholine binding sites in Alzheimer's disease. *Brain Research, 371*, 146–151.

Wonnacott, S., Irons, J., Rapier, C., Thorne, B., & Lunt, G. G. (1990). Presynaptic modulation of transmitter release by nicotinic receptors. In A. Norderg, K. Fuxe, B. Holmsteat, & A. Sundwall (Eds.), *Progress in brain research* (pp. 157–163). Amsterdam: Elsevier.

Wood, J. L., & Allison, R. (1982). Effects of consumption of choline and lecithin on neurological and cardiovascular system. *Federation Proceedings, 41*, 3015–3016.

Wright, C. I., Geula, C., & Mesula, M-M. (1993). Protease inhibitors and indolamine selectively inhibit cholinesterase in the histopathologic structures of Alzheimer's disease. *Annals of the New York Academy of Science, 695*, 65–68.

Wurtman, R. J., Hirsch, M. J., & Growdon, J. H. (1977). Lecithin consumption raises serum free-choline levels. *Lancet, 2*, 68–69.

Yamamoto, Y., Nakano, S., Kawashima, S., Nakamura, S., Urakami, K., Kato, T., & Kameyama, M. (1990). Plasma and serum G_4 isoenzyme of acetylcholinesterase in patients with Alzheimer-type dementia and vascular dementia. *Annals of Clinical Biochemistry, 27*, 321–326.

Yankner, B. A., Duffy, L. K., & Kirschner, D. A. (1990). Neurotropic and neurotoxic effects of amyloid beta protein: Reversal by Tachykinin Neuropeptides. *Science, 250*, 279–282.

Yasuda, R. P., Ciesla, W., Flores, R., Wall, S. J., Li, M., Satkus, S. A., Weisstein, J. S., Spagnola, B. V., & Wolfe, B. B. (1992). Development of antisera selective for M_4 and M_5 cholinergic receptors: Distribution of M_4 and M_5 receptors in rat brain. *Molecular Pharmacology, 43*, 149–157.

CHAPTER **13**

Management of Families Caring for Relatives With Dementia: Issues and Interventions

**Donna Cohen
Blake Andersen
Richard Cairl**

Estimates are that by the year 2040, the number of people with Alzheimer's disease and related dementias will be approximately 10 million (Brody & Cohen, 1989). With a projected census of 300 million people in the United States in 2040, that means 1 in 30 Americans will suffer from dementia! These projections, however, may be conservative. They are based on 1980 mortality rates, and mortality rates for the entire population, including the older population, are dropping.

The implications of these numbers are profound in human and socioeconomic terms. Alzheimer's disease and related disorders are long-term illnesses characterized by progressive deterioration of mental capacities and self-care, and the experience tortures and humiliates those who suffer with it as well as those who are caregivers (Cohen & Eisdorfer, 1986). Although the progression of the disease is variable, the time from onset to death averages 7 years (Gustafson, 1992). Direct medical costs such as long-term care can be calculated, but other costs such as lost productivity of the individual and family caregivers, altered family lifestyle, and increased health care costs for caregivers are difficult to determine accurately. The annual national costs for the care of people with Alzheimer's disease range from $70 to $90 billion (Cohen, 1993; Hay & Ernst, 1987).

Family members provide most of the care for relatives (Brody, 1985; Doty, 1986), and for some caregiving can be a satisfying experience (Lawton, Kleban, et al., 1989). Even when family members are distressed, caregiving provides opportunities for improving relationships, increasing family cohesiveness, and enhancing personal growth (Gatz, Bengtson, & Blum, 1990; Toseland & Smith, 1991). However, family members must learn to take care of themselves as well as the identified patient, because the intense demands of caregiving puts them at risk for a wide range of personal, family, and lifestyle problems. Over the long years of what Eisdorfer has called ''interminable care,'' healthy family functioning will be affected negatively, even in the most resourceful families, unless a balance is found meeting the needs of everyone in the family. The dynamics of the family system as well as subsystems, such as spouses, siblings, children, and parents, are affected by the demands of caregiving (Cohen & Eisdorfer, 1995; Pruchno, Peters, & Burant, 1995).

The negative consequences of caring for family members are well documented. Caregivers are at risk for depression, anger, anxiety, poor physical health, immunological dysfunction, low levels of life satisfaction, and exhaustion (Cohen & Eisdorfer, 1988; Gallagher et al., 1989; Kielcolt-Glaser et al., 1988; Light, Niederele, & Lebowitz, 1994; Schultz, O'Brien, Bookwala, & Fleissner, 1995). Furthermore, the level of distress in family members is mediated by behavioral disturbances in the patient (Deimling & Bass, 1986; Miller, 1990), satisfaction with social supports (Cliff & George, 1995), and linkages with formal caregiver services (Toseland & Rossiter, 1989).

A number of intervention programs have been developed to alleviate the stresses of caregiving, including family support groups, respite care programs, community and home services, and psychoeducational programs. However, these interventions often are not available, and their effectiveness to promote mental health and well-being is equivocal (Zarit &

Teri, 1991). Despite efforts to make formal interventions available to caregivers, only about 10% to 25% of caregivers utilize them (Collins, Stommel, Givens, & King, 1991). Numerous explanations have been offered for the remarkable disuse of service, and most have focused on caregiver beliefs about several issues. They alone can and should provide exclusive care without informal or formal assistance (Brody, 1985; Gwyther, 1989). It is preferable to use family and friends rather than rely on formal community-based services (Gwyther, 1989). Certain cultural and ethnic groups (e.g., African Americans) view help-seeking outside the family as unacceptable (Henderson, 1993; Hinrichsen & Ramirez, 1992). Use of formal help will relinquish family control over caregiving (Gwyther, 1989). It is difficult to discuss emotional problems in face-to-face interactions with strangers (Montgomery & Borgatta, 1989). Finally, services often are not available or accessible.

The majority of caregivers avoid or delay use of community-based services because of strong personal, family, and cultural belief systems about motivations and styles of providing care. Using community-based interventions that involve face-to-face meetings with professionals or other caregivers as well as travel may be perceived as invading privacy and cause anxiety or fear about revealing emotional issues to others (Burgeon & Walther, 1990). Thus caregivers may be reluctant to reveal family conflicts and problems as well as emotional reactions to others and therefore avoid such interactions.

Family members often look to physicians and other health professionals for information and support, but it is a challenge for clinicians to deal with the complex needs of family caregivers, especially in managed care settings. Reimbursement is limited, and clinicians vary in their interest, motivation, experience, and resources to work with family. It takes time to listen to family members tell the emotional story of a dehumanizing illness. It takes time to provide information and to answer questions, deal with multiple family members, and sometimes mediate patient or family conflict, counsel caregivers to manage emotions, and help them find a balance between caregiving and other life demands. It takes time to teach families how to cope with patient problems, for example, behavioral disturbances, swallowing problems, as well as their own problems, for example, depression and the need for respite. However, not to develop a care plan incorporating the needs of family members as well as of the patient is to violate the fundamental clinical and ethical principle of nonmalfeasance—to do no harm (Cohen, 1991).

This chapter introduces a primary clinical framework for family care, reviews the effect of dementia on the patient, and suggests guidelines for discussions of difficult and sensitive issues such as marital problems, institutionalization, violence and abuse, and genetic risk. General principles of primary care have been published elsewhere (Cohen, 1994). Clinicians do not have to be family specialists, but there is a responsibility to provide technical clinical information (Roth, 1993), as well as create a professional relationship to support patient and family efforts to sustain hope, that is, not let hope die too far ahead of the patient, prepare for losses over the course of the illness, and feel a sense of effectiveness doing the best they can in an impossible situation. A number of excellent practice-oriented references for family counseling and therapy for older persons and their families are available for mental health specialists (Bumagin & Hirn, 1990; Cohen & Eisdorfer, 1995; Hargrave & Anderson, 1992; Neiderhardt & Allen, 1993).

A PROCESS MODEL FOR CLINICAL CARE

The problems families face through the course of dementia encompass every aspect of life, and many of the decisions and actions required in caring are ambiguous, painful, and confusing. The clinician's role is to guide the patient and family members through a process of identifying and dealing with the multiple problems associated with caregiving. There are no easy prescriptions, but a great deal can be done if the clinician acts as a coordinator, focusing family members on a process of compartmentalizing the complexities of caregiving into manageable parts. Not all problems of caregiving can be solved, but identifying and discussing issues provides a "framing process" for families. Open discussions and shared decision making can assist families to maintain a sense of limited mastery in the face of the unrelenting losses that accompany dementia. Cohen and Eisdorfer (1995) have described this concept of limited control in caregivers' tasks as "effectivity."

The clinical framework for family intervention is a three-stage process of assessment: care-plan development, followed by resolution and implementation. There are specific tasks for the clinician in each of the three stages. In the assessment phase, the tasks are to investigate and characterize issues, concerns, or problems, determine the decision capabilities of the patient, and identify the individual needs of the patient, family caregivers, and other family members affected but not necessarily involved in direct caregiving, for example, young children. It is important, where possible, to convene all involved family members to identify and clarify each person's perceptions of the problem(s), clarify unmet needs of the patient and other family members, and facilitate discussions to reach relative agreements on the most important problem(s) at that time. Even when family members live far away, or there is a history of conflict, group meetings or conference calls may be needed to clarify family dynamics and move toward the best care plan.

In the care plan, the tasks are to identify reasonable goals within each of the problem areas, clarify various options the family has to reach these goals, and ensure that family members understand the effect of solving these problems on everyone in the family. It is important to identify resources the family needs to meet goals, such as community-based services or information about drugs, medical conditions, and treatment. A major challenge in care-plan development is helping the identified patient explain his or her values and preferences, where possible, to other family members.

The resolution and implementation stage efforts should encourage the family to think through their options, arrive at workable solutions, develop a checklist of tasks for implementation, and identify which family members will be responsible for each task. It also is important during this stage to reaffirm that as the dementia progresses, the care plan also will have to change.

This model prescribes a framework to guide and support family members, blending the value of the clinician's technical and formal caregiving role. Through the course of dementia, families will face different dilemmas, from emotional ambiguities in the early diagnostic phase through work and lifestyle changes as caregiving demands increase in later phases, and finally decisions regarding humane palliative care during the terminal phase. There is enormous variation in the ways families respond and adapt because of historical, cultural, and economic factors, and effective strategies in one family may be ineffective in others. The value of the model is to prescribe a way of thinking about caregiving as a process of solving problems. Thus in families who are willing and able to sustain responsibilities for caregiving, who are coping well with most situations, and who have family and community support, the clinician plays a consultative role, using the model to give the family feedback, encouragement, and support. In contrast, families who are unable or unwilling to sustain caregiving because of deterioration in the patient, declining caregiver health, family conflict, or a host of other issues, the clinician either plays a coordinating role, using the model to work with the family, or refers the family for specialized mental health care.

When working with families, there are several areas to be evaluated to use the clinical model effectively:

1. the presence of depression or other psychiatric problems in family caregivers;
2. knowledge of how the family operates;
3. knowledge of family members about medical and psychological problems;
4. family belief systems; and
5. cultural and ethnic influences.

The Presence of Depression in Family Caregivers

There are brief depression self-report screening tests that can be administered to family members in the waiting room. One of the best is the Center for Epidemiological Studies—Depression Test (CES-D). Primary care diagnostic and treatment guidelines have been developed and are available for practitioners (Department of Health and Human Services, 1993). A clinical interview should focus on changes in mood, thinking, behavior, and body functions. To be diagnosed with a major depressive disorder with current diagnostic criteria, individuals must display five of the following nine symptoms:

1. depressed mood or dysfunction;
2. loss of interest in usual activities;
3. loss of appetite with significant weight loss or increase of appetite with weight gain;
4. insomnia;
5. slow thinking and movement or agitation and restlessness;
6. loss of energy;
7. feelings of worthlessness and hopelessness;
8. decreased ability to concentrate; and
9. suicidal thoughts or actions.

Caregivers also may present significant anxiety and hostility with the depression. Furthermore, depression also exists in disguise with other medical conditions. If the depression is detected, diagnosed, and treated appropriately, the family caregiver will be a more active and effective partner in care.

How the Family Operates

Every family has a characteristic way of doing things, and family members usually react to each other around the demands of caregiving as they have around other family issues. For example, most siblings coordinate their efforts to help impaired parents, but siblings who have had strong conflicts and rivalries seldom cooperate concerning the care of a parent who has Alzheimer's disease.

Not every family works well together or even wants to work together. The size and composition of the family, factors such as divorce, proximity, economic security, and previous conflicts, as well as the willingness of family members to help each other, have an impact on how well family members will cooperate. The goal of the clinician is to help the primary family members develop reasonable expectations about help from others and, where desirable, refer the family for therapy.

Individual family members may solve problems effectively but may have difficulty working with other members. Families can be characterized in five general styles: denial, cooperation, alternating leadership, contentiousness, and chaos (Cohen & Eisdorfer, 1995). Families in denial do not see problems and, therefore, always seem to be in crisis. Referral to a specialist in family mental health counseling is the best course of action. Cooperative families communicate well, solve their problems together, and handle the responsibilities of caregiving reasonably well. A third style is one in which members of the family alternate leadership rather than collaborate. Members do well as long as they agree about who is in charge and when. Contentious families usually have a long history of conflict and find it impossible to work together. Finally, some families are chaotic. Relationships are formulated and dissolved rapidly with the consequence that as a family unit, it is disorganized and people are engaged in hurting each other. Caring for a cognitively impaired relative creates numerous opportunities to attack and belittle other family members, including the patient. In some cases, family members may use the caregiving consultation as an opportunity to draw the clinician into the family system in an attempt to defend their usual way of operating. It is critical that the clinician maintain neutrality by acknowledging the perceptions of individual family members but returning to the concrete issues of caregiving.

If family members have serious problems with denial, conflict, and anger, help from a specialist in psychiatry, psychology, or social work is important. When families have serious fights, the feuds are often not about what they seem. They may stem from personal rivalries that are typically embedded in family history as well as from perceived pain and injury. Mental health professionals will be useful to clarify whether family caregivers can separate emotions about prior perceived insults from emotional reactions to caregiving tasks.

Knowledge About Medical and Psychological Problems

Family members, including the identified patient, do best when they understand what happens during the course of dementia. Clinicians need to educate family members about how physical illness, drugs, and pain affect the behavior of people with dementia, as well as learn about the main effects and side effects of drugs. It often is helpful to refer family members to appropriate self-help books, nursing, and pharmacy guides. There are excellent consumer references for dementia caregiving (Cohen & Eisdorfer, 1986, 1995; Coughlan, 1993; Mace & Rabins, 1981), drugs (Gorman, 1990), mastering emotions (Klein & Wender, 1993; Lerner, 1985; Ryan, 1986), management of behavior problems (Cairl, 1995), conflict resolution (Weeks, 1991), exercise and diet (McIllwain, Steinmeyer, Bruce, Fulghum, & Bruce, 1990), housing (Golant, 1992), nursing homes (Goldsmith, 1990), living wills (Flynn, 1992), and medical care decisions (Dubler & Nimmons, 1992).

Family Belief Systems

The beliefs that family members have about what influences events and circumstances during the course of dementia are powerful forces in determining how well individuals cope as well as how effectively they participate in treatment decisions. Beliefs can range from views that external forces are influencing the situation, for example, "It's in God's hands," to internal forces, for example, "It's our problem, and we'll handle it," or families may attribute changes to chance. However, these attributions affect the way family members interpret changes, declare their involvement in caregiving, and guide how willing they are to take care of themselves, and how successfully they will form partnerships with professionals. Families with a strong internal locus of control tend to be highly invested in caregiving and are at high risk for responding with guilt, anger, and blame. For these families, deterioration in the patient implies failure. Families with an internal locus tend to hold onto the patient, whereas families with an external locus of control are more apt to give up on the patient, for example, not keep medical care visits, consider early institutionalization.

Effect of Cultural or Ethnic Influences

Practitioners need to be sensitive to the effect of ethnicity on the way family members provide care (McAdoo, 1993). The challenge is to stay focused on present caregiving problems and also recognize that ethnic history, beliefs, and customs affect the way family members perceive problems, use services, and develop solutions.

Professionals should be careful about their assumptions regarding who is a member of the family to be involved in caregiving. There are ethnic variations in the definition of family and family membership, real or fictitious, that is, nonblood but valued individuals. Fictive kin may play important support roles in the support of older people in many cultures. In fact, in some families the older adult is a fictive member of the family. Serious problems may occur if the dementia evaluation and care plan do not include such individuals or do not acknowledge their importance in the family.

It also is important to understand cultural expectations for independence and dependence of family members as well as expectations for intergenerational roles and responsibilities. In contrast to traditions of self-sufficiency and independence in white Protestant families, other ethnic groups such as Italian and Mexican-Americans have strong generational traditions of committed caregiving to relatives. African American families are usually large and extended networks of family members who often share the many caregiving demands. Cultural sensitivity to the complexities of different families will avoid misinterpretations of family motivations and will maximize the cooperation of families in an effective care plan.

Immigration and assimilation are associated with problems of language, economics, and education as well as disruptions of personal and family life. The demands of caring for parents with dementia may cause intergenerational distress between older immigrant parents and children, who may be torn between two worlds and experience conflicts about values, loyalties, and responsibilities. It is essential to sort through this type of conflict carefully to avoid exacerbating family problems. It may be necessary to find knowledgeable religious or family allies to help adult child caregivers sort through role confusions. The clinician acts as a broker to help family members reframe the problems of caregiving as a cultural issue, not to discuss the shortcomings of any family members or psychopathology in the family.

There also are significant ethnic variations in what is regarded as a medical problem needing treatment. Many ethnic groups such as African Americans, Koreans, and Vietnamese do not define dementia as a disease and therefore do not seek help. For example, the criteria for deciding whether to seek help for a medical problem in many African American families are impaired activities of daily living. Thus African Americans often delay seeking a diagnosis or other treatment interventions. Ethnic variations in attitudes toward pain, suffering, and death also affect health care utilization. Mexican American, Irish, and African American families caring for relatives with dementia may not appear for the patients' regular checkups or adhere to treatment recommendations. Clinicians will be best served to find professional allies within the ethnic group of the family being cared for.

HOW DEMENTIA AFFECTS THE PATIENT

One of the most important principles of family caregiving is to keep the person with dementia as active a participant as possible. Over time, individuals with Alzheimer's disease lose cognitive capacities and abilities to do things for themselves and others, but not all skills and abilities deteriorate at the same rate. Furthermore, "individuals-turned-patients" have needs, preferences, and desires to be expressed and understood, and they can do so even in late stages of the disease (Cairl, 1995; Cohen, 1991). To the extent possible, individuals need and want to be involved in making decisions about their care and how they will continue to function as part of the family. Personal alliances with family members and health care providers are necessary to preserve the patient's dignity and serve his or her comfort and welfare. The goal is to empower individuals early in the illness when many cognitive capacities remain and involve them in discussions about health care, finances, legal issues, and other matters.

Although the progressive cognitive losses during the course of dementia compromise memory, judgment, reasoning, and decision making, these changes do not occur overnight. During early and middle phases, the individual can participate in legal, financial, and health care decisions to prepare for the future. Encourage the patient and family members to discuss two documents: a living will and a durable power of attorney for health care decisions. These advanced directives specify an individual's preference in advance. This can be a family affair because a living will is something everyone should have. A values history form is an effective tool to give the family to stimulate discussion about the many possibilities that may occur. Determining the patient's wishes and preferences takes time because the subject includes some difficult and painful issues. Several books contain the values history form to guide family discussions (Cohen & Eisdorfer, 1995; Dubler & Nimmons, 1992).

Discussions with family members and the identified patient require active listening. A stressed, well-intentioned family may talk for the patient and act as if they had synthesized the patient's preferences. Likewise, relatives may be good facilitators in the exchange of information, interpreting technical details to the patient and providing emotional support. When family members are trying to work together, this shared discussion can lead to increased mutual comfort and intimacy. This cooperation also creates the foundation for future care when medical decisions have to be made and the patient is incapacitated.

As the disease progresses and patients become more impaired, efforts should be made to maintain involvement in decision making, if only to sit in the room during discussions. It is a challenge to learn what individuals think and feel in order to involve them appropriately, especially when deficits make communication difficult. The most important rule of thumb is to take the time to listen and observe carefully.

Changes in physical health affect the patient's behavior and ability to communicate: There is no evidence that individuals with Alzheimer's disease have more physical health problems than older persons without dementia, but medical problems, such as infections, cancer, and heart problems occur, and chronic health problems are exacerbated. Unfortunately, as the dementia progresses, the ability to describe feelings as well as pain and discomfort may be difficult. Physical illness, pain, and especially drug effects often cause behavioral problems because the individual cannot translate thoughts and feelings into words.

How the individual adapts to the illness has been described as a series of six psychological changes (Cohen, Kennedy, & Eisdorfer, 1984). These six phases of change describe the subjective experiences of the illness—how individuals perceive and react to their illness before and during the diagnosis as well as into later stages:

- Recognition and concern ... "Something is wrong."
- Denial ... "Not me."
- Anger, sadness, or shame ... "Why me?"
- Coping ... "In order to go on, I must do ... "
- Maturation ... "Living each day until I die."
- Separation from self ...

Not every person with Alzheimer's disease experiences these changes in the order described, but all have thoughts and feelings about what is happening as the disease robs them of their humanity. Individuals need opportunities and encouragement to talk. Gentle, persistent probing often will reveal many issues that the patient has not discussed for fear of upsetting other family members. Many family members are uncomfortable and fearful of upsetting the patient by talking about personal issues, precisely at the time when most individuals with Alzheimer's disease want to talk. It is a major challenge for family members to sort out their own reactions to the diagnosis, the disease, and the deterioration of their relative (the patient) to be an effective caregiver. Although people differ in their ability to accept the diagnosis, in most cases, the identified patient should be told what the diagnosis is and what the immediate future may hold. In other cases, the information needs to be titrated to help patients assimilate their circumstances. It is important to answer questions truthfully and to give the clear message that you will be there for them.

It can be harmful to withhold information because this begins a pattern or limited disclosure and distrust. Trust is a key issue in a disease where feelings of safety, comfort, and support are based on trust and attachment as cognitive abilities wane. Trusting someone who has withheld information creates suspicion and distrust even in healthy people!

It is not uncommon for people to deny their problems, and this is not unique to dementia. Denial can be an effective way to deal with the shock of bad news if the denial does not last too long. Family members and the identified patient need to be encouraged to listen to each other and be supportive. It is not uncommon to observe that the patient has accepted the circumstances much better than the rest of the family.

Strong emotions always are present following the diagnosis, and allowing the person to express them is therapeutic. Many individuals struggle to find an explanation for what has happened to them, and anger, sadness, shame, anxiety, and agitation are natural responses. The goal is to help them acknowledge their losses, identify human strengths still present, and to accept increasing dependency.

The coping phase is a period in which ways to deal with the impairments are established, and the patient develops some sense of safety and limited, structured involvement in his or her world. The maturation phase is one in which the patient is less able to learn coping strategies and requires more constant companionship and increasing structure. Although dependency is increasing and losses become more disabling, patients are still people who need to feel intimacy, acceptance, and safety, as well as to be active. The last phase, separation from self, is one in which individuals are reactive rather than active and extremely difficult to communicate with in most situations. As individuals eventually become frail, bedbound, and wasted, their major needs are to be comfortable, secure, and free of pain.

One of the most difficult issues for practitioners to discuss is the wish of many patients with dementia to die. It is common for patients to express a desire to be dead, and it is also common for families to wish them dead rather than endure the humiliating loss of self. This issue became a national issue in 1990 when Janet Atkins, a woman diagnosed with Alzheimer's disease in her 50s, flew to Michigan to seek assistance from Dr. Kevorkian. He used his homemade suicide device to help her die. An anonymous survey of geriatric internists in four geographic regions of the country revealed that most would not consider assisting individuals with dementia to die (Watts, Howell, & Prieter, 1992). Two thirds thought Dr. Kevorkian's assistance was not appropriate, whereas 14% believed it was morally justifiable. A total of 57% were in opposition to changing restrictions on physician-assisted suicide, whereas 26% were in favor. If restrictions were eased, two thirds would not help a competent dementia patient commit suicide, whereas 21% would consider it. However, 41% of these geriatricians indicated that they would consider suicide if they had dementia.

These wide-ranging responses reflect a combination of religious beliefs, professional values and ethics, and personal experiences. Watts et al. (1992) interpreted the diversity of responses and the high percentage of physicians who would consider suicide if diagnosed with dementia as reflecting a sense of the loss of control with the progression of the disease. It is important for clinicians to be vigilant when communicating with families, *not* to convey hopelessness because it reinforces their helplessness. Supportive communications regarding this issue are essential. Families of patients need to express their feelings and have someone listen to them. Listening often is the best medicine in these circumstances.

There is one important rule to keep in mind. Patients with dementia are people, first, last, and always! Throughout the course of illness needs vary, caregiving demands change, and the patient's ability to communicate deteriorates. The overall clinical challenge is to empower the patient's participation in the family and to represent his or her interests. Even in late stages of the disease, it is possible to discern patients' interests and preferences if we watch and listen carefully as well as look for opportunities, however fleeting, to make contact.

HOW DEMENTIA AFFECTS INTIMACY AND MARRIAGE

Through the course of dementia, intimacy and sexual relations are disrupted in stable marriages, and conflict and rejection, for example, institutionalization, of the patient occur in unstable marriages. Intimacy is defined as the ability to form a relationship characterized by mutuality and reciprocity, open communication, effective and thoughtful conflict resolution, passionate attachment, and emotional commitment. All of these are affected by the very nature of Alzheimer's disease and related disorders, and the challenge for caregiving spouses, who are at the highest risk for depression, are many. Results of interviews with 516 caregivers comparable to national samples by sociodemographic characteristics showed that 63% of wives and 39% of husbands reported significant levels of depressive symptoms (Cohen et al., 1990). The high rates of depression and depressive symptoms in spouse caregivers may reflect not only the emotional distress of caregiving, but also psychological distress with the dissolution of the marital bond.

A few studies have examined the quality of the marriage in relation to the assumption, maintenance, and abandonment of the caregiver role. Shorter duration of the marriage, poor marital adjustment prior to the diagnosis, and age have been reported to be associated with depression in spouse caregiving (Schultz & Williams, 1991). Conversely, an intimate marriage prior to the illness is associated with a lower perceived burden (Williamson & Schulz, 1990), less perceived stress (Horowitz & Shindelman, 1983), lower levels of depression (Schulz & Williamson, 1991), increased caregiver satisfaction (Cairl & Kosberg, 1993), and less willingness to institutionalize the spouse (Wright, 1991, 1994).

When interviewing the caregiving spouse, it is important to determine what gives him or her satisfaction during caregiving as well as what causes the most distress. Most couples cope reasonably well as long as the caregiving spouse feels a sense of doing the best he or she can with the circumstances. It is common for spouses, especially wives, to feel that they cannot do enough, and they often lack insight into how much they are actually doing. Stress and depression often cloud clear judgment, and it is a clinical challenge to help spouses set limits on what they can do and still feel good about themselves. A useful technique is to ask the spouse caregivers to make a list of all they do for their husband or wife and what they also have done for themselves during the past week. This provides an opportunity to review how much the caregivers actually are doing, how well they are taking care of themselves, and reward them through support and encouragement.

Sexual relations may be satisfying for some couples until the middle or even later stages, if the patient does not have significant behavioral disturbances or hypersexual needs. Sleeping in the same bed even without sexual intimacy may be comforting to the patient. However, at some point, separate sleeping arrangements usually become necessary because the patient is restless, combative, and disruptive.

It is not uncommon for the healthy spouse to develop intimate relations with another partner, especially when the husband or wife is significantly deteriorated and in a nursing home or assisted living facility. Adult children, neighbors, and friends may be angry and upset by the perceived infidelity and withdraw support from caregiving responsibilities. These are times when the spouse needs understanding and support from clinicians. Frequently, the affair occurs with another caregiver or a longtime friend, and the motivations are the need for comfort, love, and support. Shuttle diplomacy with family and friends may help them understand and accept the situation. This topic is clearly a sensitive one, but Alzheimer support groups can be particularly useful because such relationships are not unusual.

Homicide-suicides appear to be increasing in older couples when the husband is depressed, despondent about separation, institutionalization, or a future with little hope (Cohen & Eisdorfer, 1995). Depressive thinking is fueled by constant demands of caregiving, persistent mounting losses, social isolation, and decreased opportunities for rest and pleasurable activities. Individuals with few outside supports or those without a strong sense of identity may be particularly vulnerable.

Husbands are usually the perpetrators, perhaps because they do not have the social networks or friendships that many older women have, and they have become isolated and withdrawn from others because of the burdens of caregiving. Even older men who have contact with other people, including health professionals, usually do not talk about suicide. Older couples who have been together a long time and are suffering from dementia or other chronic illnesses have reasons to be upset and depressed. It is common for spouses to wish a wife or a husband who is very sick with dementia, cancer, or another chronic illness to be dead, but most are afraid or unwilling to talk about these wishes. If one or both have talked about the desire to die, even as a joking reference, and there is a gun in the house, the risk for homicide-suicide may be real.

Clinicians should probe older couples about suicide and a desire to die. Most people do not know that these feelings are normal or that talking with someone can relieve the distress and sense of being alone to bear the pain. The more detailed the plan or the more concrete the details, the more likely it is that the event may happen. Although little is known about the antecedents of homicide-suicide, the following circumstances merit review during a clinical interview: depression; alcohol abuse; isolation; a deterioration in the caregiver's health or the patient; pending institutionalization; complaints of burning out; hopelessness; pain; and isolation (Cohen & Eisdorfer, 1995).

Clinicians are well advised to probe for suicidal and homicidal-suicidal ideation, while conveying a clear message of support and of availability to help the spouse. In the late phases of dementia, when spouse caregivers feel helpless and hopeless watching their loved one deteriorate and waste away, acknowledging the reality of the situation but communicating that you are there for them can help. Words of support are a lifeline for spouses who need to know someone shares their anguish.

COPING WITH A MOVE FROM THE HOME

The decision to find an alternative living arrangement or a nursing home often is agonizing for most families who have exhausted their options to maintain a relative at home. Spouses are especially reluctant to move their marriage partner into a long-term care setting, but the physical demands of personal care, including dressing and feeding, dealing with incontinence, wandering, and behavioral disturbances, usually precipitate a move to an assisted living facility or nursing home. Unfortunately, the move usually occurs after multiple stressful events overwhelm the family or lead to deterioration in the patient, for example, falls, strokes, or injuries.

Most families perceive institutionalization as a failure and feel guilty for years, even after the patient has died. Assisted living facilities and nursing homes are legitimate options for care that allow the family to get on with their lives and also maintain involvement with the patient. It is appropriate to take a relative to the hospital or medical setting when he or she needs acute medical care, and, likewise, it is legitimate to move a relative into another setting when the demands of care outstrip family capabilities or are affecting the caregiver's health.

Long-term care needs to be reframed as a technical rather than a moral issue. Family members should be encouraged to talk with others who have made the decision, visit assisted living and nursing homes, and contact caregivers' organizations that know about long-term care resources in the community. The latter include the local agency on aging and Alzheimer support groups.

Assisted living facilities are appropriate supportive homes where individuals can live in a structured environment with meals, assistance with medications, activities, transportation, and the social support of their peers. Nursing homes become placement options when community-based services are not available, the patient is difficult to manage because of functional impairments, and family caregivers are exhausted, ill, and unable to care for themselves or their relative. Family members need to be encouraged to find the right placement or residence for their relative. Books and guides on the subject can be helpful (Cohen & Eisdorfer, 1986, 1995; Goldsmith, 1994).

A move out of the home is a sensitive and complex issue. Clinicians can help families by raising the issue and validating caregiver feelings about loss of control as their loved one deteriorates and logistical, emotional, or financial resources are exhausted. Family members commonly are resistant to talk about "the forbidden" after vowing "never" to send their relative to a nursing home. The move often is perceived as abandonment, accompanied by guilt, anger, and sadness. These emotions can immobilize a caregiver spouse and also provoke arguments among adult children, who may force the issue with their parents.

Family members can overcome feelings of abandonment if the clinician helps them see the assisted living facility or nursing home as an extension of the family home. The patient and the family need reassurance that they are working toward the "best of both worlds" by scheduling weekend visits for the patient in the family home or holiday homecomings. Family members should be encouraged to keep family traditions and other rituals that increase their relative's sense of belonging in the family although he or she is separated geographically.

One of the most difficult challenges is helping family members to develop a reasonable visitation schedule. They need active support and suggestions to reactivate a life for themselves, in and out of the nursing home. It is not uncommon for impaired relatives to adapt well to the nursing home move, and family members need to be reminded this is a likely result. Over time, as patients deteriorate with the ravages of the dementia, families find great comfort when clinicians maintain contact with them through visits and telephone contact. Being there to support the family, answer questions about medications, health and behavioral problems, and comfort them is a critical role.

ABUSE AND VIOLENCE IN FAMILIES

Abuse and violence are common in families caring for a relative with dementia when they are depressed and overwhelmed with the demands of caregiving (Paveza et al., 1992). Severe violence may occur in 17% of the families (Paveza et al., 1992), and other forms of abuse such as financial, psychological, and neglect may affect up to 75% of older persons (Paveza, 1995).

There are several forms of neglect, abuse, and violence: passive neglect, active neglect, physical abuse, psychological abuse, financial abuse, violation of individual rights, and self-abuse (Kosberg & Garcia, 1995). Passive neglect is the unintentional failure to provide help or resources and occurs when the patient is left alone or forgotten. The caregivers are usually depressed and not aware of what they are doing (or not doing). Depressed caregivers may forget medications and physician visits. Active neglect is intentional, and the caregiver may withhold food, medicine, and assistance to punish or hurt the patient.

Physical abuse ranges from physical restraint to severe violence, that is, hitting, kicking, shooting, or stabbing. The family member may be responding adversely because of cumulative stress, or depression, or the actions may be premeditated, where the infliction of pain, injury, or confinement results in bodily harm. Psychological abuse characterized by insults, name-calling, humiliation, and infantilization may be intentional or reflect the aberrant behavior of a depressed or angry caregiver overwhelmed by the situation. Financial abuse, which includes monetary or material theft, can be perpetrated by relatives but more commonly by individuals who are involved with a cognitively impaired older person as a case manager or paid caregiver.

Violation of the patient's rights occur more commonly than recognized. Most family members are motivated to do what they think is in the best interest of their relative. However, family members may overstep their boundaries by making medical, financial, and material decisions, as well as by forcing a cognitively impaired relative into a nursing home with no preparation or explanation.

Cognitively impaired older persons who live alone or are geographically distant from relatives may not be able to care for themselves adequately. Friends and neighbors, for whatever reason, may be unwilling to intervene, and the individual may deteriorate, lose weight, wander from home, or live in squalor, unaware of how serious his or her condition really is. It is difficult to intervene when older persons are neglecting themselves because of the denial of the seriousness of their condition. Sometimes family members or neighbors unknowingly assist in the self-abuse by purchasing alcohol or drugs for the cognitively impaired person.

When interviewing older persons and their family members, evaluate the possibilities of elder abuse. Sensitivity to the issue is the first step in detection, and it is the key to prevention. Family members usually welcome the opportunity to discuss such impulses. Caregiving takes its toll on the family, and a desire to hurt the patient or wish for the patient to die may occur occasionally in the most normal circumstances. Acting on the impulse is not. There are several family situations that may create a high-risk environment for abuse:

1. Family caregivers develop depression or other psychiatric problems and hurt the patient;
2. Family members are resistant to caring for the patient because of previous disagreements, hostility, dislike for the parents, intergenerational conflict, or unwillingness to provide care; and
3. Some families already have a significant caregiving burden because of alcoholism, mental illness, a handicapped or chronically ill child, delinquency, domestic violence, or unemployment.

The following guidelines are important considerations during a family interview: screen for depression in caregivers, be direct in asking caregivers if they have ever wanted to hurt the patient or if the patient has ever hurt them, and assess how dysfunctional the family is. If abuse is a problem, there are several clinical and legal options. Certain forms of elder abuse are a crime, and legal action is necessary. It may be possible to avoid legal avenues by referring the abusing family members for individual or family therapy, treating depression when it is present in family caregivers, finding community services such as day care, respite care, or home care, or helping the family find alternative housing. However, all states except Colorado, Illinois, New Jersey, New York, North Dakota, South Dakota, Pennsylvania, and Wisconsin have mandatory reporting laws. There are several organizations to contact for information about intervening in elder abuse (the American Bar Association, Commission on Legal Problems of the Elderly; and the National Center on Elder Abuse, both in Washington, D.C.).

PERCEPTIONS OF GENETIC RISK

Rapid advances are being made in our understanding of the molecular genetics of Alzheimer's disease. At the present time, genetic testing for Alzheimer's disease is most informative for individuals who have several affected relatives, whose onset occurred prior to 65 years of age—clues that may suggest a known mutation on chromosome 14 or 21, for which markers are available. For some forms of early-onset Alzheimer's disease, and for the more common late-onset Alzheimer's disease, genetic testing likely is to be much less informative. APOE testing for late-onset Alzheimer's disease is currently available but probably will not provide family members with useful information regarding risk of Alzheimer's disease. Given the heterogeneous etiology of late-onset Alzheimer's disease, Apo E typing will, at least with current technology, provide an incomplete estimate of future risk.

For high-risk families who choose to participate in genetic testing, genetic counseling is necessary to inform and disseminate genetic risk information (Mullan, Crawford, & Buchman, 1994). As patterns of familial transmission are clarified, family caregivers are likely to experience added distress as they witness deterioration in the patient and a preview of what the future may hold for siblings, children, as well as for them. Many myths and misconceptions exist in Alzheimer families. At-risk individuals may cope with their fears by trying to gain some illusion of control over the unknown and frightening possibilities of future illness, for example, assigning risk to family members based on their resemblance to an affected parent. Some families develop an identity around the certainty that they will or will not develop the disease.

Family transmission patterns, particularly for late-onset Alzheimer's disease, often are difficult to explain to families (Mullan, Crawford, & Buchman, 1994). Describing the range of possibilities to family members often leads to a tendency to reduce complex risks to binary form, that is, "I will (won't) get Alzheimer's disease" (Lippman-Hand & Fraser, 1979). Many family members view genetic information in a fatalistic fashion regardless of the evidence for heterogeneity in Alzheimer's disease.

Technical questions may conceal deeper fears and concerns about the implications of the fact that "Alzheimer's runs in the family." Not only must family members cope with the present reality of a family member with the disease, but also the future reality of themselves, a partner, or a child being affected. Discussions of factual information often will provide family members with opportunities to work through their feelings about these issues and give clinicians a chance to provide support and validation, while normalizing these emotional reactions.

SUMMARY

The objective of this chapter was to describe a clinical model for primary care practitioners to care for the patient within the family and discuss complex and sensitive issues such as marital problems, alternative living arrangements, clarification of abuse and violence, and clarification of genetic risk. A great deal can be done to help the family and patient cope, but as the dementia progresses, caring becomes more difficult and wearing on caregivers. Listening and "being there" can be the best medicine that provides a lifeline for families living with the disease.

REFERENCES

Brody, E. M. (1985). Patient care as a normative family stress. *Gerontologist, 25,* 19–29.

Brody, J., & Cohen, D. (1989). Epidemiologic aspects of Alzheimer's disease: Facts and gaps. *Journal of Aging and Health, 1,* 139–147.

Bumagin, V. E., & Hirn, K. F. (1990). *Helping the aging family: A guide for professionals.* New York: Springer.

Burgeon, J. K., & Walther, J. B. (1990). Nonverbal expectancies and the evaluative consequences of violations. *Human Communications Research, 17,* 232–267.

Cairl, R. (1995). *Somebody tell me who I am.* St. Petersburg, FL: Caremor.

Cairl, R., & Kosberg, J. (1993). The interface between burden and competence among caregivers of Alzheimer's Disease patients. An examination of clinical profiles. *Journal of Gerontological Social Work, 19,* 133–151.

Cohen, D. (1991). The subjective experiences of Alzheimer's disease: The anatomy of an illness as perceived by patients and families. *American Journal of Alzheimer's Care, 6,* 6–11.

Cohen, D. (1993). The 1990's: The decade of the brain and the family. *Behavior, Health, and Aging, 3,* 63–64.

Cohen, D. (1994). A primary care checklist for effective family management. *Medical Clinics of North America, 78,* 795–809.

Cohen, D., & Eisdorfer, C. (1986). *The loss of self: A family resources for Alzheimer's disease and related disorders.* New York: W. W. Norton (Hardback), 1986, Plume (Softback), 1987.

Cohen, D., & Eisdorfer, C. (1988). Depression in family members caring for a relative with Alzheimer's disease. *Journal of the American Geriatric Society, 36,* 885–889.

Cohen, D., & Eisdorfer, C. (1995). *Caring for your aging parents: A planning and action guide.* New York: Jeremy Tarcher/Putnam.

Cohen, D., Kennedy, G., & Eisdorfer, C. (1984). Phases of change in the patient with Alzheimer's dementia: A conceptual dimension for defining health care management. *Journal of the American Geriatrics Society, 32,* 11–15.

Cohen, D., Luchins, D., Eisdorfer, C., Paveza, G., Ashford, W., Gorelick, P., Hirschman, R., Freels, S., Levy, P., Semla, T., & Shaw, H. (1990). Caring for relatives with Alzheimer's disease: The mental health risks to spouses, children and other family caregivers. *Behaviors, Health and Aging, 1,* 165–182.

Collins, C., Stommel, M., Givens, C. W., & King, S. (1991). Knowledge and use of community services among family caregivers of Alzheimer's disease patient. *Archives of Psychiatric Nursing, 5,* 84–90.

Coughlan, P. B. (1993). *Facing Alzheimer's: Family caregiving speak.* New York: John Wiley.
Deimling, G. T., & Bass, D. M. (1986). Symptoms of mental impairment among elderly adults and their effects on family caregivers. *Journal of Gerontology, 41,* 778–784.
Department of Health and Human Services (1993). *Depression in primary care: Detection, diagnosis and treatment* (AHCPR Publication No. 930552). Washington, DC: Department of Health and Human Services.
Doty, P. (1986). Family care of the elderly: The role of public policy. *The Milbank Quarterly, 67,* 485–506.
Dubler, N., & Nimmons, D. (1992). *Ethics on call: A medical ethicist shows how to take charge of life-and-death choices.* New York: Harmony Books.
Flynn, E. P. (1992). *Your living will: Why, when and how to write one.* New York: Citadel Press.
Gallagher, D., Wrabetz, A., Lovett, J., Del Maestro, & Rose, J. (1989). Depression and other negative effects in family caregivers. In E. Light & B. Liebowitz (Eds.), *Alzheimer's disease: Treatment and family stress: Directions for research* (pp. 218–244). Rockville, MD: National Institute of Mental Health.
Gatz, M., Bengtson, V. L., & Blum, M. J. (1990). Caregiving families. In J. E. Birren & K. W. Schaie (Eds.), *Handbook of psychology of aging* (3rd ed., pp. 404–426). San Diego, CA: Academic Press.
Golant, S. M. (1992). *Housing America's elderly: Many possibilities/few choices.* Newbury Park, CA: Sage.
Goldsmith, S. B. (1990). *Choosing a nursing home.* New York: Prentice-Hall.
Gorman, J. M. (1990). *The essential guide to psychiatric drugs.* New York: St. Martin's Press.
Gustafson, L. (1992). Clinical classification of dementia conditions. *Acta Neurologica Scandinavica* (Suppl. 139), *17,* 16–20.
Gwyther, L. P. (1989). Carfing and Alzheimer's disease. A social perspective. In G. C. Gilmore, P. J. Whitehouse, & M. L. Wykle (Eds.), *Memory, aging, and dementia: Theory, assessment and treatment* (pp. 234–242). New York: Springer.
Hargrave, T. D., & Anderson, W. T. (1992). *Finishing well: Aging and reparation in the intergenerational family.* New York: Brunner/Mazel.
Hay, J. W., & Ernst, R. L. (1987). The economic costs of Alzheimer's disease. *American Journal of Public Health, 77,* 1169–1175.
Henderson, Z. P. (1993). Racial poverty gap exists among elderly. *Human Ecology Forum, 21,* 31.
Hinrichsen, G. A., & Ramirez, M. (1992). Black and White dementia caregivers: A comparison of their adaption, adjustment and service utilization. *Gerontologist, 32,* 126–130.

Horowitz, A., & Shindelman, L. W. (1983). Reciprocity and affection: Past influences on current caregiving. *Journal of Gerontological Social Work, 5,* 5–20.

Kielcott-Glaser, J., Dura, J., Speicher, C. (1991). Spousal caregivers of dementia victims: Longitudinal changes in immunity and health. *Psychosomatic Medicine, 53,* 354.

Klein, D., & Wender, P. (1993). *Understanding depression.* New York: Oxford University Press.

Kosberg, J., & Garcia, J. (1995). Confronting maltreatment of elders by their family. In *Strengthening aging families* (Vol. 4, pp. 63–79). Sage.

Lawton, M. P., Bordy, E. M., & Saperstein, A. R. (1989). A controlled study of respite services for caregivers of Alzheimer's patients. *Gerontologist, 29,* 8–16.

Lerner, H. G. (1985). *The dance of anger.* New York: Harper and Row.

Light, E., Niederehe, G., & Lebowitz, B. (1994). *Stress effects on family caregivers of Alzheimer's patients.* New York: Springer.

Lippman-Hand, A. L., & Fraser, F. C. (1979). Genetic counseling: Provision and reception of information. *American Journal of Medical Genetics, 3,* 113–127.

Mace, N., & Rabins, P. (1981). *The 36-hour day.* Baltimore: Johns Hopkins University Press.

McAdoo, H. P. (Ed.). (1993). *Family ethnicity: Strength in diversity.* Newbury Park, CA: Sage.

McIlwain, H. H., Steinmeyer, C. F., Bruce, D. F., Fulghum, R. E., & Bruce, R. G. (1990). *The 50+ Wellness Plan: A complete program for maintaining nutritional, financial, and emotional well-being for mature adults.* New York: John Wiley.

Miller, B. (1990). Gender differences in spouse caregiver strain—Socialization and role explanations. *Journal of Marriage and the Family, 54,* 311–321.

Montgomery, R. J. V., & Borgatta, E. F. (1989). The effects of alternative support strategies on family caregiving. *Gerontologist, 29,* 457–464.

Mullan, M., Crawford, F., & Buchman, J. (1994). Technical feasibility of genetic testing for Alzheimer's disease. *Alzheimer Disease and Associated Disorders, 8*(2), 102–115.

Neiderhardt, E. R., & Allen, J. A. (1993). *Family therapy with the elderly.* Newbury Park, CA: Sage.

Paveza, G. (1995). What factors place elders at risk for elder abuse? *Patient Care Advisor,* 7–9.

Paveza, G., Cohen, D., Eisdorfer, C., Freels., S., Semla, T., Ashford, J., Gorelick, P., Hirschman, R., Luchins, D., & Levy, P. (1992). Severe family violence and Alzheimer's disease. Prevalence and risk factors. *Gerontologist, 32,* 493–497.

Pruchno, R. A., Peters, N. D., & Burant, C. J. (1995). Mental health of coresident family caregivers: Examination of a two-factor model. *Journal of Gerontology: Psychological Science, 50B,* 247–256.

Radloff, L. (1997). The CES-D Scale: A self-report depression scale for research in the general population. *Applied Psychological Measurement, 1,* 385–401.
Roth, M. E. (1993). Advances in Alzheimer's disease: A review for the family physician. *Journal of Family Practice, 37,* 593–607.
Ryan, R. S. (1986). *The fine art of recuperation: A guide to surviving and thriving after illness, accident or surgery.* Los Angeles: Jeremy P. Tarcher.
Schultz, R., O'Brien, A., Bookwala J., & Fleissner, K. (1995). Psychiatric and physical morbidity effects of dementia caregiving: Prevalence, correlates, and causes. *Gerontologist, 35,* 771–791.
Schulz, R., & Williamson, G. M. (1991). A 2-year longitudinal study of depression among Alzheimer's caregivers. *Psychology & Aging, 6,* 569–578.
Toseland, R. W., & Rossiter, C. M. (1989). Group interventions to support family caregivers: A review and analysis. *Gerontologist, 31,* 217–233.
Toseland, R. W., & Smith, G. C. (1991). Family caregivers of the frail elderly. In A. Gitterman (Ed.), *Handbook of social work practice with vulnerable populations* (pp. 549–583). New York: Columbia University Press.
Watts, D. T., Howell, T., & Priefer, B. A. (1992). Geriatricians' attitudes toward assisting suicide of dementia patients. *Journal of the American Geriatrics Society, 40,* 878–885.
Weeks, D. (1991). *Eight essential steps to conflict resolution.* Los Angeles: Jeremy P. Tarcher.
Williamson, G. M., & Schulz, R. (1990). Relationship orientation, quality of prior relationship, and distress among caregivers of Alzheimer's patients. *Psychology & Aging, 5,* 502–509.
Wright, L. K. (1994). Alzheimer's disease afflicting spouses who remain at home: Can human dialectics explain the findings? *Social Science and Medicine, 38,* 1037–1046.
Zarit, S. H., & Teri, L. (1991). Intervention and services for family caregivers. In K. W. Schaie (Ed.), *Annual review of gerontology and geriatrics* (Vol. 2, pp. 287–310). New York: Springer.

CHAPTER **14**

Community Care of Alzheimer's Disease

Kathleen Peterson
Vinod Kumar

Alzheimer's disease (AD) is an age-dependent neurodegenerative disorder, and more than 4 million Americans suffer from this devastating illness. It is projected to affect 14 million people by the year 2040, with similar increases expected in other developed countries (Alzheimer's Disease Education and Referral Center, 1993).

Although the majority of AD patients live in the community with their families, more than half of the 1.6 million nursing home residents suffer from Alzheimer's disease and other dementias (Rovner & German et al., 1990). Caring for individuals with Alzheimer's disease is challenging within institutional settings in spite of trained staff and structural modifications within the environment. Caring for individuals who wander, become confused, agitated, and who experience a decline in their functional ability can be even more challenging in the natural environment at home.

In fact, a substantial proportion of AD patients living with their family caregivers resemble nursing home residents in the severity of illness and the presence of psychiatric symptoms. Managing dementia patients in the home requires that families become educated about the illness of AD, learn behavior management techniques, and become aware of the array of support services available in the community. This knowledge can help delay and even prevent premature institutionalization. It is essential that physicians and professional care providers become aware of the number of available support services and encourage families to accept help from these services.

This chapter will give an overview of available services and describe an in-home-based intervention program that helped reduce the rate of premature institutionalizations of community-residing AD patients.

COMMUNITY SERVICE UTILIZATION

It is imperative that family physicians treating patients with AD understand the importance of family members and caregivers becoming knowledgeable about AD, understand behavior and other symptoms associated with the disease, and be aware of effective management of these behaviors. Referring families to services available in their communities is an important part of effective management of this devastating illness. Several years ago, Cohen, Hegarty, and Eisdorfer (1983) published the "Desk Directory of Social Resources" in the *Journal of the American Geriatric Society*. They recommended a guide to be available to physicians and professional care providers for appropriate referrals in the community. This type of list is very helpful in spite of reluctance on the part of some caregivers to seek help from such services. The unwillingness of AD patients and caregivers to use social supports and services is well documented in the literature (George & Gwyther, 1986; McCabe et al., 1995). Families often persist in providing care at the risk of jeopardizing their own physical and mental health (Demling & Bass, 1986; Fitting, Rabins, Lucas, & Eastham, 1986; George & Gwyther; Maritz).

It is our experience that family caregivers are more inclined to use community services as they become more educated about local resources and receive ongoing professional support to use these services.

Some training programs for primary care physicians that are designed to include lectures, seminars, case presentations, and use of social interventions in the treatment of AD can contribute a great deal toward improving the quality of life of both patient and care provider.

AVAILABLE COMMUNITY SERVICES

Governmental and nongovernmental private services are available in most communities in the United States to help with care of the elderly population. The Administration on Aging is a federal agency that oversees the Older American Act, which is responsible for providing services to the elderly population in the United States. Each state has an Area Agency on Aging (AAA) that provides services to the aged through their affiliations or branches at the community and municipal levels. Examples of services funded through AAA are nutrition programs, lunches at religious centers, Senior Centers, meals on wheels, transportation, and homemaker services (Eisdorfer, 1994).

Other services available to seniors include day care, home health care, partial hospitalization programs, assisted living facilities, and nursing homes with or without special care units. Adult day care centers provide a supervised environment, allowing the caregiver much needed respite while providing meaningful activity and socialization for AD patients. Many home health care agencies employ a variety of health care professionals to assist caregivers with providing service. Registered nurses who provide nursing care usually are available through agencies such as the Visiting Nurse Association. Hospital and home health social workers can help with referrals to appropriate agencies following an initial evaluation and often are available for counseling when necessary.

In addition to skilled care, home health agencies' staffs can assist with medication monitoring, take and record vital signs, and assist with the patient's personal care. Homemakers are able to help caregivers with general household duties, such as cleaning and doing the laundry, and are available through most home health agencies. The resources described in this section are available in many communities in the United States. These programs contribute a great deal to improving care of the AD patients and lifting at least some of the burden from the shoulders of their care providers. It is not uncommon to find a family unaware of these resources. The professional team providing treatment should assess the family's knowledge of support services and individualize a plan to help address each family's needs. Often those caregivers who are aware of services do not have the skills or resources to locate appropriate services. We as professionals should undertake the responsibility of counseling our patients and their families to use these resources.

It is important for care providers to recognize that they do not have to provide all necessary care alone to the point of exhaustion. The agencies and associations described earlier are excellent starting points when looking for health-related care. However, much of the work to care for AD patients does not require skilled professionals and can be provided by a support network. The benefits of attending support groups cannot be overemphasized. Support groups can help many distressed care providers who need support and guidance in providing care to their loved ones.

CAREGIVER ATTITUDES TOWARD COMMUNITY SERVICES

Caregivers, spouses, and other family members often are shocked and distressed after hearing the results of the diagnostic work. This time provides the opportunity for professionals to begin working with families to help them deal with clinical, psychosocial, financial, and legal problems associated with AD. Most families need at least some services but are reluctant to accept them partially because of continued denial, guilt feelings, and, to some extent, the acceptance of help being interpreted as weakness or inadequacy of the caregiver. Professionals should deal with these issues on an individual basis. Caregivers should be encouraged to accept help that is offered by family, friends, and various agencies in the community. In our experience (Kumar et al., 1990) a survey of caregivers indicated that caregivers welcome outside help provided it is not a complicated process and only a few people are involved. Caregivers, especially elderly spouses, are so overwhelmed by the physical, medical, and daily needs of their patient that they do not have the time or energy to think and plan for the needs of their patient or themselves. Intensive case management services often can help with the coordination of care for AD patients and are described in the next section.

CASE MANAGEMENT

Historically, there has been a lack of coordination of needed services, and care often has seemed haphazard and fragmented. Recently, there has been a tremendous growth of skilled professionals known as case managers. Case management is not a new concept. It has been used successfully for years with individuals requiring coordination of multiple services. It was used primarily in the provision of multidisciplinary care of the chronically mentally ill in both Europe and the United States. Case managers not only provide and coordinate care of AD patients living in the community, but also help in the evaluation of mental, physical, and financial needs of the patients and care providers. The case manager's role often includes contacting hospital emergency rooms, family practitioners, psychiatrists, internists, and other professionals whose services may be needed. They serve as the points of contact for patient(s) or care providers and help ensure a coordinated continuum of care.

Many case managers work under the auspices of home health care agencies and case coordination units. These agencies usually have nurses, social workers, and physical therapists to provide various types of medical and nursing services to patients. Some of the services provided by home health care agencies are reimbursable by third-party payers. The intervention by case managers and home health care agencies provides much needed services and possibly improves the quality of care of patients. It was evident from our study (described later in this chapter) that "in-home" evaluation and coordination of community care for AD patients significantly reduced the rate of admission to nursing homes (Kumar et al., 1990).

FINANCIAL AND LEGAL SERVICES

Ideally, couples or individuals should have completed estate planning and legal arrangements when they were enjoying their golden years. All too often, however, adequate financial planning has not occurred prior to the diagnosis of AD. The care of an Alzheimer's patient can be very costly. It is not uncommon to find families or spouses of AD patients in financial trouble because of lack of adequate planning and absence of legal management of their estate. Several factors need to be considered by families to assess their abilities to manage this costly disease.

It is imperative that professionals inform families of what to expect and link them with legal assistance to explore available options. Initially, families need to understand the illness and the corresponding decline in functional ability that accompanies the illness. This understanding is necessary to enable families to plan for potential medical and household expenses. Families need to explore the cost of medical care such as visiting nurses, medications, and physicians. Exploring the cost of respite care also should be encouraged. Commonly used respite services include general housekeeping, day care, nursing care, and someone to stay with the person on an as-needed basis. In addition, structural changes may need to occur to make the existing environment safe for the AD patient (e.g., installing grab bars, new locks, wheelchair ramps). These additional costs are not always anticipated and can be distressing to fixed income seniors. Families also should be encouraged to explore the cost of long-term care should this need arise as the illness progresses. The disease may progress to the point where the individual is no longer able to manage finances or give permission for necessary medical care.

If families have not considered financial planning, appropriate referrals should be made by the treatment team. Laws vary from state to state, but an elder law attorney should be suggested. Families could be directed to the National Academy of Elder Law Attorneys for a listing of attorneys in their geographical areas specializing in elder law. Elder law attorneys will be well versed in guardianship, living wills, and durable powers of attorney.

SAFETY ASSESSMENT AND STRUCTURAL MODIFICATION OF HOMES

As mentioned previously, it often is necessary to make structural changes to the existing home to meet the physical needs of a declining patient. In addition, minor changes in the environment often can make behavior management of the AD patient less difficult. It is important for the families of AD patients to seek expert advice to evaluate the safety and the convenience of the home to provide an accident-free environment. Often the mobility of AD patients and care providers is restricted due to arthritis or other medical problems. Homes should be evaluated, and necessary structural changes should be made in the bathroom, kitchen, and bedrooms to prevent falls. The main modifications required include safety lights, railings, and space to wander.

It is possible to find local agencies to help fund some of the minor structural changes in the AD patient's home. These minor structural changes not only improve the quality of life of patients, but improve the care provider's ability to continue to provide care at home for a longer time. These types of modifications can help to decrease the risk of premature institutionalization because of caregiver exhaustion.

HEALTH OF THE CARE PROVIDERS

The constant stress associated with care giving is well documented in the literature. Chronic fatigue, anger, guilt, frustration, and depression are common feelings reported by caregivers (Kiecolt-Glaser et al., 1987; Rabins, 1982; Zarit, Orr, & Zarit, 1985). The prevalence of depression in care providers ranges from 30% to 80% (Cohen & Eisdorfer, 1988; George & Gwyther, 1986). Caregivers have been called the "hidden patients" by some investigators, suggesting care giving duties may have negative effects on the health status of caretakers (Fengler & Goodrich, 1979). Caregivers report mental and physical health problems and a feeling of being overwhelmed as the reasons for institutionalization of their AD patient rather than the patient's level of illness (Colerick & George, 1986; Zarit et al., 1985). Caregivers receiving support from family, friends, and professionals report lower levels of burden and stress associated with caregiving. Development of community programs to support caregivers in the natural environment is essential. In addition, family physicians should be trained to monitor the health of the family in addition to the health of the AD patient.

The current literature is filled with studies describing the emotional and physical distress that is typical of AD caregivers. An important message to send to caregivers is the need to care for themselves in addition to their loved ones. Professionals need to impress upon caregivers how essential it is to remain healthy themselves. Basic stress management techniques can provide some balance in the caregiver's life (Tuebsing, 1985). Encourage caregivers to work at staying healthy with proper diet and exercises. Moderate exercise such as brisk walking can help reduce caregiver stress. In addition, it can burn off excess energy and encourage restful sleep in AD patients who are able to participate with caregivers. Advise caregivers to work at arranging personal time for themselves. Simple things like calling a friend or continuing a hobby can provide a much-needed break in the caregiver's day. Relaxation tapes, especially those involving classical music, can be very calming to both caregiver and patient (Epstein, 1989). Individuals who are religious should be encouraged to continue to pray, since the power of prayer for many is a source of comfort (Benson, 1992).

RESEARCH IN THE COMMUNITY CARE OF AD PATIENTS

Our professional experiences as clinicians in both clinic and research settings support the notion that informed and supported family members are able to function more effectively as caregivers when they are linked with appropriate community resources. Several years ago, we studied the effect of "in-home" evaluation and interventions provided to individuals with AD living with caregivers in the semirural midwestern community of Springfield, Illinois.

We hypothesized that linkage with existing community resources, timely case management, education about the illness, and appropriate medication management would increase the caregiver's ability to cope with the illness, thus resulting in fewer institutionalizations of community-residing AD patients.

To test this hypothesis, we randomly assigned 47 community-dwelling, dementia patient and care provider pairs to experimental and control groups after initial baseline evaluations in their homes. Patients and care providers in the experimental group received monthly contact with a member of the research team while the control group received no contact except for evaluation with research instruments every 6 months. During monthly home contacts, the research team provided education about the illness, assistance with problem solving, and supportive counseling as necessary. In addition to scheduled monthly contact from the research team, caregivers were instructed to call the geriatric nurse as often as needed. Topics addressed during monthly visits included a review of the symptoms of AD and effective behavioral management techniques for addressing each individual's concerns (Aronson, 1988; Mace & Rabins, 1991). In addition, nursing consultation included helping the caregiver conduct a safety evaluation of the home and suggest gradual changes to the environment to meet the progressing needs of each patient for both indoor and outdoor safety (Raschko, 1984; Ronch, 1989). The geriatric team completed regular functional assessments and educated caregivers with practical suggestions for assisting with bathing, grooming, toileting, dressing, eating, and nutrition. Communication patterns were routinely assessed. Steps to improve communication were addressed by the team as necessary with modeling and suggested readings (Carroll, 1990; Jarvik & Small, 1988). Much of the case management involved linking family care providers with existing medical and social service agencies.

Analysis of the data at a 24-month follow-up found that 52% (13/25) of the control group and only 23% (5/22) of the experimental group were admitted to nursing homes. This was a significant difference (see Figure 14.1).

Group demographic and clinical indicators were essentially equal. No significant differences were found between groups on any of the demo-

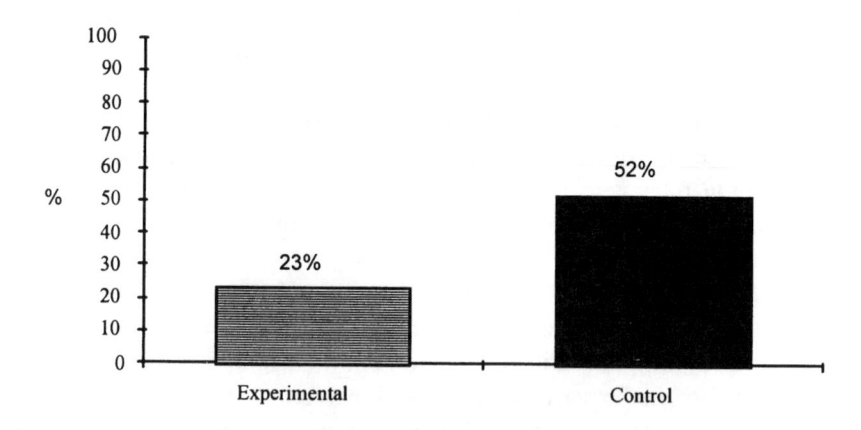

FIGURE 14.1 Nursing home admissions.
Source: From the study, "Community Care of Alzheimer's Disease." Supported by Illinois Department of Public Health, P. I. V. Kumar, 1987–1989.

graphic variables measured, including sex, age, duration of illness, education, caregiver age, and caregiver sex (see Table 14.1).

No significant differences were found between control and experimental group patients on any of the various neuropsychiatric scales at baseline

TABLE 14.1 Demographic Data on Patients and Care Providers of Two Groups

Item Description	Control ($n = 25$)	Experimental ($n = 22$)	Sig
Sex (M/F)	9/16	9/13	NS
Age	75.3 ± 7.1	77.2 ± 8.8	NS
Duration of illness	5.0 ± 2.7	5.1 ± 2.4	NS
Education	11.1 ± 3.1	10.1 ± 3.6	NS
Caregiver sex (M/F)	5/20	4/16	NS
Caregiver age	62.1 ± 13.1	63.7 ± 11.1	NS

Community care of Alzheimer's disease. Supported by Illinois Dept. of Public Health. P. I. V. Kumar, 1987–1989.

or at 24-month retesting. These findings verify equivalent severity of illness, psychiatric symptomatology, and level of functioning for both groups (see Table 14.2).

More than half of the control group was admitted to the nursing home after 2 years in the study, while less than a quarter of the experimental group was admitted to the nursing home during that same period. Further evaluation of the data yielded no clinical differences between individuals or caregivers of the patients admitted to nursing homes versus those remaining in the community (see Table 14.3).

Anecdotal information on these patients suggested that continuous support and information regarding agency standards and licensing did encourage caregivers to use help. Furthermore, encouraged "assertiveness" by professionals to ask friends and family for help seemed to give some caregivers "permission to request assistance." Caregivers did report that a feeling of "community support," including family, friends, and the research team, did build a hopeful attitude and increased their ability to manage effectively the illness in spite of continuing patient decline.

RELATIONSHIPS OF CARE PROVIDERS TO PATIENTS

The majority of care in our "In-home Care" study was provided by the spouses and daughters of the dementia patients. There was no significant difference between control and experimental groups concerning the rela-

TABLE 14.2 Baseline Neuropsychiatric Test Mean Scores for Control and Experimental Group Patients

Scales	Control ($n = 25$)	Experimental ($n = 22$)	Sig
Haycox	12.2 ± 10.7	13.2 ± 9.5	NS
Ham-D	7.9 ± 4.6	9.0 ± 3.5	NS
MMSE	15.6 ± 8.8	14.1 ± 7.4	NS
BPRS	37.6 ± 11.5	36.4 ± 6.6	NS
ADL	34.5 ± 12.6	36.3 ± 12.0	NS

Community care of Alzheimer's disease. Supported by Illinois Dept. of Public Health. P. I. V. Kumar, 1988–1990.

TABLE 14.3 Demographics of Patients Admitted to Nursing Homes and Patients Remaining in the Community

Item Description	Admission ($n = 18$)	Nonadmission ($n = 29$)	Sig
Age	76.0 ± 5.8	76.3 ± 9.0	NS
Sex (M/F)	6/12	12/17	NS
Duration of illness	5.6 ± 2.7	4.7 ± 2.4	NS
Education	10.1 ± 3.2	11.0 ± 3.4	NS
Number with spouse as caregiver	9 (50%)	15 (52%)	NS
Caregiver age	59.5 ± 12.3	65.0 ± 11.7	NS
Caregiver sex (M/F)	4/14	5/22	NS

Community care of Alzheimer's disease. Study supported by Illinois Department of Public Health. P. I. Vinod Kumar, 1987–1989.

tionship of the care provider to the patient, as shown in Figure 14.2. It has been suggested that the relationship of the care provider to the AD patient may be an important variable affecting the likelihood of admission to long-term care facilities, with spouses being less likely than children to admit their AD spouse to a nursing home. However, this was not evident in our study.

Although the level of depression measured in control and experimental caregiver groups in our pilot study did not differ significantly, approximately 80% of the study's caregivers scored in the depressed range as measured by the Zung Self-Rating Scale for Depression (Zung, 1965). A score of 50+ on this scale is indicative of depression. A breakdown of mean scores and ages of our caregiver population is shown in Table 14.4. The high incidence of depression scores prompted the research team to construct a survey to investigate caregivers' needs. Our primary goal was to assess what services the caregivers felt would help them cope with the stresses of caregiving. Listed next in order of occurrence are the types of services caregivers reported would be beneficial. Ninety-four percent of our sample returned completed surveys.

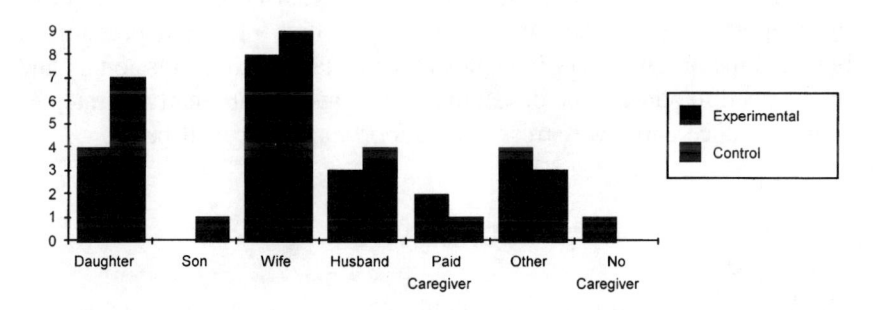

FIGURE 14.2 Caregiver relationship.
Source: From the study, "Community Care of Alzheimer's Disease." Supported by Illinois Department of Public Health, P. I. V. Kumar, 1987–1989.

1. individual supportive counseling and stress management techniques (70%);
2. more information about coping with patient behavior (64%);
3. help finding assistance with patient care (55%); and
4. more frequent visits from the research team (55%).

It is evident from the results of our pilot data that in-home interventions have a positive effect on the institutionalization rate of the cognitively impaired elderly person. It seems that the intervention provided in the "In-Home Care" study increased caregiver coping abilities enough to

TABLE 14.4 Caregiver Depression Scores

Age Group	%	Zung Mean Score
41–50	13	57.6
51–60	20	55.9
61–70	36	55
71–80	26	54
>80	5	58

Community care of Alzheimer's disease. Supported by the Illinois Dept. of Public Health. P. I. V. Kumar, 1987–1989.

deal with the tasks of caregiving, but were not extensive enough to improve the mental health of the care provider. The high rate of depression in both groups of caregivers indicates that mental health professionals and others need to address the development of low-cost alternative strategies to help reduce caregiver stress and support caregiver well-being.

SUMMARY

The first step toward providing quality community care involves a thorough evaluation of the patient and the care provider. The evaluation of the caregiver's understanding of Alzheimer's disease, knowledge of financial planning and available community resources should be completed. During and following this evaluation process, education about AD and the techniques for managing the illness should be provided to family members and care providers. Appropriate referrals and linkages should be made to existing community resources.

As suggested by Kumar et al. (1990) by our pilot data, these interventions can reduce the probability of premature admission of dementia patients to nursing homes. A coordinated family and community support system can help caregivers deal with the arduous task of caregiving. We feel this much-needed support will help improve the quality of life for both AD patients and care providers.

REFERENCES

Alzheimer's Disease Education and Referral Center. (1993). *Progress report on Alzheimer's disease.* Silver Spring, MD: Alzheimer's Disease Education and Referral Center.

Aronson, M. K. (1988). *Understanding Alzheimer's disease.* New York: Scribner's.

Benson, H., & Stuart, E. (1992). *The wellness book.* New York: Fireside.

Carroll, D. L. (1990). *When your loved one has Alzheimer's: A caregiver's guide.* New York: Harper and Row.

Chenowith, B., & Spencer, B. (1986). Dementia: The experiences of family caregivers. *The Gerontologist, 26,* 267–272.

Cohen, D., & Eisdorfer, C. (1988). Depression in family members caring for a relative with Alzheimer's disease. *Journal of the American Geriatric Society, 36,* 885–889.

Cohen, D., Hegarty, J., & Eisdorfer, C. (1983). The desk directory of social resources: A physicians' reference guide to social and community services for the aged. *Journal of the American Geriatrics Society, 31,* 338–341.

Colerick, E. J., & George, L. K. (1986). Predictors of institutionalization among caregivers of patients with Alzheimer's disease. *Journal of the American Geriatrics Society, 41,* 493–498.

Deimling, G., & Bass, D. (1986). Symptoms of mental impairment among elderly adults and their effects on family caregivers. *Journal of Gerontology, 41,* 778–784.

Eisdorfer, C. (1994). Community resources and the management of dementia patients. *Medical Clinics of North America, 4,* 869–875.

Epstein, G. (1989). *Healing visualizations: Creating health through imagery.* New York: Bantam.

Fengler, A. P., & Goodrich, N. (1979). Wives of elderly disabled men: The hidden patients. *The Gerontologist, 19,* 175–183.

Fitting, M., Rabins, P., Lucas, M., & Eastham, J. (1986). Caregivers for dementia patients: A comparison of husbands and wives. *Gerontologist, 26,* 248–252.

George, L. K., & Gwyther, L. P. (1986). Caregiver well-being: A multidimensional examination of family caregivers of demented adults. *Gerontologist, 26,* 253–259.

Jarvik, L., & Small, G. (1988). *Parentcare: A commonsense guide for adult children.* New York: Crown.

Kiecolt-Glaser, J., Glaser, R., Shuttleworth, E. C., Dyer, C. S., Ogrocki, P., & Speicher, C. E. (1987). Chronic stress and immunity in family caregivers of Alzheimer's disease victims. *Psychosomatic Medicine, 49,* 523–535.

Kumar, V., & Peterson, K. (1990). Update: Diagnosis and treatment of Alzheimer's disease. (Abstract). Lecture Presented at the Annual Meeting of the Hospital and Community Psychiatry Convention, October 1990, Denver, Colorado.

Mace, N., & Rabins, P. (1991). *The 36 hour day.* Baltimore: Johns Hopkins University Press.

McCabe, B. W., Sand, B. J., Yeaworth, R.C., & Nieveen, J. L. (1995). Availability and utilization of services by Alzheimer's disease caregivers. *Journal of Gerontological Nursing, 21,* 14–22.

Rabins, P. V., Mace, N. L., & Lucas, M. J. (1982). The impact of dementia on the family. *Journal of the American Medical Association, 248*(3), 333–335.

Raschko, B. (1984). *Housing interiors for the disabled and elderly.* New York: Van Nostrand Reinhold.

Ronch, J. (1989). *Alzheimer's disease: A practical guide for those who help others.* New York: Cross and Continuum.

Rovner, B. W., German, P. S., Broadhead, J., Morriss, R. K., Brant, L. J., Blaustein, J., & Folstein, M. F. (1990). The prevalence and management of

dementia and other psychiatric disorders in nursing homes. *International Psycho geriatrics, 2,* 13–24.
Tuebsing, D. (1981). *Kicking your stress habits.* Duluth: Whole Person Associates.
U.S. Department of Health and Human Services. (1990). *Guide to health insurance for people with medicare.* Baltimore, MD: Health Care Financing Administration.
Zarit, S., Orr, N., & Zarit, J. (1985). *The hidden victims of Alzheimer's disease: Families under stress.* New York and London: New York University Press.
Zarit, S. H., Reever, K. E., & Bach-Peterson, J. (1980). Relatives of the impaired elderly: Correlates of feelings of burden. *Gerontology, 20,* 649–655.
Zung, W. K. (1965). A self-rating depression scale. *Archives of General Psychiatry, 12,* 63–70.
Zung, W. K. (1967). Depression in the normal aged. *Psychosomatics, 8,* 287–292.

CHAPTER 15

Ethical and Medicolegal Issues in Alzheimer's Disease Treatment

**Panagiota V. Caralis
Edwin J. Olsen**

As our population ages, Alzheimer's disease (AD), which is well recognized to be an increased risk with aging, will become a significant public health concern. Currently, an estimated 4 million Americans are afflicted, and the cost of diagnosis, management, and caring for AD patients is estimated at over $80 billion annually (Selkoe, 1992). In the 21st century, 10 million Americans may be affected; 10.3% of people over 68 and 47.2% of those over 85 will suffer from this disease (Office of Technology Assessment, Congress of the United States, 1987).

With this background, it is understandable that research on AD has become a central concern. The National Institute on Aging, as well as other international funding agencies, have prioritized the urgent need for such research (Trent, 1989). The benefits of this research will go beyond the specific disorder and should provide new insights into genetic testing and quality of life issues for victims who suffer chronic diseases. Since no animal model currently exists, this research must be conducted on human subjects. The ethical and legal challenges of conducting research on vulnerable people and populations are among the most significant for investigators and biomedical research institutions today. The traditional concerns in biomedical research have been the protection of research subjects and the furtherance of scientific knowledge. Research with AD patients opens up new challenges for international codes of conduct and national and local laws governing research. This chapter will explore the most common ethical and legal dilemmas investigators and institutions encounter in AD research: (a) federal and state regulations and institutional review process; (b) assessment of competency and informed consent; (c) the use of proxy decision makers and advance directives; (d) guidelines on risk and benefit analysis and limitations on research.

HISTORICAL BACKGROUND AND CURRENT REGULATION OF RESEARCH

Ethical principles for the protection of human subjects in clinical research are now well recognized and rooted in the inherent worth of human life and the dignity of the individual. At the heart of all guidelines and regulations of biomedical research on human subjects has been the collective memory of previous horrific abuses and the potential for new ones, especially in vulnerable patient populations (e.g., the Nazi experiments, the Tuskegee syphilis study, the Willobrook hepatitis study). Many of the existing constraints on research come from knowledge of the Nazi atrocities committed in World War II. The Nuremberg Code formalized a worldwide acceptance of fundamental ethical obligations to respect the life and dignity of human subjects in biomedical research (Annas & Grodin, 1992). These ethical principles of respect for a person's beneficence (do good) and nonmaleficence (do no harm) and justice have been codified in national statutes and regulations. They help support self-autonomy, protect the vulnerable, and promote the welfare and equality of human subjects. Research ethics expanded significantly from the Nuremberg Code through the Helsinki Declaration in 1964 (revised by the World Medical Association in 1975 and 1983) and the World Health Organization Geneva Accord in 1982 (World Medical Association, 1984). The latter two provided guidelines for conduct of research and allowed for proxy consent and even a waiver of consent if in the subject's best interest.

In this country, the National Commission for Protection of Human Subjects of Biomedical and Behavioral Research published the Belmont

Report in 1978, which focused on the need for advance information on research methods, objectives, benefits, and risks to allow an informed choice (National Commission, 1978). Not every human subject can give a competent and voluntary consent to research. The commission believed that respect for people with diminished capacity, those who are not entirely free to choose, or those with heightened risk present special ethical problems in conducting research. Strict criteria are required to protect vulnerable subjects from potential harm. The commission specifically addressed research involving incompetent subjects (including infants and young children, the mentally disabled, the terminally ill, and the comatose individuals) and prescribed that special justification was required prior to conducting research on these individuals. Research is permissible only if it is of very low risk or has a direct prospect of therapeutic benefit for the subjects. Additionally, the commission prescribed that a third party should be appointed to take action on behalf of the subject, adhering to the subject's wishes to the greatest extent possible.

In 1983, the President's Commission for the Study of Ethical Problems in Medicine and Biomedical and Behavioral Research issued a report on the problems of conducting important studies in areas such as "Senile Dementia of the Alzheimer's type," resulting in the publication of federal regulations for the protection of human subjects (President's Commission, 1983; Department of Health and Human Services, 1983). Although the regulations permitted legally effective consent to include an "authorized representative of the subject," they remained vague as to the specific requirements for effecting proxy consent.

Since then, other national guidelines have been developed for conducting research with impaired human subjects (see Table 15.1). In 1985, the National Institutes of Health (NIH) instituted a trial policy for intramural programs (1986). It adopted the "Durable Power of Attorney for Clinical Center Research Protocols" as a legal instrument that could be executed prior to incapacity, appointing a proxy who could consider participation in research for the subject when the subject became decisionally incapacitated. The American College of Physicians' (ACP) position paper in 1989 endorsed advance consent to research participation, accepted proxy consent, and proposed Institutional Review Boards (IRBs) establish special protections for institutionalized subjects to fully protect against abuses (American College of Physicians, 1989). In 1993, the FDA guidelines included informed consent by a legally authorized representative (FDA "Informed Consent of Human Subjects" Guidelines, 1993). Despite the

TABLE 15.1 Guidelines for "Vulnerable Subjects" Research

Agency	Subjects Covered	Process	Advance Directives (AD)	Risk/Benefit Analysis	Incomplete Revocation of Previous Consent
NIH Clinical Center Policy 1985	"Cognitively impaired"	1. Guidelines for institute clinical review subpanels to review special cases 2. Surrogate consent 3. Proposed legislation for proposal review by ethics committee and to establish national ethics committee to oversee them	Restricted to appointment of durable power of attorney or court-appointed guardian Review of surrogate appointment through ethics consultation	Prohibits non-therapeutic research with more than minimal risk	Assent of subject is necessary

394

ACF Position Paper 1989	"Cognitively impaired, including Alzheimer's patients	1. Use of AD and proxy to carry out intent by supervising subject's participation 2. Local IRBs should develop special protections for institutionalized patients 3. National review board to review protocols which do not fit these guidelines	In cases with no AD, legally authorized proxy can consent using mixed SJ and BI standards*	Prohibits consent to non-therapeutic research with more than minimal risk Proxy may consent to therapeutic research if in patient's BI and patient would not have refused	Proxy must withdraw subject if continuation would cause "substantial distress"

(continued)

TABLE 15.1 (continued)

Agency	Subjects Covered	Process	Advance Directives (AD)	Risk/Benefit Analysis	Incomplete Revocation of Previous Consent
FDA Guidelines 1993	"Vulnerable subjects include...those incapable of giving consent"	Accepts "legally effective consent of subject or the subject's legally authorized representative"		IRBs must include one person primarily concerned with welfare of subjects	

*SJ = Substituted judgment.
*BI = Best interests.

national recognition and proliferation of writing regarding the subject, consistency and practical guides remain elusive. Compounding the problems for researchers are a variety of local practices, regulations, and state laws governing research with impaired subjects. Although most national experts emphasize the importance of local institutions and IRBs in providing specific protection for individual human subjects, they recognize the need to develop national consensus on ethical and legal prescriptions on research of vulnerable people and populations (Berg, 1996; Fletcher, Dommel, & Cowell, 1985).

Some of the issues of concern about the conduct of research involving AD patients are discussed next. These are of particular importance not only for IRBs and investigators evaluating and implementing protocols, but also for physicians and other health care professionals and the families caring for these patients.

ASSESSING COMPETENCY AND INFORMED CONSENT

Autonomy and individual consent are fundamental principles that allow competent persons to keep control of their health and research decisions. Ethical research and the principle of consent help to prevent abuse (President's Commission, 1982). This formal requirement evolved from the Anglo-American legal doctrine of informed consent and is universalized in the explicit process of IRB approval and written consent process. However, as in everyday medical practice, true informed consent to research requires vigilant safeguarding to avoid abuses. Numerous problems can interfere with a truly informed and voluntary consent, not the least of which is the complexity of the written forms and the desperate hope of patients and their families. For a full expression of autonomy, a patient must understand the information and be able to manipulate the information rationally, come to a decision on a voluntary basis, and be able to express that decision in some fashion (President's Commission, 1982). This may seem to be an incongruous notion for AD patients, in view of their deteriorating cognitive abilities. Indeed, dementia patients may have significant difficulties with the elements required for autonomous decision making. It should not be automatically assumed, however, that AD patients are not capable of making decisions about their health care.

Practicing physicians make assessments of decision-making capacity daily. Decisional capacity is not an "all-or-none" determination. Neither are the determinants of decision-making capacity for those of court-determined incompetence. In fact, "competence" is a legal concept, whereas "capacity" is a medical assessment and varies with each clinical situation (Appelbaum & Roth, 1982; Emanuel, 1993; Sprung & Winick, 1989). Although patients may not have the functional ability to handle legal or monetary matters, they may still have adequate capacity for decisions related to medical treatments. Numerous tests are used to assess capacity, ranging from simple communication to more objective screening analysis, such as the Folstein Mini-Mental State Exam (Folstein, Folstein, & McHugh, 1975; Roth, Meisel, & Lidz, 1977). The definitive test of decision-making capacity does not yet exist (High, 1992; Roth et al.; Stanley, Stanley, Guido, & Garvin, 1988).

Patient interviews, however, can follow practical guidelines that acknowledge that capacities are decision specific (ranging from simple, routine treatments to complex medical interventions with risk) and must be assessed several times in several settings. Patients can be asked to repeat the information or paraphrase it. They should be asked if they understand their role in the decision. The patients must grasp what the information means for them and place their own values on the risks, benefits, and options. What are the reasons for their choices? Alzheimer's patients, especially early in their disease, are certainly capable of making decisions. They may not know the date exactly, but if they understand the benefits and risks of the treatment contemplated, they are capable of giving consent. A sliding scale model has been proposed that applies increasingly stringent standards to different medical decisions, depending on their complexity (Drane, 1995). Other attempts at measuring decision-making functions have found that the understanding of information can be assisted with modified consent procedures designed to improve comprehension by the subjects (Tymchuk, Ouslander, Rahbar, & Fitten, 1988).

Inherent in the assessment of decision-making capacity are ethical pitfalls, which the physician must avoid. Physicians must be particularly vigilant of their paternalistic tendencies when caring for AD patients. Decisional capacity must be determined objectively and linked to the situation at hand. If patients refuse recommended treatment and choose a different course that threatens their well-being, this does not mean they are incompetent and their decision should be unilaterally ignored "for their own good." The reverse is also true: when an incompetent patient consents to treatment, this does not authorize the physician to treat. When a patient's condition has deteriorated and the patient is clearly incompetent to make decisions about treatments, a proxy decision maker must be found (Caralis, 1994). The perplexing issue is how to deal with AD patients who have borderline or fluctuating capacity to consent to research. In research, the protection of the patient is the primary concern. Some experts contend that mildly impaired elderly patients generally should be avoided since their consent may not be reliable (Rozovsky, 1990). Others have called for more rigorous assessment of decisional capacity coupled with consultation from the patient's physician and family (Cassel, 1988). Still others go beyond assessment of the capacity to consent to a determination of risk, applying a sliding scale approach, similar to that used for medical treatments, for example, the greater the risk or intrusiveness of the research, the greater the need for certainty of the subject's capacity to consent (Berg, 1996; Cassel). The ethics of allowing vulnerable patients to consent, even if capable, to greater than minimal risk research is debated (Cruzan, 1990). Presumably, subjects of questionable capacity should be excluded from such research.

PROXY CONSENT AND ADVANCE DIRECTIVES FOR RESEARCH

Specific planning for future contingencies of severe illness is important in patients with mild and moderate dementia because these patients will develop progressive cognitive impairment. When severe illness develops, the dementia may have advanced beyond the point where meaningful patient-based decisions can be made. A series of federal court decisions have focused on enhancing communication between physicians and patients. In the highly publicized *Cruzan* case (1990), the United States Supreme Court, while acknowledging incompetent patients' rights to treatment decisions, emphasized the importance of evidence of their wishes before allowing surrogates to authorize termination of life-sustaining treatment. The justices cited advance directives, both living wills and durable powers of attorney, as important documents that may help resolve legally and ethically troubling cases. All 50 states have enacted advance directive legislation, and as of December 1992, the federal Patient Self-Determination Act (PSDA) requires all hospitals, health maintenance organizations, and health care institutions receiving Medicare and Medicaid funds to: (a) provide information regarding patients' rights; (b) to ask patients if they have advance directives; (c) to document the patients' directives; (d) to provide education on these issues; and (e) to maintain institutional policies and procedures with regard to advance directives (Omnibus Reconciliation Act of 1990). Because media attention has placed a national spotlight on these issues, the public in general has become more knowledgeable of advance directives. Many believe that this process will benefit patients and physicians by improving the communication between them and by increasing the understanding about patients' ultimate wishes. Little is known, however, about the attitude of AD patients toward establishing advance medical directives. One study evaluated whether being asked specific questions about future severe illness was burdensome to patients with early dementia and measured the consistency of patients' responses (Finucane, Beamer, Roca, & Kawas, 1993). Although this was a small study, it revealed that asking patients with mild or moderate dementia to discuss their plans for possible future illness did not lead to any serious adverse consequences. All of the patients and their caregivers thought it was a "good idea" to talk about the subject, and 50% of both groups that were interviewed spontaneously reported enjoying the process. Although not all patients were able to decide, several patients had clear, constant, and convincing preferences regarding the use of life-support treatments during specific illnesses. Knowledge of the patient's personal values is always useful to physicians and families to assist them in making difficult treatment decisions.

The ACP and NIH policies have borrowed from the concept of advance directives for treatment decisions and advocated this process as a vehicle to enhance opportunities for impaired patients to participate in research. Potential AD subjects could execute advance directives while competent, allowing research to occur even if they became incapacitated. A duly appointed surrogate (durable power of attorney under the NIH policy) would be authorized to exercise consent under the patient's initial concurrence. The ACP position goes even further by recommending that in those instances where there is no advance directive and no proxy appointed by the subject, a legally authorized representative could act as a surrogate. The representative could be a guardian, a designated health care proxy, or a family member authorized by applicable law for medical treatment decisions. Specific guidelines are in each policy for indicating when surrogates could decide and when further protections are available (Table 15.1). Although not fully in agreement, these policies offer insight into the difficulties in developing an appropriate approach to research. Furthermore, it is unclear if State Advance Directive Laws apply to research, since they are drafted to address treatment concerns (Berg, 1996; De Renzo, 1993). Some states explicitly exclude guardians from consenting to research, or only allow consent with prior court approval. Some laws may allow surrogates to consent to life-saving potentially therapeutic experimental treatments, but not to nontherapeutic research. Other states either explicitly or implicitly allow surrogate consent to experimental treatment or research and may distinguish nontherapeutic treatments only if there is minimal risk. The process of using advance directives for research remains unresolved. Additionally, specific questions regarding its validity remain unanswered:

1. Can it be valid in advance of knowledge of a specific research protocol?
2. How can broadly written directives be interpreted to cover the subject's intent with particular protocols?
3. How should subsequent refusals by incapacitated patients be dealt with in light of their advanced consent when they were lucid?

Each state has laws that govern who and how substitute decisions for incapacitated patients are made. Surrogate or proxy decision makers range from hierarchical schemes of the next-of-kin, to court-appointed legal guardians, to durable powers of attorney for health care. Proxy deciders are accepted because society and the law have determined that they are generally the most knowledgeable about what the patient would have wanted (substituted judgment standard) and are the most likely to want what is best for the patient (best-interest standard) (Hardwig, 1990). In the social system, which values autonomy, often codified by laws, the patient's own directives (living wills) are considered better for proxy decisions, followed by substituted judgment and best-interest standards (durable power of attorney, next-of-kin) (Buchanan & Brook, 1989). Proxy decisions should be guided by what is known about the patients' wishes and values. Written documents are most helpful, but remembered conversations about treatment preferences under various conditions are useful and allow the proxy to "step into the shoes" of the patient and decide as the patient would have decided. Lacking information about the patient's preferences, the proxy should act to weigh the burdens and benefits of treatment in the patient's best interests. The ethical dilemmas related to proxy medical decision making in incapacitated patients are common

(Emanuel & Emanuel, 1992; Freer, 1993; Gutheil & Appelbaum, 1982). The family or caregiver's role is so essential to the care of AD patients that it is difficult to separate the interests of each. Physicians must be aware that proxy decisions for AD patients may involve multiple interest layers, represent multiple stakeholders, and may not be patient centered. Into this complex milieu step the proxy decision makers for research. There are few guidelines and many unanswered questions to guide researchers and proxies through the ethical difficulties related to proxy decisions (Miller, 1982).

The first question is, who would be the appropriate surrogate decision maker for research? Some state statutes, when there is no advance directive, designate a hierarchy of decision makers (ranging from close family and next-of-kin to close friends). Should the presumption favoring family and next-of-kin consent be regularized for research decision making when no other has been specified? It would seem that they are in the best position to know the patient's values and desires. NIH policy recommends that a court-appointed guardian be sought on such occasions for greater "legitimacy." Regardless of who the surrogate decision makers are, there need to be guidelines for the standards they apply to make their decisions: pure substituted judgment, best interests, or a hybrid of the two. Substituted judgment allows surrogates to give voice to the incompetent subject's already expressed consent or refusal. Both the ACP and NIH policies allow research in this context. If there is no previous evidence of a patient's willingness to consent to specific research, both policies still allow research but provide different additional requirements. The NIH policy requires ethics committee consultation to ensure the families' understanding. Others propose oversight of the proxy consent process by a disinterested third party, such as a "consent auditor" appointed by the IRB (Bierbaum, 1991; Dworkin, 1987; Fletcher et al., 1985). The ACP proposal permits use of other evidence of what a patient's wishes would be and only permits consent to research that is in the patient's best interest. Thus the use of the best-interest standard would be limited to previously competent subjects who have left no specific evidence or always to incompetent patients (Berg, 1996; Cruzan, 1990). Others have called for the use of national review committees (American College of Physicians, 1989). In some instances, these committees would function purely as advocates of the impaired subjects, others, in contrast, would act to endorse or prohibit protocols. What roles local IRBs would have in this context have not been worked out.

SPECIAL CIRCUMSTANCES FOR RESEARCH ON VULNERABLE GROUPS; RISK AND BENEFIT ANALYSIS

Traditional ethical principles require justifications before research is conducted on vulnerable subjects. In general, there is consensus that participation of vulnerable patients in protocols involving greater than minimal risk without the possibility of direct therapeutic benefit is not permissible (American College of Physicians, 1989; Berg, 1996; Gostin, 1991; National Institutes of Health, 1986). It is felt that although this research may provide good for the community and provide benefit by finding a cure for the disease, prohibition protects vulnerable patients. Our societal ethic has placed particular importance on individual rights. Although overly strict ethical and legal limits on research of vulnerable patients may be "paternalistic" and "inhibitory" of progress, they provide consistent protections.

The extent of protection afforded cognitive impaired subjects should depend on the balance of the risk of harm and the likelihood of therapeutic benefit (National Commission for the Protection of Human Subjects, 1978). Much like the sliding scale assessments of decision-making capacity, the greater the risk and the less the potential for therapeutic benefit, the greater the protections necessary. When research involves minimal risk and there is a potential for direct therapeutic benefit if the patient is competent, no further protections are required, even if the patient is incompetent or incapable of executing a durable power of attorney. The NIH policy allows next-of-kin to act as surrogates following consultation with a bioethicist or ethics committee. The ACP policy also would allow a surrogate to consent to therapeutic research if participation is in the patient's best interest. It recommends that the surrogate not consent to any research the subject would have refused or to any nontherapeutic research presenting more than minimal risk. Others have recommended that as risk increases, in light of potential therapeutic benefit, local IRBs should take more active oversight roles in assessing competency, adequacy of the consent process, education of proxy decision makers, and appropriateness of risk and benefit balance (Berg, 1996; Cassel, 1988; High, 1992; Robertson, 1982). IRBs can improve the consent process in a variety of ways (special educators, customized consent forms, video consent) and take additional steps to ensure noncoerced recruitment, adequate understanding, and protection of cognitively impaired subjects (Benson, Roth, &

Winslade, 1985; Robertson). Some IRBs have taken specific steps requiring investigators to adhere to certain guidelines to provide local review. As an example, the Miami Veterans Administration Medical Center Policy is as follows:

1. The Miami VAMC Human Studies Subcommittee is concerned about protection of research subjects who are members of "vulnerable populations." These are generally psychiatric, geriatric, emergency and pediatric patients. Your study includes subjects from at least one of these groups. It is especially important that the following precautions be taken:

I. *Determination of competence.* It is necessary that subjects be competent to consent to participate in the study. If you are in doubt about an individual's competence it might be necessary to obtain a professional consultation to assess competence and/or to seek consent from a valid surrogate or proxy. Note that competence is not a global concept and that competence in one aspect of life does not imply competence in another; and that incompetence in one area does not necessarily imply incompetence in others.

II. *Providing sufficient information.* It is vital that any documents and conversations explaining the study and its risks be easily understandable *and* that the subjects in fact understand what they have been told, or that their surrogates do. This means that all documents, especially the informed consent form, must be written simply and clearly. Also, mere presentation and signing of a form is generally regarded as insufficient for informing subjects about a study: it is also necessary to talk with them about it and make it easy for them to ask and receive answers to their questions, especially about risks of participation.

III. *Elimination of coercion or manipulation.* Few if any researchers would intentionally force or trick a subject into participation in a research protocol. Nevertheless, it is possible (perhaps because of disparities in social status or education, or mistaken fear of consequences of refusal) for potential subjects to be intimidated into thinking they have an obligation to participate in a study. It is imperative that investigators and subjects or their surrogates be aware that consent must be freely given. Researchers must always be mindful of the potential conflicts that arise when one's patients are (potential) research subjects.

CONCLUSIONS

As we enter the 21st century, the growth of the elderly population, the costs of care, and the need for advances of medical science and technology will require the development of a clear framework of ethical and legal principles for research on AD patients. The rules of conduct should balance the need to protect vulnerable patients and the need to provide them the benefit of therapeutic innovation. We need to continue to refine our efforts to assess competency. We can further the ethical principle of autonomy and respect for individual rights in AD research by facilitating the ability of patients who are early in their disease and still capable of providing consent, even for future research, through Advance Directives. We must further the capabilities of proxy decision makers through better education, use of research auditors, or advocates to assist them in making research decisions. IRBs must develop institution-specific processes to monitor research and ensure that participation is appropriate. As scientific zeal and social pressure requires research and investigators to cure the disease and reduce the suffering of those afflicted, special care on the part of all of us is required to meet the ethical challenges and to establish research goals that are consistent with reasoned, compassionate medical care and that respect the inherent dignity of human beings.

REFERENCES

American College of Physicians. (1989). Cognitively impaired subjects. *Annals of International Medicine, 3,* 843–883.

Annas, G., & Grodin, M. (Eds.). (1992). *The Nazi doctors and the Nuremberg Code: Human rights in human experimentation.* New York: Oxford University Press.

Appelbaum, P., & Roth, L. (1982). Clinical issues in the assessment of competency. *American Journal of Psychiatry, 138,* 1462–1487.

Benson, P., Roth, L., & Winslade, W. (1985). Informed consent in psychiatric research: Preliminary findings from an ongoing investigation. *Social Science and Medicine, 20,* 1331–41.

Berg, J. W. (1996). Legal and ethical complexities of consent with cognitively impaired research subjects: Proposed guidelines. *Journal of Law, Medicine and Ethics, 24,* 18–35.

Bierbaum, R. (1991). Doctor proposes new ethics protocol for Alzheimer's research. *Canadian Medical Association Journal, 144*(3), 335–338.

Buchanan, A. E., & Brook, D. W. (1989). *Deciding for others: The ethics of surrogate decision making.* Cambridge: Cambridge University Press.

Caralis, P. (1994). Ethical and legal issues in the care of Alzheimer's patients. *Medical Clinics of North America, 78*(4), 877–893.

Cassel, C. K. (1988). Ethical issues in the conduct of research in long-term care. *Gerontologist, 28*(Suppl., June), 90–96.

Cruzan v. Director, Missouri Department of Health, 497 U.S. 261 (1990).

Department of Health and Human Services. *Rules and regulations for the protection of human research subjects*, 45 C.F.R. §46 (1983), at 101–409.

De Renzo, E. (1993). Surrogate decision-making for severely cognitively impaired research subjects: The continuing debate. *Cambridge Quarterly of Healthcare Ethics, 3,* 543.

Drane, J. (1995). The many faces of competency. *Hastings Center Report, 15,* 17–21.

Dworkin, G. (1987). Law and medical experimentation of embryos, children and others with limited legal capacity. *Monash University Law Review, 13,* 189–208.

Emanuel, E. J., & Emanuel, L. L. (1992). Proxy decision-making for incompetent patients: An ethical and empirical analysis. *Journal of the American Medical Association, 267,* 2067–2071.

Emanuel, L. (1993). Advance directives: What have we learned so far? *Journal of Clinical Ethics, 4,* 8–16.

FDA "Informed consent of human subjects" guidelines, 21 C.F.R. §50 (1993), at 20–48.

Finucane, T. E., Beamer, B. A., Roca, R. P., & Kawas, C. H. (1993). Establishing advance medical directives with demented patients: A pilot study. *Journal of Clinical Ethics, 4,* 51–54.

Fletcher, J. C., Dommel, F. W., Jr., & Cowell, D. D. (1985). Consent to research with impaired human subjects. *Institutional Review Board, 7,* 1–6.

Folstein, M., Folstein, S. E., & McHugh, P. R. (1975). The "Mini-Mental State": A practical method for grading the cognitive state of patients for the clinician. *Journal of Psychiatric Research, 2,* 189–198.

Freer, J. (1993). Decision-making in an incapacitated patient. *Journal of Clinical Ethics, 4,* 55–58.

Gostin, L. (1991). Ethical principles for the conduct of human subject research: Population-based research and ethics. *Law, Medicine and Health Care, 19*(3–4), 191–201.

Gutheil, T. G., & Appelbaum, P. S. (1982). Substituted judgment: Best interests in disguise. *Hastings Center Report, 13,* 8–11.

Hardwig, J. R. (1990). What about the family? The role of family interests in medical treatment decisions. *Hastings Center Report, 20,* 5–10.

High, D. (1992). Research with Alzheimer's disease subjects: Informed consent and proxy decision-making. *Journal of the American Geriatric Society, 40,* 950–957.

Melnick, V. L., Dubler, N. N., Weisbard, A., & Butler, R. N. (1984). Clinical research in senile dementia of the Alzheimer type: Suggested guidelines addressing the ethical and legal issues. *Journal of the American Geriatrics Society, 32,* 531–536.

Miller, B. (1982). Autonomy and proxy consent. *IRB: A Review of Human Subjects Research, 4*(10), 1–7.

National Commission for the Protection of Human Subjects of Biomedical and Behavioral Research. (1978). *The Belmont Report: Ethical principles and guidelines for the protection of human subjects in research.* Washington, DC: U.S. Government Printing Office.

National Institutes of Health, Clinical Center Policy. (1986). *Research involving impaired human subjects: Clinical center policy for the consent process.* Bethesda, MD: National Institutes of Health.

Office of Technology Assessment, Congress of the United States. (1987). *Losing a million minds: Confronting the tragedy of Alzheimer's disease and other dementias.* Washington, DC: U.S. Government Printing Office.

Omnibus Reconciliation Act of 1990, Pub. L. No. 101-508.

President's Commission for the Study of Ethical Problems in Biomedical and Behavioral Research. (1983). *Implementing human research regulations: The adequacy and uniformity of federal rules and their implementation.* Washington, DC: U.S. Government Printing Office.

President's Commission for the Study of Ethical Problems in Medicine and Biomedical and Behavioral Research. (1982). *Making health care decisions: The ethical and legal implications of informed consent on the patient-practitioner relationship* (Vol. 2). Washington, DC: U.S. Government Printing Office.

Robertson, J. (1982). Taking consent seriously: IRB intervention in the consent process. *IRB: A Review of Human Subjects Research, 4*(5), 1–5.

Roth, L., Meisel, P., & Lidz, C. W. (1977). Tests of competency to consent to treatment. *American Journal of Psychiatry, 134,* 279–284.

Rozovsky, F. A. (1990). *Consent to treatment: A practical guide* (2nd ed.). Boston: Little, Brown.

Selkoe, D. J. (1992). Alzheimer's disease: New insights into an emerging epidemic. *Journal of Geriatric Psychiatry, 25,* 211–227.

Sprung, C. L., & Winick, B. J. (1989). Informed consent in theory and practice: Legal and medical perspectives on the informed consent doctrine and a proposed reconceptualization. *Critical Care Medicine, 17,* 1346–1354.

Stanley, B., Stanley, M., Guido, J., & Garvin, L. (1988). The functional competency of elderly at risk. *Gerontologist, 28*(Suppl.), 53–58.

Trent, B. (1989). Alzheimer's research: Physicians begin to tread in an ethical minefield. *Canadian Medical Journal, 140*(6), 726–728.

Tymchuk, A. J., Ouslander, J. G., Rahbar, B., & Fitten, J. (1988). Medical decision-making among elderly people in long-term care. *Gerontologist, 28*(Suppl.), 59–63.

World Medical Association Declaration of Helsinki. (1964). *Recommendations guiding medical doctors in biomedical research involving human subjects.* World Health Organization and Council for International Organizations of Medical Sciences. (1982). *Proposed international guidelines for biomedical research involving human subjects.* (Reprinted in *Medical ethics declarations, 1984 World Medical Journal, 31*, 4.)

CHAPTER 16

Future Directions for the Research in Alzheimer's Disease

Vinod Kumar
Carl Eisdorfer

Alzheimer's disease (AD) is a complex, heterogeneous, neurodegenerative disorder. In this volume, experts in the field focus on issues ranging from etiology through diagnosis and treatment, point to tremendous strides in understanding the pathophysiology, clinical presentation, therapeutics, and effect of this illness on family members and the society. Despite the great increase in knowledge that has occurred during the past decade, we have not yet been able to define its etiology nor successfully prevent, cure, or slow the course of this illness.

The foci of the research in AD are changing. It is noteworthy that in the United States the National Institute of Aging, which supports much of the research in AD, has begun to pay attention to clinical issues related to the disease. Until 5 years ago, virtually all of the efforts of this crucial agency were devoted to basic research related to the etiology and pathophysiology of the illness. At the present, the National Institutes of Health (NIH) is supporting three multicenter initiatives:

1. Drug Discovery Units;
2. Consortium of Alzheimer's Disease Treatment Units; and
3. Consortium of the Intervention at the Family and Care Provider Level, now referred to as REACH (Research Enhancing Caregiver Health).

These efforts in clinical research will answer some questions that may be beneficial to our patients and their families in the immediate future. An estimate of the money spent on AD research at the present in the United States should be at least a half billion dollars per year from various sources, but not even 10% of that money is spent on research related to the clinical treatment of the millions of patients and their families. There is a pressing need for the development of new treatments for the AD patient and for research into the psychosocial and behavioral interventions to improve the quality of life of patients and care providers. To date, much of the research related to the treatment of AD has been sponsored by the pharmaceutical industry in search of new medications and this, in view of the profit potential of an effective drug treatment for disease. From this background, we will suggest a research agenda for the next century; for convenience, we have divided this chapter into several sections related to distinguishable bodies of research.

EPIDEMIOLOGICAL STUDIES

Epidemiological studies focus not only on the incidence and prevalence of AD in various populations, as described in chapter 1 of this volume, but also on the possible risk factors such as genetic, head injury, alcoholism, high aluminum levels, depression, and educational achievement. It is important for us to study these factors among the various ethnic groups. Such studies will provide the opportunity to assess the contributions of various risk factors to the genesis of the illness and may uncover new factors not yet appreciated, for example, education, sex interactions, paternal age, and diet.

GENETICS OF ALZHEIMER'S DISEASE

There have been tremendous advances in understanding the genetics of AD, as discussed by Dr. Matsuyama in chapter 4. We know that at least four chromosomes (21, 19, 14, 1) and several genes are involved in AD, related primarily to the development of amyloid plaque formation. The exact mechanisms of these genes, producing pathophysiological changes in AD patients, are still under investigation as is the comparative role of plaques opposed to tau protein and neurofibrillary tangle.

The reports of one new gene or chromosome linked to AD always raise our hopes of finding a new mechanism to prevent and treat, but the issue is far more complex. The complexity of genetic research becomes apparent when one considers Familial Alzheimer's disease (FAD) as a subset of Alzheimer's disease and contrasts this with sporadic, late-onset disorder. The genetic mechanisms are focused upon the mechanisms leading to the formation of amyloid precursor protein (APP), eventuating into so-called senile or amyloid plaques believed to be pathonomic of the disease. Ongoing research in this field will be directed not only to finding other genes and chromosomes but also to understanding the mechanisms that are consequences of these genetic structures. This type of research is not only crucial for our understanding of the substrata of AD, but it contains the promise of leading to medication that may help stop the progression or even prevent the disease. It also contains the possibility that we will significantly improve our understanding of the nature of AD. Eisdorfer and Wilkie (1995) have discussed the possibility that AD represents a syndrome and that there are different etiologies suggesting that disaggregation of the disease may lead to more precise diagnosis and treatment strategies.

ETIOLOGY AND PATHOGENESIS OF ALZHEIMER'S DISEASE

Dr. Wisniewski and colleagues have provided an overview of the etiology and pathogenesis of AD in chapter 2. Recent understanding of the possible role of amyloid precursor protein in AD has been encouraging. Two different forms of Aβ (nonfibrillar Aβ and fibrillar Aβ) seem to have different cellular origins. The nonfibrillar amyloid plaques appear to be produced by neurons, whereas microglia perivascular and muscle cells appear to produce fibrillar amyloid (Wisniewski & Wegiel, 1995). Aβ is secreted as a product of proteolytic cleavage of βAPP, and several forms of βAPP are generated by alternative splicing of mRNA from the single gene on chromosome 21 (Ashall & Goat, 1994). Further research is needed to understand the APP secretion in normal humans and the point at which it becomes abnormal. This understanding already has increased enthusiasm in basic scientists that we may be able to control APP secretions and subsequently abnormal production and aggregation of Aβ in AD brains. It also may be that some of the cholinesterase inhibitors modify the APP secretion (Giacobini, personal communication, 1996). This, in turn, may result in the slower progression of the illness; however, there are as yet no convincing clinical data to support this hypothesis. Once again, it is clear that an understanding of the pathogenesis of AD is a significant area for the effects of new compounds on APP expression, abnormal Aβ production, and aggregation of Aβ.

The efficacy of inflammatory medications in AD has received some attention in the past 5 years, but the time of onset of purported inflammatory response in AD patients and its cause or effect in the pathogenesis of AD is not well understood. This represents another possible research venue of interest not only in patients but in at-risk relatives of AD patients compared to a non-at-risk population. Since it is not a difficult task to control the inflammatory process by several steroidal and nonsteroidal preparations, its effect on the course of AD could be valuable. This raises another significant area of investigation, namely, the course of the disease and what factors may influence this course.

The role of increased blood level of aluminum in AD has never been proven to be a contributing factor in the cause or progression despite much peripheral information. Other data suggest that head injury also may be a risk factor for AD, and it is interesting to note that none of the environmental and dietary risk factors gets mentioned in the literature. We should be vigilant in studying such environmental and psychosocial risk factors that may help us to understand the disease process, since not every person with a strong genetic predisposition or even brain changes indicative of AD will develop the cognitive dysfunctions associated with AD. Those who will develop the illness are likely to have some other predisposing factors. There are a number of studies suggesting that little or no education, particularly among women, may be a risk factor or that higher education may protect a person from developing AD. This finding is very interesting and creates a new area for research. We do not know whether education at early age is of more significance than education gained at a later age. Is it useful to continue educational activities after retirement? Are there definitive biological processes involved in learning that are preventing the disease process? Does early stimulation have a lifelong protective effect on us? There clearly is brain reserve capacity, a significant concept that has implications for other disorders as well as AD. While we are considering genetics, protein molecules, and transport mechanisms, we also should devote resources to evaluating the significance and role of other possible risk factors that may be affecting the onset or course of AD. The role of depression opens up the issue of subsets of AD and the role of later maternal age but younger paternal age again leads to questions of genetic abnormalities as yet poorly understood.

Clinical Diagnosis and Intervention Research

Even in the absence of knowledge regarding exact etiology, it is imperative for us to develop simpler, more cost-sensitive diagnostic measures and new treatments to improve cognition and behavioral symptoms associated with AD. Strides have been made in developing drugs to treat memory deficits in AD patients, and these efforts have resulted in the approval of Tacrine (COGNEX) by the FDA in 1993 and approval of E2020 (Aricept) in 1996, and probably of ENA713 (Exelon) in 1997. All of these drugs are able to help at least some of the patients (see chapter 12 by Kennedy). In the instances of E2020 (Pfizer/Eisai) and ENA713 (Sandoz), they have fewer side effects than Tacrine. However, these medications are largely stabilizing and questionable neuroprotective agents, and the need for medications with greater efficacy remains.

Several drug trials are in progress to evaluate the efficacy of other types of medications, for example, antioxidants (vitamin E, deprenyl, idebenon), anti-inflammatory, and other neuroprotective agents in hopes of slowing down the progression of the illness and possibly being able to prevent or delay the onset of the illness. The recent drug research focusing on the treatment of the symptoms of AD has been challenging in view of the variable albeit progressive course of the illness. Even a modest improvement in symptoms or slowing the course of the illness may be very expensive. Although we can do Apo E typing and can identify other genes involved in FAD, the expense is high, the probability of disease expression is uncertain, and we do not have the drugs to prevent the illness in the at-risk population at this time. However, it is encouraging to know that the next few years will see the discovery and development of the compounds designed to prevent AD among those at high risk.

Virtually every AD patient manifests psychiatric or behavioral symptoms requiring specific treatments during the course of the illness. The most common psychiatric symptoms and syndromes include depression, psychosis, agitation, wandering, aggressiveness and sleep problems (see chapters 9 and 10 by Dr. Myers and Dr. Thadlake). The etiology and treatments of symptoms and syndromes are not well understood. Indeed, as we suggested earlier, it is not clear whether they represent subtypes of the disease. Future research should answer the questions regarding the comparative efficacy and tolerability of various medications and of nonpharmacologic interventions. Of particular relevance is the effect of social and environmental factors on the symptomatology and course of illness, and such outcomes as family distress and the utilization of short-term and long-term care institutions.

The need for research into treatment programs affecting the psychiatric and behavioral symptoms of the AD patient is critical since these are the most frequently identified issues in caregiver depression, probability of institutionalization, and virtually by definition of the quality of life of the patient and those close to the patient.

There appears to be a tendency both in the government and in the pharmaceutical industry to put research into ongoing clinical care on the back burner. While this is understandable, given the limited economic perspective once drugs are approved, it seems crucial, perhaps by government agencies in partnership with the industry, to organize and fund joint protocols to answer important clinical management questions faced by the patients' families and clinicians in their everyday practices. This is particularly relevant in view of the long-term changes occurring with the disease and the increasing consequences as the disease progresses. Since most current medications are symptomatic (i.e., improve cognition and behavior), an understanding of the course of the illness becomes even more crucial because cognition and behaviors continue to deteriorate, and as the disease progresses, the effectiveness of the medications disappears. Eisdorfer and Wilkie (1995) have suggested that the course of the illness may be reliable to subtype, and we need to establish parameters of the disease progression (the course of the illness needs to be established more firmly with an appreciation of concurrent mediating risk factors and other variables).

There is, by now, an extensive literature on the effect of caregiving (see chapter 13 by Dr. Cohen) on the caregiver, including depression, use of psychotropic medication effects, on physical health, including the immune function. While new research initiatives are under way, it should be recognized that there is no clearly demonstrated intervention that has served to ameliorate caregiving distress.

Studies of direct behavioral intervention with Alzheimer patients, including cognitive methods, control of environmental stimulation, and contingency management approaches, are needed.

There also is a need to continue to increase our efforts in the area of service research related to the management of AD patients in the community and nursing home. The initiation of OBRA regulations has had the salutary effect of reducing overmedication with neuroleptics and the overuse of physical restraints, but has done little to help establish positive treatment parameters. This type of research may provide improved critical pathways to manage these patients in various settings that will not only save money but also improve the quality of life of the patient and care provider.

In closing, one overriding issue is noteworthy: Increasingly, there are data that support the idea that AD is an eponym that includes several subtypes of conditions. As Eisdorfer has proposed, the conditions for assessing the heterogeneity of a phenomenologically (i.e., signs and symptoms) appearing state could be tested by showing variations in *Etiology, Risk Factors, Treatment Specificity, Clinical Course,* and *Outcome*. The study of the heterogeneity of AD is imperative for predicting the course of the illness and the response to differing treatment strategies. It will help clinicians to answer the commonly asked question after diagnosis, "What should we expect now and for how long?" Unfortunately, we do not have the exact answers to this question.

REFERENCES

Ashall, F., & Goat, A. M. (1994). Role of the β-amyloid precursor protein in Alzheimer's disease. *Trends in Biochemistry and Science, 19,* 42–46.

Eisdorfer, C., & Wilkie, F. (1995). The dementias of Alzheimer's and AIDS. In S. H. Koslow, R. S. Murthy, & G. V. Coelho (Eds.), *Decade of the Brain: India/U.S.A. research in mental health and neurosciences* (pp. 127–137). Rockville, MD: National Institute of Mental Health.

Wiesniewski, H. M., & Wegiel, J. (1995). Commentary—Do neurofibrillary tangles initiate plaque formation or is it β-amyloiclosis that leads to N.F.T. pathology. *Neurobiology Aging, 16,* 341–343.

Index

ABT-418 therapy, 332
Abuse and violence in families, 368–370
Acetyl coenzyme A in acetylcholine synthesis, 302, 305
Acetyl group donors, therapeutic effects of, 305–306
Acetyl-L-carnitine therapy, 306
　in memory problems, 265–269
Acetylcholine, 298–299
　compounds promoting release of, 306–307
　deficiency in AD, 60, 64–65
　medications affecting synthesis and release of, 303–307
　muscarinic receptors, 319–328. See also Muscarinic receptors
　nicotinic receptors, 329–332. See also Nicotinic receptors
　synthesis of, 302–303
Acetylcholinesterase, 299–300, 307–308
　in Alzheimer's disease, 310–313
　inhibitors of, 303, 313–319, 333
　in neuritic amyloid plaques, 311
　in normal humans, 308–310
Activities of Daily Living tests, 126
Acute phase proteins in AD, 40–41, 221
Administration on Aging, 378
β-Adrenergic blockers in behavioral problems, 257–258
Advance directives for research, 399–400
African-Americans
　neuropsychological assessment of, 159, 162
　prevalence of dementia in, 11
Age
　and depression in AD, 235
　maternal, at birth of child, and occurrence of AD, 13
　and neuropsychological assessment scores, 158
　as risk factor for AD, 9
Aggressive behavior in AD, 136
Agitation in AD, 134, 248
　assessment of, 250–251
Alaproclate in memory problems, 266, 269–270
Alcohol consumption as risk factor for AD, 17
Aluminum
　in neurofibrillary tangles, 73
　role in AD pathogenesis, 18–19, 76–77, 113, 412
Alzheimer's Disease Assessment Scale, 239
American College of Physicians guidelines for "vulnerable subjects" research, 395, 400
γ-Aminobutyric acid neurons colocalized with somatostatin, 60, 66
Amygdala, cholinergic innervation of, 300
Amyloid-β, 69–71, 215
　accumulation in neuropils, 32
　complex with Apo E, 36
　decreased levels in cerebrospinal fluid, 71

417

fibrillar, 32, 33–36, 411
iron affecting, 77
neurotoxicity of, 38–39
nonfibrillar, 32, 411
precursor protein, 32, 33, 69, 215, 412
  abnormal cellular processing of, 332
  derivatives in plasma and CSF, 216–221
  gene mutations, 42, 68, 96–99
  and related APLP1 protein, 101
soluble, 33
vascular, 34, 35
Amyloid component P, 35, 41
  in blood and CSF, 221
  in plaques, 40
Amyloid plaques, 32, 215
  cholinesterases in, 311
  diffuse, 34, 215
  fibrillized, 33–36
  neuritic, 33–34, 57, 215
Angular gyrus syndrome, 130
α_1-Antichymotrypsin
  in amyloid plaques, 40, 41
  in blood and CSF, 221
Anticonvulsants in behavioral problems, 254, 258–259
α_1-Antitrypsin
  in amyloid plaques, 40
  in blood and CSF, 221
Aphasia, tests of, 155
Apolipoprotein E
  cerebrospinal fluid levels in AD, 221
  complex with amyloid-β, 36
  e4 allele association with AD, 13–14, 32, 42, 68, 76, 101–102, 221
    and parietal metabolic deficits, 195
    and right hippocampal atrophy, 186
  genotypes of, 101, 119
  role in AD pathology, 72
Apoptosis, and cell loss in AD, 38–39
Arecoline therapy, 326
Argyrophilic grain disease, 128
Aricept therapy, 315–316, 413
Assisted-living facilities, 367, 378

Behavioral disorders, 247–260, 414

assessment tools in, 137
behavioral therapy in, 252–253
clinical importance of, 248
computed tomography in, 181
diagnosis of, 250–251
etiology of, 251
medications in, 253–260
negative effects of, 249–250
prevalence of, 248–249
psychiatric hospitalization in, 260
treatment of, 251–260
Behavioral therapy
  in behavioral problems, 252
  in depression, 240–241
Belief systems of family caregivers, 358–359
Benzodiazepines in behavioral problems, 256–257
Beta-adrenergic blockers in behavioral problems, 257–258
Bethanechol therapy, 326
Binswanger's disease, magnetic resonance imaging in, 189
Biochemical marker in AD, 214–225
Blessed Dementia Scale, 126, 131
Blood-brain barrier
  permeability in AD, 183
  PET scan studies, 197
Blood flow, cerebral, 60
  MRI studies, 191
  PET scan studies, 194
  SPECT studies, 197–198
Blood studies
  amyloid-associated proteins in, 221–222
  cholinesterase activity in, 310
  derivatives of amyloid-β precursor protein in, 216
Boston Naming Test, 116
Brain
  extracellular fluid contact with cerebrospinal fluid, 216
  imaging of, 59–60, 72, 119, 123–125, 170–201
  reserve capacity of, 413
    education affecting, 12

Index

Buflomedil in memory problems, 266, 270–271
Buspirone in behavioral problems, 256
Butrylcholinesterase, 307–308
  in Alzheimer's disease, 310
  inhibitors of, 313–319
  in normal humans, 309

Calbindin D-28K in cholinergic cells, 300
Calcium, intracellular, homeostasis in AD, 39, 64, 70–71, 74, 77
Carbamazepine therapy in behavioral problems, 254, 258
Caregivers, 414–415
  affected by behavioral problems of patients, 249
  assessment of patient's behavior, 250
  in community services, 376–388, 415
  in families, 351–371
Case management to coordinate care of patients, 379–380
Caudate nucleus, magnetic resonance imaging of, 183
Ceranapril in memory problems, 266, 271–272
Cerebral blood flow, 60
  MRI studies, 191
  PET scan studies, 194
  SPECT studies, 197–198
Cerebral cortex
  cholinergic innervation of, 300
  nicotinic receptors in, 330
  pathology in AD, 58
Cerebrospinal fluid, 123
  acetylcholinesterase in, 223
  amyloid-associated proteins in, 221–222
  amyloid-β levels in, 71, 123
  cholinesterases in, 309
  in Alzheimer's disease, 311–312
  contact with brain extracellular fluid, 216
  derivatives of amyloid-β precursor protein in, 216–221
  neurofibrillary tangle-related proteins in, 222

  tau levels in, 71, 123
Cerebrovascular disease, dementia in, 129–131
  computed tomography in, 181
Chlordiazepoxide in behavioral problems, 256–257
Choline
  availability for acetylcholine synthesis, 302–303
  therapy with, 303
Choline acetyltransferase, 299–300, 302
  activity modulation as therapy, 306
  deficiency in AD, 60, 63, 64–65, 223, 310
Cholinergic system, 298–301
  therapy in AD, 301–336
Cholinesterases
  in Alzheimer's disease, 310–313
  in amyloid plaques, 311
  characteristics of, 307–308
  inhibitor therapy, 303, 313–319, 333
  in normal humans, 308–310
  in red blood cells, 310, 312–313
Chromosome defects in AD, 13, 32, 42, 68, 96. *See also* Genetic factors in AD
CI-979 therapy, 326–327, 333
Cigarette smoking, and reduced risk for AD, 16–17, 334
Circadian rhythm disruption, 136
Citalopram in depression, 240
Cognex. *See* Tacrine therapy
Cognitive impairment
  depression in, 236–237
  functional assessment in, 156, 162–164
Cohen-Mansfield Agitation Inventory, 250
Community care, 376–388, 415
  attitudes toward services in, 358–360, 379
  available services in, 377–379
  case management in, 379–380
  financial and legal services in, 380–381
  and health of care providers, 381–382
  research in, 382–385

safety assessment and structural changes of homes in, 381
Complement system in AD, 40, 41
Computed tomography, 124, 171–183
  in behavior disorders, 181
  blood-brain barrier in, 183
  loss of brain tissue in, 179–181
  periventricular white matter in, 181–183
  in vascular dementia, 181
Connectivity mechanisms in AD pathology, 66–67
Consortium to Establish a Registry in Alzheimer's Disease (CERAD), 157–158
Cornell Scale for Depression in Dementia, 238
Corpus callosum, magnetic resonance imaging of, 183
C-reactive protein
  in amyloid plaques, 40
  in blood and CSF, 221
Creutzfeldt-Jakob disease, 123, 127, 128
Cultural and ethnic groups
  biases in assessment of, 158–162
  effects on family caregivers, 359–360
  as risk factors for AD, 11
Cycloserine in memory problems, 266, 272–273
Cytokines produced in AD, 40, 41

Day care centers for adults, 378
Decision-making capacity of patients, assessment of, 397–399
Delusions in AD, 249
Dementia
  affecting intimacy and marriage, 364–366
  of Alzheimer's type, 4, 112
  effects on patient, 360–364
  family history of, 12–13
  multi-infarct
    MRI studies in, 189, 191
    PET scans in, 194
  reversible, depression with, 237
  vascular, 129–131

computed tomography in, 181
Dementia Mood Assessment Scale, 239
Denial of dementia, 362
Depression
  associated with AD, 15–16, 113, 134, 233–242
    course of, 241
    diagnosis of, 233–238
    dimensional scales for, 238
    incidence of, 235–236
    prevalence of, 234–235
    problems in measurement of, 237–238
    risk factors for, 235
    treatment of, 238–242
  in family caregivers, 356–357, 364, 368, 370, 386, 388
Desferrioxamine in memory problems, 266, 273–274
Diagnosis of AD, 111–138
  assessment of severity and clinical course in, 131–133
  behavioral problems in, 250–251
  biochemical marker in, 214–225
  brain imaging in, 123–125
  clinical examination in, 110–125
  cognitive tests in, 116–119
  criteria of NINCDS-ADRDA, 142–143, 164–165
  depression in, 233–242
  description of dementia stages in, 117–118
  differential diagnosis, 122–123, 126–129
  DSM-IV criteria for, 125–126
  early recognition of problems in, 114–119
  and features of vascular dementia, 129–131
  laboratory tests in, 123
  medical history in, 120–121
  Mini-Mental State Exam in, 115–116, 155–156
  neuroimaging in, 170–201
  neurological examination in, 121–123

neuropsychological assessment in, 119, 123
  goals and issues in, 152–166
  physical examination in, 121
  in preclinical and early phase, 113–114
  psychiatric mental status examination in, 133–137
  tropicamide eyedrop application in, 325
Diazepam in behavioral problems, 256–257
Diet as risk factor for AD, 17–18
Differential diagnosis of AD, 122–123, 126–129
Dihydroergotoxin in depression, 239
Direct Assessment of Functional Status Scale (DAFS), 156, 162–163
DNA, 93
  polymerase chain reaction, 95
  restriction fragment length polymorphisms, 95
  short tandem repeat polymorphisms, 95
Donzepil hydrochloride therapy, 315–316, 413
Down's syndrome
  and development of AD, 68, 96
  family history of, 13, 121
  PET scans in, 195
Drug therapy. *See* Medications
DSM-IV criteria for diagnosis of AD, 125–126, 236
DUP-996 therapy, 306

E2020 therapy, 315–316, 413
Education
  affecting neuropsychological assessment scores, 115, 159
  and occurrence of AD, 11–12, 114, 412
Electroconvulsive therapy in depression, 239
Electroencephalography, 124–125
ELISA studies, problems in, 224–225
Embolism, brain damage in, 129–130
ENA-713 therapy, 317–318, 413
Entorhinal cortex pathology, 37, 57, 59, 67, 68

Environmental exposures as risk factors for AD, 18–19, 414
Epidemiology of AD, 3–20
  incidence studies, 6–8
  prevalence studies, 4–6
  research needed in, 410
  risk factors, 8–19
Epilepsy associated with AD, 16
Eptastigmine therapy, 317
Erythrocytes, cholinesterase activity in, 310, 312–313
Escala de Inteligencia Wechsler Para Adultos (EIWA), 159
Estrogen
  deprivation as risk factor for AD, 9–11, 75
  therapy in behavioral problems in males, 259
Ethical and medicolegal issues, 391–405
Ethnic and cultural groups
  biases in assessment of, 158–162
  effects on family caregivers, 359–360
  as risk factor for AD, 11
Etiology and pathogenesis of AD, 31–43
  research needed in, 411–413
Event-related potentials (ERP), 125
Excitotoxicity hypothesis of AD, 74–75
Exelon therapy, 317–318, 413
Eyedrops, tropicamide, as diagnostic test, 325

Familial AD (FAD) gene linkage to chromosome 21 DNA markers, 96, 113
Family caregivers, 351–371, 414–415
  abuse, neglect, and violence in, 368–370
  attitudes toward community services, 358–360, 379
  belief systems in, 358–359
  clinical framework for guidance and support of, 354–360
  cultural or ethnic influences on, 359–360
  and dementia affecting intimacy and marriage, 364–366

depression in, 356–357, 364, 368, 370, 386, 388
and effects of dementia on patient, 360–364
genetic counseling for, 370–371
health of, 381–382
knowledge of medical and psychological problems, 358
linkage to community resources, 383–385
reactions to institutionalization of patient, 366–368
types of, 357
Family history
and depression in AD, 235
as risk factor for AD, 12–13, 91–92, 121
Fetal neuronal transplants, 335
Financial and legal services available, 380–381
Food and Drug Administration guidelines for "vulnerable subjects" research, 396
Forebrain, basal
cholinergic neurons in, 300
nicotinic receptors in, 330–331
Free radicals
associated with AD, 18, 39, 73, 77
generation by amyloid-β, 69
Frontal cortex
muscarinic receptors in, 321, 322
pathology in AD, 58
Functional Activities Questionnaire, 119
Functional assessment in AD, 156, 162–164
Functional studies of brain
magnetic resonance imaging in, 191–193
PET scans in, 193–197

G protein linkage with muscarinic acetylcholine receptors, 319
Gait dysfunction, 122
Galanthamine therapy, 316–317
Gegenhalten, 122
Gender

and depression in AD, 235
as risk factor for AD, 9–11
Gene therapy, 335
Genetic counseling for families, 370–371
Genetic factors in AD, 13–14, 32, 42, 68, 90–103, 113, 121
amyloid precursor protein gene in, 96–101
apolipoprotein E gene in, 101–102
chromosome 1 in, 100, 113
chromosome 14 in, 99–100, 113
chromosome 19 in, 100–101, 113
chromosome 21 in, 96, 113
classical studies of, 91–93
familial AD (FAD) genes in, 96, 113
family studies of, 91–92
linkage analysis in, 94
and molecular genetic techniques, 94–103
research needed in, 410–411
twin studies of, 92–93
Glasgow Coma Scale, 132
Glucocorticoids in pathogenesis of AD, 75
Glucose metabolism in AD, 60, 72–73
PET scan studies, 194–197
SPECT studies, 197–198
Glutamate
deficiency in AD, 60, 63, 66
and excitotoxicity hypothesis of AD, 74–75
Glyburide therapy, 307
Gray-matter structures, magnetic resonance imaging of, 183

Hachinsky Scale, 130
Hallucinations in AD, 249
Haloperidol in behavioral problems, 254–255
Hamilton Scale for Depression, 238
Head trauma as risk factor for AD, 14–15, 76, 113, 128, 411
Helical filaments, paired
antigen in CSF, 222
in neurofibrillary tangles, 36–37, 57, 215

Hemicholinium-3 affecting acetylcholine synthesis, 304
Heptyl-physostigmine therapy, 318
Hippocampus
  cholinergic innervation of, 300
  magnetic resonance imaging of, 184–186
  muscarinic receptors in, 321, 322
  nicotinic receptors in, 330
  pathology in AD, 37–38, 58, 67, 68, 114
Home health care agencies, 378, 380
Homemaker services, 378
Homicide-suicide risks, 365–366
Hospitalization, psychiatric, 260
Huntington's disease, 122, 128
Hydergine in depression, 239
Hydrocephalus, normal pressure, 122, 127, 129
Hypochondriasis, cognitive, 236
Hypothyroidism as risk factor for AD, 15, 76

Imipramine in depression, 240
Immune system in AD, 39–41, 72
Incidence of AD, 6–8
Indomethacin in memory problems, 267, 275–276
Inflammatory response in AD, 39–41, 412
Information storage in brain, disruption of, 56–57
Informed consent, and assessment of decision-making capacity, 397–399
Institutionalization of patient, family reactions to, 366–368
Interleukins produced in AD, 39–40, 41
  in blood and CSF, 222
Iron
  and aggregation of amyloid-β, 77
  in neurofibrillary tangles, 73–74

Japanese groups, neuropsychological assessment of, 162

Laboratory tests, 123

Language biases in assessment tests, 158–162
Learning mechanisms
  impairment of, 56, 65–66
  olfactory system in, 67–68
Lecithin therapy, 303, 312, 333
Legal and financial services available, 380–381
Legal issues in research, 391–405
Leukomalacia, periventricular, 181–182
Lewy body disease, 112, 122, 128, 133
Lifestyle as risk factor for AD, 16–18
Light boxes in therapy of behavioral problems, 259
Limbic system, cholinergic innervation of, 301
Lipid peroxidation in AD, 69–70, 73
Lithium therapy in behavioral problems, 234, 259
Lod score in linkage analysis, 94
Lorazepam in behavioral problems, 256–257
Lucencies, periventricular, 181–182

α_2-Macroglobulin
  in amyloid plaques, 40
  in blood and CSF, 221
Magnetic resonance imaging of brain, 124, 181, 183–191
  contrast in, 192
  periventricular halo in, 189
  in persons with apolipoprotein E e4 allele, 186
  spectroscopic, 192–193
  in studies of functioning brain, 191–193
  volumetric studies in, 173–176
  white matter changes in, 183, 188–189, 191
Marriage, dementia affecting, 364–366
Mecamylamine as nicotine receptor antagonist, 330
Medical history as risk factor for AD, 14–16, 130–131
Medications
  in behavioral problems, 253–260

anticonvulsants, 254, 258–259
benzodiazepines, 256–257
beta-adrenergic blockers, 257–258
buspirone, 256
lithium, 254, 259
neuroleptics, 254–255
trazadone, 255–256
cholinergic system therapy, 298–336
acetyl group donors, 305–306
choline acetyltransferase activity modulation, 306
cholinesterase inhibition, 313–319
direct receptor modulation, 319–332
muscarinic receptor agonists, 325–328
nicotinic receptor agonists, 331–332
precursors and reuptake enhancers, 303–305
promotion of acetylcholine release, 306–307
reducing rate of AD progression, 332–335
in memory problems, 264–287
acetyl-L-carnitine, 265–269
alaproclate, 266, 269–270
buflomedil, 266, 270–271
ceranapril, 266, 271–272
cycloserine, 266, 272–273
desferrioxamine, 266, 273–274
indomethacin, 267, 275–276
milacemide, 267, 276–278
monosialoganglioside (GM-1), 267, 274–275
nerve growth factor, 267, 278–279
nimodipine, 268, 279–281
phosphatidylserine, 268, 281–282
thiamine, 268, 282–285
zimeldine, 268, 285–286
Medicolegal issues in research, 391–405
Melatonin therapy in circadian rhythm disorders, 136–137
Memory
impairment of, 56, 65–66
treatment with noncholinergic drugs, 264–287
olfactory system in, 67–68
tests of, 155
Metabolism in brain, 59–60, 72–73
PET scan studies, 194–197
SPECT studies, 197–198
Metanicotin therapy, 332
Metrifonate therapy, 317
Milacemide in memory problems, 267, 276–278
Mini-Mental State Exam (MMSE), 115–116, 155–156
Mitochondrial activity in AD, 38
Molecular genetic techniques, 94–103
Molecular mechanisms in AD, 68–77
Monoamine oxidase inhibitors in depression, 240
Monosialoganglioside (GM-1) in memory problems, 267, 274–275
Muscarinic receptors, 299–300, 319–328
agonist therapies, 325–328, 333–334
arecoline, 326
bethanechol, 326
CI-979, 326–327
oxotremorine, 326
pilocarpine, 326
RS-86, 326
Xanomeline, 327–328
antagonists of, 324–325
central, 320–323
functions of, 324–325
loss of, 65
peripheral, 323–324

National Institute on Aging, 391, 409
National Institutes of Health guidelines for "vulnerable subjects" research, 394, 400
Neglect and abuse in families, 368–370
Nerve growth factor
production affected by nicotine, 334
receptor in cholinergic cells, 300
therapies with, 335
in memory problems, 267, 278–279
Neurofibrillary pathology, 32–33
formation of tangles in, 36–37, 57, 71, 215
region-specific, 32, 37, 57

neuron-specific susceptibility to, 38
   staging of changes in, 37–38
Neuroimaging, 170–201
   computed tomography, 171–183
   magnetic resonance imaging, 183–191
      contrast in, 192
      spectroscopic, 192–193
      in studies of functioning brain, 191–193
   PET scans, 193–197
   SPECT studies, 197–199
Neuroleptic therapy in behavioral problems, 254–255
Neurological examination, 121–123
Neuronal loss, patterns of, 37–38, 114, 222–223
Neuronal transplants, 335
Neuropeptide-Y deficiency, 60, 63
Neuroplasticity, and vulnerability to AD pathology, 68
Neuropsychological assessment, 119, 123
   extent of, 154–157
   goals and issues in, 152–166
   and prediction of AD development, 158
   selection of tests in, 157–158
Neurotransmitters, 60–66
   in brain and CSF, 222
   cholinergic system, 64–65
   cortical systems, 66
   cortically projecting systems, 64–66
   role in behavioral problems, 253–254
Neurotrophic factors in AD, 75
Nicotine therapy, 331–332
Nicotinic receptors, 299–300, 329–332
   agonist therapies, 331–332, 334
      ABT-418, 332
      metanicotin, 332
      nicotine, 331–332
   in Alzheimer's disease, 330–331
   loss of, 65
   in normal humans, 329–330
Nimodipine in memory problems, 268, 279–281
NINCDS-ADRDA guidelines for diagnosis of AD, 142–143, 164–165, 215, 223

Norepinephrine deficiency, 60, 63, 65–66
Nortriptyline in depression, 239, 240
Nucleus basalis
   cholinergic neurons in, 300
   muscarinic receptors in, 321, 322
Nursing care available, 378
Nursing homes, 367

Object Memory Evaluation (OME), 156, 161–162
Occipital cortex
   muscarinic receptors in, 321, 322
   pathology in AD, 58
Olfactory bulb, cholinergic innervation of, 300
Olfactory system in AD, 59, 67–68, 122
Opercular region, cholinergic innervation of, 301
Oxazepam in behavioral problems, 256–257
Oxidative stress in AD. *See* Free radicals
Oxotremorine therapy, 326

Paired helical filaments
   antigen in CSF, 222
   in neurofibrillary tangles, 36–37, 57, 215
Paranoia in AD, 134, 136, 248
Parietal area
   cholinergic innervation of, 301
   muscarinic receptors in, 321, 322
   pathology in AD, 58
Parkinson disease, 112, 122, 128
   family history of, 13
Parkinsonism in AD, pathophysiology of, 198
Pathogenesis of AD, 31–43
   research needed in, 411–413
Peripheral medical factors in AD, 76
PET scans of brain, 124, 193–197
   blood-brain barrier in, 197
   in classification of patients, 196
   and postmortem findings, 197
   regional metabolic deficits in, 194–196
Pharmacologic therapy. *See* Medications

Phosphatidylcholine in acetylcholine synthesis, 303
Phosphatidylserine therapy in memory problems, 268, 281–282
Physical examination, 121
Physostigmine therapy, 314, 315
  compared to heptyl-physostigmine, 318
  in reversal of scopolamine-induced cognitive deficits, 324
Pick's disease, 128
  computed tomography in, 181
Pilocarpine therapy, 326
Pindolol in behavioral problems, 257
Plastic mechanisms in AD pathology, 68
Praxis, assessment of, 155
Prevalence studies of AD, 4–6
Propranolol in behavioral problems, 257
Protease activity in AD, 41
Proxy consent for research, 400–402
Pseudocholinesterase, 307
Pseudodementia, 236–237
Psychiatric mental status examination, 133–137
Psychosocial systems in AD, 54–57
Psychotic symptoms, 136, 249, 414
  etiology of, 251–252
Putamen, muscarinic receptors in, 321, 322

Race as risk factor for AD, 11
Reflexes, examination of, 122
Research
  in community care of AD, 382–385
  ethical and medicolegal issues in, 391–405
  future directions for, 409–415
  guidelines for, 392–397
  informed consent for, and assessment of competency, 397–399
  proxy consent and advance directives for, 399–402
  risk and benefit analysis in, 403–404
Respite care, cost of, 380
Risk factors for AD, 8–19, 41–42
  environmental exposures, 18–19
  family history/genetic factors, 12–14

lifestyle, 16–18
medical history, 14–16
sociodemographic characteristics, 9–12
Risperidone in behavioral problems, 255
RS-86 therapy, 326

S182 protein mutations in AD, 42
Scopolamine, cognitive deficits from, 324–325
Serotonin
  deficiency in AD, 60, 63, 66
  reuptake inhibitors in depression, 240
Severe Impairment Battery, 132
Sex
  and depression in AD, 235
  as risk factor for AD, 9–11
Silver, role in AD pathogenesis, 77
Sleep disorders, 135, 248
Smoking, and reduced risk for AD, 16–17, 334
Snout reflex, 122
Social systems affected by AD, 54–57
Somatostatin
  colocalized with GABA neurons, 60, 66
  deficiency in AD, 60, 63
Spanish-speaking groups, neuropsychological assessment of, 158, 159–161
SPECT images of brain, 124, 197–199
Spectroscopy, magnetic resonance, 192–193
Steroid hormones in pathogenesis of AD, 75
Striatum
  cholinergic neurons in, 299–300
  muscarinic receptors in, 321
Strokes, and vascular dementia, 129–131
Suicidal thoughts in dementia, 363, 365–366
Sundowning in AD
  bright-light therapy in, 259
  management of, 253
Support groups, benefits of, 379
Synapses, loss of, 58, 59–60

Tacrine therapy, 306–307, 313–315, 413

compared to other agents, 317, 318, 332
  trials of, 303
Tau
  abnormal phosphorylation of, and formation of neurofibrillary tangles, 36–37, 38, 57, 71–72, 102
  in cerebrospinal fluid, 222
  in paired helical filaments in neurofibrillary tangles, 216
Telencephalic systems affected by AD, 57–60
Temazepam in behavioral problems, 256–257
Temporal area
  cholinergic innervation of, 301
  muscarinic receptors in, 321, 322
  pathology in AD, 57–58
Testing
  in assessment of disease severity, 131–133
  in behavioral problems, 250–251
  in diagnostic screening, 116–119
  functional assessment in, 156, 162–164
  and issues in neuropsychological assessments, 119, 123, 152–166
  neurological examination in, 121–123
  problems in assessment of mood symptoms in, 237–238
  for psychiatric mental status, 134–137
Thalamus, magnetic resonance imaging of, 183
Thiamine in memory problems, 268, 282–285
Thyroid disease as risk factor for AD, 13, 76, 113
Time course of AD, 133
Tolbutamide therapy, 307
Trauma to head as risk factor for AD, 14–15, 76, 113, 128, 412
Trazadone in behavioral problems, 255–256
Treatment
  in behavioral problems, 251–260
  community care in, 376–388
  in depression, 238–242
  ethical and medicolegal issues in, 391–405
  family caregivers in, 351–371
  future directions for, 413–415
  in memory problems, 264–287
  new strategies in, 43
Trisomy 21. *See* Down's syndrome
Tropicamide eyedrop testing for AD, 325
Tumor necrosis factor produced in AD, 40, 41
Twin studies of AD, 92–93

Ubiquitin in paired helical filaments in neurofibrillary tangles, 215–216
Ungulate gyrus, cholinergic innervation of, 301

Valproate sodium in behavioral problems, 254, 258–259
Vascular alterations in AD, 75–76
Vascular dementia, 129–131
  computed tomography in, 181
Vasopressin deficiency in AD, 60, 63
Violence and abuse in families, 368–370
Vitamin B-1 in memory problems, 268, 282–285
Vitamin deficiencies as risk factor for AD, 17–18

Wanderings in AD, 248
  management of, 252–253
Wechsler Adult Intelligence Scale–Revised (WAIS-R), 160
White matter changes
  computed tomography of, 181
  magnetic resonance imaging of, 183, 188–189, 191
  significance of, 129

Xanomeline therapy, 327–328, 333

Zifrosilone therapy, 316
Zimeldine in memory problems, 268, 285–286
Zinc role in hippocampus, 77

Springer Publishing Company

Hospice Care for Patients with Advanced Progressive Dementia

Ladislav Volicer, MD, PhD and
Ann Hurley, RN, DSNc, GRECC

Caring for patients with a progressive dementia provides many challenges for both family and professional caregivers. The editors and contributors demonstrate how hospice care leads to improved quality of life for patients with terminal dementia and their families. Many of the chapters in this volume are based on the successful 10-year experience of the E.N. Rogers Memorial Veterans Hospital, where the first palliative care program for the management of patients with advanced dementia was developed.

The book describes Alzheimer's Disease and other progressive dementias and reviews the clinical problems encountered including infections, eating difficulties, and behavioral problems. This volume is of importance to nurses, physicians, and social workers involved in hospice care or who care for patients at the terminal stage of dementia, as well as policy makers.

Partial Contents:

Part I. Alzheimer's Disease and Other Progressive Dementias • Intercurrent Infections • Overcoming Eating Difficulties in the Severely Demented • Quality of Life in Late Stage Dementia

Part II. Ethical Foundations for Treatment Limitations in the Care of People with Advanced Dementia • Palliative Care for Alzheimer Patients • Nursing Staff as Moral Agents • Advance Proxy Planning

Part III. Acceptance of Hospice Care for Dementia Patients by Health Care Professionals • Effects of Hospice Interventions on Behaviors, Discomfort, and Physical Complications of the End-Stage Dementia Nursing Home Residents

Springer Series on Ethics, Law, and Aging
1998   320pp   0-8261-1162-9   hardcover

536 Broadway, New York, NY 10012-3955 • (212) 431-4370 • Fax (212) 941-7842

Ŝ *Springer Publishing Company*

Research and Practice in Alzheimer's Disease

Bruno J. Vellas
J. L. Fitten, Editors

Advances on the latest research findings about Alzheimer's Disease and related dementias continue to be of the utmost importance to practitioners as well as the general public. In this impressive international volume, Bruno Vellas has assembled the most important researchers in the field to present their latest research results. Contributions are made from: the United States, France, Japan, Switzerland, Italy, Finland, England, and Israel. Topics range from biological advances, to behavioral outcomes, to services implications and much more.

Partial Contents: Several Questions About Zinc: The Role of Zinc in Alzheimer's Disease, *A. Law, G. Grossberg* • Protective Factors in Alzheimer's Disease: A Review, *E. McDonough, J. Grossberg, G.T. Grossberg* • Measurement of Outcomes in Alzheimer's Disease, *G. Lussignoli, et al* • Depressive Symptoms in Alzheimer's Disease: A Cross-Ethnic Comparison of Cuban-American and White Non-Hispanic Patients, *D. Harwood, et al* • Individual Quality of Life Assessment in Healthy Elderly and Early Dementia Patients, *D. Meier, D. Ermini-Fünfschilling, H. Stähelin* • Education and Heterogeneity in Alzheimer's Disease, *C. Garcia, M. Guerreiro* • Neuropsychiatric Symptoms in Frontotempora Dementia, *F. Lebert, F. Pasquier* • The Relationship Between Functional Ability and Cognitive Ability Among Elderly People, *L. McInnes, P. Rabbitt* • Medical Management and Non-Cognitive Aspects of Alzheimer's Disease, *F. Nourhashemi, P.J. Ousset, J. Fitten, B.J. Vellas, J.L. Albarède*

1998   400pp (est)   0-8261-1194-7   *softcover*

536 Broadway, New York, NY 10012-3955 • (212) 431-4370 • Fax (212) 941-7842

⑤ Springer Publishing Company

Treating Alzheimer's and Other Dementias
Clinical Application of Recent Research Advances

Manfred Bergener, MD
Sanford I. Finkel, MD, Editors

This volume's international scope provides a comprehensive overview of the most current knowledge on Alzheimer's Disease. Based on the 6th Congress of the International Psychogeriatrics Association, the prestigious editors have included contributions ranging from prevention, diagnosis, and treatment to the latest activities in clinical Alzheimer's research. This volume will appeal to geriatricians, psychogeriatricians, gerontologists, and researchers in the field of aging.

Partial Contents:

- Perplexing Problems in the Assessment of Cognitively Impaired Older Persons, *M.G. Weisensee, D.K. Kjervik, & J.B. Anderson*
- Further Developments in the Molecular Biology of Alzheimer's Disease with Special Reference to the Development of New Methods of Treatment, *C.M. Wischik, et al.*
- Latest Advances in Alzheimer's Drug Research, *A.Q. Bungash & G.T. Grossberg*
- Electroconvulsive Therapy for Agitated Dementia Patients, *D.P. Hay, L. Hay & G.T. Grossberg*
- Social Ties and Social Support Among Alzheimer's Disease Caregivers, *J.C. Stuckey*
- Diagnostic Criteria for Vascular Dementia, *T. Erkinjuntti*

1995   576pp   0-8261-8930-X   hardcover

536 Broadway, New York, NY 10012-3955 • (212) 431-4370 • Fax (212) 941-7842

Ṣ *Springer Publishing Company*

JOURNAL

INTERNATIONAL PSYCHOGERIATRICS

Official Journal of the International Psychogeriatric Association

Robin Eastwood, MD, FRCP, FRCPsych, Editor-in-Chief

This multidisciplinary international publication features refereed contributions from the full spectrum of the mental health field, and from the health professions in general. In addition to reports of original research—or reviews of research—each issue spotlights psychogeriatric advances in specific countries. Serving as a forum for advances in practice, *International Psychogeriatrics* includes informative supplements dedicated to current research on important topics.

Partial Contents:

- Diagnosis of Alzheimer's Disease, *B. Reisberg and A. Burns*
- Diagnosing Alzheimer's Disease in the Presence of Mixed Cognitive and Affective Symptoms, *B. Reifler*
- A Guide to the Standardized Mini-Mental State Examination, *D.W. Molloy and T.I.M. Standish*
- Alzheimer's Disease Assessment Scale–Cognitive in Clinical Practice, *J. Peña-Casanova*
- The SKT–A Short Cognitive Performance Test for Assessing Deficits of Memory and Attention, *H. Lehfeld and H. Erzigkeit*
- Use of the Colombia University Scale to Assess Psychopathology in Alzheimer's Disease, *D.P. Devanand*
- Functional Disability in Alzheimer's Disease, *S. Gauthier, I. Gélinas, and L. Gauthier*
- Discriminant Analysis of Brain Imaging Data Identifies Subjects with early Alzheimer's Disease, *S.I. Rapoport*
- Neurological Markers of the Progression of Alzheimer's Disease, *E.H. Franssen and B. Reisberg*

ISSN 1041-6102 • 4 issues annually (plus supplements)

536 Broadway, New York, NY 10012-3955 • (212) 431-4370 • Fax (212) 941-7842